Mosby's Review Series

MATERNITY NURSING

Mosby's Review Series

MATERNITY NURSING

Paulette D. Rollant, PhD, MSN, RN, CCRN
President, Multi-Resources, Inc.
Grantville, Georgia

Karen A. Piotrowski, RNC, MSN
Assistant Professor of Nursing
D'Youville College
Buffalo, New York

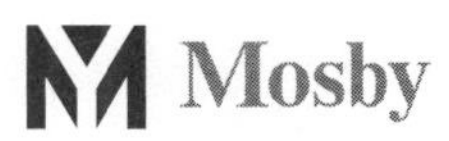

St. Louis Baltimore Boston Carlsbad Chicago Naples New York Philadelphia Portland
London Madrid Mexico City Singapore Sydney Tokyo Toronto Wiesbaden

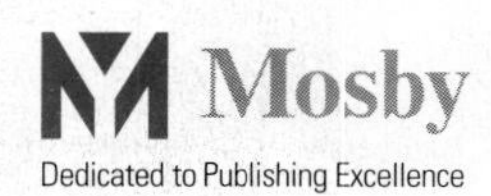

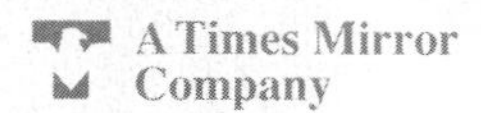

Vice-President and Publisher: Nancy L. Coon
Senior Editor: Susan R. Epstein
Associate Developmental Editor: Laurie K. Muench
Project Manager: Carol Sullivan Weis
Designer: Sheilah Barrett
Manufacturing Supervisor: Karen Lewis
Cover Illustrator: Susan Swan

Printed in the United States of America
Composition by Shepherd, Inc.
Printing/binding by R.R. Donnelly

Mosby–Year Book, Inc.
11830 Westline Industrial Drive
St. Louis, MO 63146

International Standard Book Number 0-8151-7246-X

95 96 97 98 99 / 9 8 7 6 5 4 3 2 1

REVIEWERS

Bette B. Hammond, RN, BSN, MSN
Assistant Professor
St. Charles County Community College
St. Peters, Missouri

Tina Weitkamp, RNC, BSN, MSN
Associate Professor of Clinical Nursing, University of Cincinnati
Staff Nurse-Maternity, Mercy Hospital Anderson
Cincinnati, Ohio

To Dan, Mom, Dad, Joanne, Joe, Alan, and Amy
Paulette Rollant

To Edward and Lottie Piotrowski
Karen Piotrowski

HOW CAN *MOSBY'S REVIEW SERIES* BE USED?

Mosby's Review Series is designed to help you obtain the most from your preparation and study time for your nursing exams. These books should be used to review essential concepts, theory, and content prior to nursing courses, challenge, certification, or licensing examinations. The review series can be used to prepare for clinical experiences and as a quick reference when providing care of clients. Mosby's Review Series consists of five books:

Maternity Nursing
Medical-Surgical Nursing
Mental Health Nursing
Pediatric Nursing
Nursing Pharmacology

The series is designed to highlight important information related to the specific content. It is not meant to provide a comprehensive, in-depth coverage of the selected area of nursing. The reference list at the end of each book is a compilation of resources used to develop these books. These references as well as other texts should be consulted when a more comprehensive discussion of a particular topic is desired. Use these books to jog your memory, to reinforce what you know, to guide you to identify what you don't know, and to lead you to appropriate sources for more details. If you are in a formal education setting, these books are not intended to be considered as a substitute for attending classes or completing required reading assignments.

Used correctly these books can help you:

1. Increase your ability to prioritize in clinical situations while using the nursing process.
2. Increase your ability to remember essential content.
3. Increase your productivity in studying to leave some time for you and your family.
4. Apply new behaviors for improvement of your testing skills.
5. Evaluate your strengths and weakness related to content areas or testing situations.

WHAT IS UNIQUE ABOUT *MOSBY'S REVIEW SERIES?*

1. Computer disks of exams
2. Comprehensive rationales
3. Test-taking tips
4. Chapter format
5. References for further reading

Computer Disk

Each book in the series has a comprehensive exam on computer disk. For your convenience, the exam is also included in the book. The answers for the comprehensive exams, like the end of the chapter questions, include the answers, comprehensive rationales, and test-taking tips.

Comprehensive Rationales

These include answers and rationales for each option in each test question.

Test-Taking Tips

These tips aid in your decision-making and facilitate the development of your logical thinking for the selection of the correct answers, especially if you have narrowed your choice to two options.

Chapter Format

Each chapter contains an easy-to-follow format divided into five sections:

Study Outcomes: provides an advanced organizer approach to what is in each chapter

Key Terms: includes the most common difficult terms to recall

Content Review: is organized and structured by the nursing process to help you identify what is most important

- All information within each heading is prioritized
- Nursing diagnoses are prioritized
- Goals are client-centered
- Client teaching content is focused for in-hospital and at-home clinical settings
- Home care content is included
- Older adult alerts are included where applicable
- Evaluation criteria includes decision-making tools concerning which actions to take when client's clinical status shows improvement or deterioration
- Many tables, charts, and figures contrast, cluster, and simplify information for ease of remembering

Review Questions: stand-alone, 4-option multiple choice

Answers, Rationales, and Test-Taking Tips:

- Comprehensive rationales: given for each option to explain why it is correct or incorrect

- Test-taking tips: give strategies to use in situations such as when options are narrowed to two or when you have no idea of a correct answer

References

Current references are suggested for further study if more in-depth discussion is needed.

WHAT'S IN *MOSBY'S REVIEW SERIES: MATERNITY NURSING?*

Mosby's Review Series: Maternity Nursing begins with coverage of the pregnant woman and her support system during periods of the antepartal, labor, and birth of the fetus. The needs of the postpartal woman and her support system during the fourth trimester are then emphasized. The processes of recovery and adaptation, and the resolution of problems during the puerperium are included.

The remaining chapters focus on the needs of the newborn. The physiologic adaptations to extrauterine life, alterations in the newborn's health status, and application of the nursing process to the needs of the newborn are presented.

ACKNOWLEDGMENTS

I express my heartfelt gratitude to those who have endured with me throughout this publication opportunity for a nursing review series: an adventure from idea to reality.

I especially want to thank the following people:

Beverly Copland, who thought that I had the potential to complete this project and who eagerly gave me tons of strong support in the initial and ongoing book development phases.

Laurie Muench, who picked up the ball in the middle of manuscript preparation and persisted with me through the process to completion of book publication. The response "OK . . . when *can* I expect it?" provided silent encouragement and sometimes comic relief when my mental and physical energies ran quite low. Laurie's thoughtfulness and guidance to help me set priorities were invaluable! I am very grateful and fortunate to work with Laurie.

Suzi Epstein, who was full of enthusiasm and total support from the birth of the idea for a nursing review series to the final publication of the books. Suzi's creativity and suggestions provided essential building blocks in the overall development of the series.

My *coauthors,* for their enormous efforts to produce manuscript content in a short period of time. Their nursing expertise was helpful for the development of the unique aspects of each book.

My wonderful husband, *Dan,* for his patience, humor, support, and love. His faith in my abilities has sustained my energies and maintained my sense of self.

My parents, *Joseph and Mildred Demaske,* for their love, encouragement, and prayers.

Paulette D. Rollant

I wish to acknowledge with special thanks: my parents, *Edward and Lottie Piotrowski* for their unwavering encouragement and support; *Irene M. Bobak* and *Beverly J. Copland* for providing me with the first opportunity to write professionally; *Paulette D. Rollant* and *Laurie Muench* for their invaluable guidance during the preparation of this book.

Karen A. Piotrowski

CONTENTS

HOW CAN I USE THIS BOOK?

This book is designed to work for you—at your convenience. Read the following guidelines first to help save you time and energy during test preparation. The chapters are designed for short, quick intervals of review. Carry this book with you to catch the times when you are stuck and have nothing to do.

The directions will help you to:

- **Maximize your individual performance in review and testing situations.**
- **Identify your personal priorities in preparation for testing.**
- **Sharpen your thinking and discrimination skills for testing.**

DIRECTIONS ON HOW TO REVIEW

I. Identify your routine for reviewing: the best days, the best time of day
   A. Write the days and times on the inside front cover of this book and on your personal calendar and the calendar at home. This communicates to your family or support systems that you will be unavailable to them at these times. It is also a nice reminder every week to yourself that this is important to you.
   B. Refer to section V for specific directions on how to develop your routine
II. Scan the table of contents
   A. Put a check mark in front of the content with which you are comfortable
   B. Circle the content in which you think you are weak
   C. Prioritize the weak content with #1 being the weakest content area. Put these numbers in front of your circles.
   D. Prioritize the strongest content areas in the same manner
III. When you are feeling a high-energy day
   A. Go to the #1 chapter of the weakest content area for review
IV. When you are having a low-energy day
   A. Go to the #1 chapter of the strongest content area for review

V. General guidelines for the development of a routine for reviewing
   A. Develop a system of review that meets your needs
   B. Set aside time when you are least tired or stressed both mentally and physically
   C. Limit your review time to a maximum of 90 minutes for the most effective, efficient retention of reviewed content
   D. If possible, relax and take a nap after reviewing to further place the information into long term memory. Some research reveals that sleeping for 2 to 3 hours after studying results in a 70 to 80% retention rate of content into long term memory in contrast to 30 to 40% retention when you are active after studying.
   E. Use at least one relaxation technique *at the onset* and *at the end* of your review time. Deep breathing that is slow with a concentration on the air movement going in and out is one of the best ways to relax physically and mentally.
   F. Use at least one relaxation technique *during* the time you review.
   G. If your time is limited, use 10 to 15 minute intervals to review small portions of the content. For example, you may want to review the different aspects of hypertension in one study session.
   H. Use a theme per week or per day approach. For example, if there is enough time between your test and when you begin to study, every Monday review something on sodium from the book. Then at work find clients with sodium imbalances, review their charts, and discuss their situations with colleagues or with the clients' physicians. Continue with themes for the day such as:
      1. Tuesdays are potassium
      2. Wednesdays are calcium
      3. Thursdays are magnesium
      4. Fridays are acidosis situations
      5. Saturdays are alkalosis days
      6. Sundays are fun days. Don't forget to keep one day to relax and have fun. This allows your mind to work for retention and reorganization of the content that you reviewed during the week.
      7. Weekly themes also might be of help. Do one system per week such as pulmonary, endocrine and so forth.

DIRECTIONS ON HOW TO USE THIS BOOK FOR SUCCESS

I. Suggested study sequence #1 for each chapter
   A. Read the objectives
   B. Complete the key terms

C. Complete the content review
D. Complete the review questions
E. Review the answers, rationales, test-taking tips

III. Suggested study sequence #2 for each chapter
A. Complete the review questions
B. Review the answers, rationales, test-taking tips
C. Review the missed content areas
D. Review the unfamiliar and the familiar content areas
E. Complete the key terms
F. Complete the objectives to evaluate your level of understanding

III. Suggested study sequence #3 *after* doing #1 or #2 suggested sequence
A. Complete the comprehensive exam in the book
B. Correct comprehensive exam answers with review of the rationales and test-taking tips
C. List content areas missed, then cluster them in terms of similar content
D. Prioritize these clusters with #1 being the least familiar content
E. Review additional content as directed by the questions you missed

IV. Suggested study sequence #4 *before* doing #1 or #2 suggested sequence
A. Complete the comprehensive exam in the book
B. Correct comprehensive exam answers with review of the rationales and test-taking tips
C. List content areas missed, then cluster them in terms of similar content
D. Prioritize these clusters with #1 being the least familiar content
E. Implement either sequence #1 or #2
F. Complete the computer comprehensive exam. Note that even though the questions are the same as in the book, you should evaluate how your reading of the questions and options differed as related to perception and consistent ability to identify key words, terms, age, and developmental needs.
G. Review content as needed and directed from your missed questions on your exam

V. Suggested techniques for use of the objectives during your review
A. Read the objectives to have them guide you where to start
B. Put a check next to the ones in which you feel the weakest
C. Prioritize them with #1 being the weakest
D. Review the weakest content first or on high-energy days
E. Review the most familiar content last or on low-energy days

VI. Suggested techniques for the use of the key terms, the content review section, and the exams
A. Key terms—suggested study techniques
1. Use a 3 x 5 index card to cover the definitions of the key terms
2. State your definition out loud

3. Uncover the definition and read the given definition out loud (speaking the content as well as seeing the content will enhance your retention)
4. Write key notes in terms of a few words on a 3 x 5 card for the information you have difficulty recalling
5. Carry the card with you for a few days to review this content again. Suggestion: put the card on your sunvisor in the car and review it at the stoplight or if stopped in traffic.

B. Content review—suggested study techniques
1. Use a 3 x 5 card to cover the content under a major heading
2. State out loud what 3 or 4 important aspects of the content under the major heading might be or ask yourself a few questions about that content heading. Try to state the items in order of priority.
3. Uncover the content under the major heading. Check your information against that given in the book. See what you forgot or added that may or may not be important.
4. Write key notes in terms of a few words on a 3 x 5 card for the information you have difficulty recalling
5. Carry the card with you for a few days to review this content again. Suggestion: carry the card with you to review whenever you get 5 to 10 minutes free.
6. When you practice prioritizing the content you will enhance your critical thinking skills

C. Exam review—suggested study techniques
1. For all tests read all the rationales and test-taking tips for missed and correct questions. These often contain pearls of wisdom on how to remember or get a better understanding of the content.
2. Remember to do a relaxation exercise before you begin your questions and repeat the exercise about every 25 questions
3. When you miss a question ask yourself
   a. Did I not know the content?
   b. Did I misread the question or option(s)?
4. If you miss questions because of a knowledge deficit
   a. Make a list on a 3 x 5 card for 3 to 4 days
   b. Group or cluster the content according to the steps in the nursing process, the content area, or a system
   c. Look up that content
   d. Do not look up content after every practice test. A better approach is to cluster the content and look it all up every

3 to 4 days. With this approach you will have better retention into long term memory and the best recall at a later time.
    e. Try to identify new ways to approach reading questions and their options
5. If you misread the question or the option(s)
    a. Try to identify what key words, timeframes, ages, and developmental stages that you may have overlooked
    b. Try to identify new ways to approach reading the questions and their options
    c. Practice, practice and practice doing questions
    d. Practice, practice, and practice doing relaxation before you begin the practice exam, after every 10 to 20 questions, and then at the end of the exam to refresh your thinking and diminish your tenseness or tiredness.
6. Be sure to do a practice exam with the exact number of questions as your real exam. Note after this exam when you were the most tired, anxious, or nervous. Plan to do a relaxation exercise at these times during the real exam.
7. Your success is directly correlated to your degree of effort to review content as well as relax during the review and exam processes.

SUMMARY

It is hoped that after you have completed your review with the use of this book as your major tool that you have:

- Maximized your individual performance in review and testing situations.
- Identified your personal priorities in preparation for testing.
- Sharpened your thinking and discrimination skills for testing.

Let this book work for you to make it easy, enjoyable, and effective to review at times that are convenient for you. The short, condensed, and prioritized chapter content may spark new ways to develop your skills in critical thinking and content recall.

It is feedback from students, graduates, and practitioners in nursing that prompted the development and publication of this book. We welcome your comments. We wish you a successful career in the nursing profession and hope that *Mosby's Nursing Review Series* has made that success a little easier to obtain!

CHAPTER 1

Essential Elements for Nursing

STUDY OUTCOMES

After completing this chapter, the reader will be able to do the following:

- Identify essential elements common to all nursing specialties.
- Discuss the priority content for each essential element.
- Incorporate the essential elements into nursing practice.

KEY TERMS

Client education	Process of meeting the client's needs for the acquisition of skills, knowledge, or attitudes to deal with a pathological condition in the arenas of primary, secondary, or tertiary health promotion as based on the prior skills, knowledge, and attitudes of the client.
Nursing process	Process used as the basis of nursing practice. It includes five steps: (1) assess, (2) select nursing diagnosis, (3) plan, (4) intervene, and (5) evaluate.

CONTENT REVIEW

ESSENTIAL ELEMENTS IN NURSING

I. The essential elements

A. Nursing process
B. Client education

II. Nursing incorporates these common essential elements irrespective of the level, environment, or client population

III. The nursing process is the priority common thread throughout nursing practice

IV. Client education facilitates clients' behavior changes in areas of primary (preventive), secondary (early diagnosis), and tertiary (restorative, rehabilitative) health promotion

NURSING PROCESS

I. The nursing process has five steps

A. Assess
B. Select nursing diagnosis
C. Plan
D. Intervene
E. Evaluate

1. Nurses follow the nursing process sequence in any initial client contact
2. Evaluation of the interventions occurs to determine effectiveness or ineffectiveness
3. If effective results, the client-nurse relationship either terminates or new priorities are set for new client problems
4. If ineffective results, nurses select the appropriate step(s); at this point in the evaluation process, the sequence of steps is a creative process by nurses as dictated by client need
5. If a client has unexpected changes during care, nurses typically do further assessment of the situation before implementing actions
6. Use of these steps is a dynamic, client-centered process
7. Communication is essential in all phases of the nursing process

II. The initial assessment process

A. **Includes subjective and objective information**

B. **Subjective information: elicited by questions such as**
   1. What is the one item that made you decide to seek help?
   2. What is your major problem today?
   3. When did this start? How long did it last? What relieved it?
   4. Do I need to know any other information that can help me better care for you?

C. **Objective information: elicited through the senses**
   1. Inspection: done initially for the client's respiratory rate, breathing effort, color, and position
   2. Inspection and touch: a handshake of the client elicits
      a. Demonstration of respect for the client; reduction of client's anxiety
      b. Level of consciousness and the motor ability/strength of client to initiate an appropriate response
      c. Pulse assessment for rate and regularity if two-handed technique is used
      d. Skin assessment for temperature, color, texture, and moisture
   3. Smell for odors: done simultaneously with inspection
   4. Hearing: asking the initial questions, then auscultating elicits
      a. Specific information about the client's perception of the problem
      b. Information about the client's emotional reaction to the situation by noting the tone and inflection of the speech
      c. Degree of influence from others based on whether they answer or clarify client's answers to questions

d. Auscultation typically includes the lungs, heart sounds, bowel sounds, and then any vascular sounds such as the carotid arteries or arterio-venous (A-V) fistulas

5. Touch: commonly the approaches to other touch techniques such as percussion or palpation are completed by starting with the problem system then moving to the respiratory, cardiac, and neurological systems followed by the other systems

D. In emergency situations, objective information may take precedent over subjective information

1. Airway, breathing, and circulation, the ABCs, may dictate assessment priorities
2. Deferment of the history and physical assessment of all body systems may take a secondary focus, with priority actions aiming to support the cardiac and respiratory systems

E. Subjective information is best obtained from the client, the primary source, or from secondary sources such as the caretaker, family, or friends

F. History can be obtained from prior documentation to expedite the initial contact and conserve client energy

G. Results of the client's assessment act as the foundation for selecting priority nursing diagnoses and the development of an appropriate plan of care

H. In acute- and home-care settings, nurses may limit priorities to two nursing diagnoses for a more realistic, attainable, efficient, and effective approach to client care

III. The selection of nursing diagnoses

A. Nursing diagnoses

1. Are clinical judgments about responses of an individual or family to actual or potential threats to health or life situations
2. Provide the basis for the selection of nursing interventions or referrals to achieve positive outcomes for evaluation
3. Are designed with a three-part statement; however, in clinical practice the first part is consistently used, but the other parts may not be required as part of the documentation
   a. The three parts, also referred to as the PES format, are
      (1) P = health problem, stated as a nursing problem
      (2) E = etiological or related factors
      (3) S = the defining characteristics or cluster of signs/symptoms as identified from the assessment data
   b. The words *related to* connect the health problem and the etiological factors

c. The words *as manifested by* connect the etiological factors and the signs/symptoms
d. Example: urinary elimination—altered *related to* loss of muscle tone *as manifested by* incontinence, nocturia, dribbling.
e. A health problem may be an actual or a risk for (formerly potential or high-risk) problem

B. Process to the selection of nursing diagnoses

1. Assessment data are analyzed and interpreted for priorities in relation to time, for an actual or risk for problem with respect to what interventions are accountable by nursing
   a. In acute care: what needs to be accomplished
      (1) In the next 30 to 60 minutes?
      (2) In the next 8 hours?
      (3) In the next 24 hours?
      (4) By discharge from the facility?
   b. In other settings such as clinic, home, and outpatient care
      (1) What was the priority in the last few visits?
      (2) What necessitated this visit?
      (3) What has changed to require a reorganization of the priorities?
2. A diagnostic label is selected with or without the phrases *related to* and *as manifested by;* institutional documentation policies guide the specific format for each agency
3. In most situations, one or two priority nursing diagnoses are appropriate
4. The ABCs are appropriate to use as a guide for setting priorities

IV. The planning process

A. Blueprint for nursing actions, also called nursing orders or planned nursing interventions, which are

1. Based on the priorities collected or clustered from the assessment data
2. Selected in reference to time and resources available
3. Safe for the client and the nurse
4. Commonly a combination of independent, interdependent, and dependent actions

B. Involves goal setting for achievement of client outcomes

C. May be done cooperatively if client is able to participate

D. Commonly involves some component of education for a client knowledge deficit

E. **Commonly dictates client outcomes, which need to be**
    1. Achieved in a set amount of time
    2. Objective
    3. Realistic
    4. Observable or measurable for changes in client's activity, behavior, or physical state
    5. Used as a standard of measure in the evaluation process
    6. Examples
        a. Client outcome: within 48 hours the client will sleep through the night without the need to void
        b. Planned interventions
            (1) Provide use of the bedside commode before bedtime
            (2) Give no liquids after 8:00 P.M.

V. The intervention process

A. **Actual execution of the planned nursing actions**

B. **Incorporates supervision, coordination, or evaluation of the delivery of care**

C. **Includes the recording and exchange of information among different disciplines**

VI. The evaluation process

A. **Based on client outcomes as identified from the planning process**

B. **Determination of the degree of effectiveness or ineffectiveness of the interventions taken to achieve the stated outcomes**

C. **Ongoing throughout the client-nurse relationship**

D. **Often performed concurrently with other phases of the nursing process rather than as a distinctly individual step**

E. **May result in the client's reassessment to reorder priorities and set new outcomes, especially if the stated time frame has been exceeded**

F. **Requires documentation of the date when revisement or resolution of the health problem occurred; may be documented as ongoing**

G. **Requires timely, accurate, and objective documentation and communication**

H. **Includes identification of the client's level of knowledge and degree of willingness to change behaviors, skills, knowledge, or attitudes in any of these areas**
    1. Diet
    2. Activity

3. Environment
4. Equipment
5. Medications: knowledge of
   a. Expected side effects
   b. Side effects that are treatable
   c. Side effects to report to the physician and within what time frame
   d. Length for the course of treatment

CLIENT EDUCATION

I. Client education: the process

A. Integral part of nursing care on either a formal or informal basis

B. Incorporates the use of the nursing process

C. Requires the use of teaching and learning principles

D. Varies with clients according to their life experiences, present situation, and age

E. Includes six main steps

1. Assessment of client education needs or wants
2. Identification of priorities
3. Identification of client goals or outcomes: what is needed
   a. Behavior changes
   b. Skill acquisition
   c. Cognitive or attitude changes
4. Development of a teaching plan
   a. Development of learner objectives
   b. Determination of the content required for the given situation
   c. Determination of the resources and how to use them
      (1) Identify the available referral support agencies
      (2) Identify the materials available for teaching/learning activities
      (3) Investigate whether there is money available for materials, courses, transportation to and from education classes
      (4) Estimate the amount of time available versus the amount of time needed to implement the teaching plan
      (5) Decide whether the nurse will initiate and complete the education or refer to another support service for the education
   d. Determination of sequence and presentation approach of the content

5. Implementation of the teaching plan over a stated time frame
6. Evaluation of outcomes with revisions or reteaching as needed

II. Client assessments for education

A. Client's knowledge base. What does the client know? What does he or she want to know? Respect that some clients desire no information and document that response.

B. Readiness

1. Emotional
    a. Which stage of loss does client exhibit?
        (1) Denial
        (2) Anger
        (3) Bargaining
        (4) Depression
        (5) Acceptance
    b. If clients are in denial or anger, education will probably be ineffective; document stage of loss
2. Motivational: intrinsic motivation, stimulated from within the learner, is preferred to extrinsic motivation, stimulated from outside the learner
3. Experiential climate
    a. Values associated with social roles
    b. Personal resources and support systems
        (1) Family, friends
        (2) Finances for medications, equipment
        (3) Environmental factors: indoor plumbing, electricity
        (4) Prior and currect exposure to interactions with the healthcare system and providers
        (5) Availability of healthcare services, time versus distance with available transportation
    c. Developmental stage
4. Physical
    a. Clinical status is stable or improved
    b. Functional abilities
        (1) Hearing, attention span, listening
        (2) Vision
        (3) Touch and manual dexterity
        (4) Reading, level of highest education
        (5) Endurance
        (6) Short-term memory
            (a) Limited in its capacity
            (b) Enhanced if distractions are avoided

(c) Enhanced if opportunities are given for repeating or rehearsing the information

(7) Long-term memory

(a) Unlimited in its capacity and duration

(b) Influenced by the rate at which new information is introduced: the best approach is to introduce one new item every 4 to 5 seconds

(c) Enhanced by 20% to 90% if material is incorporated into a story or real-life situation

5. Signs of client's readiness
   a. Beginning behaviors of adaption to the original problem
   b. Exhibits awareness of the health problem and its implications
   c. Asks direct questions
   d. Presents clues that suggest client is seeking information
   e. Begins to ask questions about how to handle situations at home
   f. Indicators during a teaching session
      (1) Client is physically comfortable; basic needs are met
      (2) Client readily gives attention; eye contact is made
      (3) Client turns off television or asks visitors to leave

III. Special needs of clients for their education

A. Interventions for low-literacy clients

1. Give only simple (basic) information
2. Present no more than three new points at a given time
3. Give the most important information first and last
4. Sequence information in the way the client will use it
5. Give information the client can use immediately
6. Use the same words when meanings are the same (e.g., medicine or drug, not both words)
7. Use small, simple words and short sentences; introduce no more than five new words in one session
8. Present information at the fifth-grade level or lower
9. Be concrete and time specific. Example: take two pills at 4:00 P.M.
10. Ask the client to repeat the information or the skill
11. Use humor appropriately; be creative
12. Avoid long explanations
13. Reward frequently—even for small accomplishments

B. Interventions for older clients

1. Priority evaluations
   a. Establish the degree of functional losses

b. Identify the degree of social support; lack of social support may be an important determinant in the decreased compliance of older adults
c. Identify their habit structures
d. Have an evaluation completed by social services or the business office for the availability of monies

2. Clients with impaired hearing
    a. Use low-pitched voice
    b. Face client when speaking
    c. Use clear, concise terms
3. Clients with impaired vision
    a. Use large print and a magnifying glass
    b. Black on white or black on yellow paper may be easier for the older clients to read
    c. Provide adequate lighting
    d. Have client use prescription glasses
4. Clients with limited endurance
    a. Keep sessions short (10 to 15 minutes)
    b. Schedule the teaching session at a time of day when clients are comfortable and their energy levels are higher
    c. Break down the information into small steps
    d. The initial session should have only survival-level information
5. Clients with memory loss
    a. Provide repeated exposure to same message
    b. Provide cues: visual, verbal, written
    c. Question frequently
    d. Use advanced organizers: "I'm going to tell you 2 ways to give your insulin," "I've told you how to give your insulin by using two methods."

IV. Learning theory

A. Learning theory for adults

1. Adult learner is defined as a self-directed, independent person who becomes ready to learn when the need to know or perform is experienced
2. Adult education is learner centered
3. Adult education is dynamic, interactive, and cooperative
4. The responsibility for success of adult learners is shared by all participants
5. Adult learners
    a. Like to participate in identification of their learning needs, formulation of learning objectives, and evaluation of learning

b. Expect a climate of mutual respect
c. Enter the learning situation with a life-centered, task-centered, or problem-centered approach
d. Are motivated internally to learn in order to increase self-esteem, self-confidence, or seek a better quality of life
e. See the educator as a facilitator rather than a director of the activity

B. Learning theory for children

1. Learning programs for children are more subject centered
2. Design of learning experiences is topic centered
3. Learning may be more of an external process with emphasis on externally sanctioned approvals for learning such as stars, happy-face stickers
4. Objective, content development, and evaluation process are teacher controlled

C. Factors that interfere with learning

1. Nervousness, anxiety, fear
2. Too much content at one session
3. Unfamiliar terms
4. Complexity of the task
5. Limited time with too much content, results in rushing
6. Background noise or other distractions
7. Fear of the task or information
8. Frequent interruptions
9. Inability of an educator to listen to the client
10. Absence of silence
11. Left-handed student's learning skills with right-handed educator
12. Client is not healthcare oriented; healthcare educator is
13. Stage of development; older adults may have the attitude that they have lived more or less successfully with their present habits and there is no reason to change now

V. Tools for teaching

A. Types of teaching

1. One to one
2. Group
   a. Homogeneous clients for a topic
   b. Heterogeneous clients for a topic
3. Programmed instruction
4. Guided independent study
5. Lecture

6. Role playing
7. Simulation
8. Case method
9. Demonstration/return demonstration
10. Computerized instruction

B. Media for teaching

1. Printed materials: pamphlets, books, crossword puzzles, study guides
2. Pictorial materials: coloring books, videotapes, cartoons, flowcharts, slides, posters, overhead transparencies, computer simulations
3. Visual representations: models, actual equipment
4. Auditory: lectures, paired and small-group discussion, one-to-one interaction, role playing, cassette tapes, simulations
5. Tactile, kinesthetic: practice with real or simulated items, manipulating or constructing models, playing games, completing worksheets, drawing, preparing charts, bulletin boards, developing a calendar of activities

C. Factors to consider in the selection of media/support materials

1. Items readily available within acceptable costs
2. Suitability: for the purpose of the teaching, to the environment in which the teaching will take place, for the availability of ancillary equipment
3. Language: appropriate, understandable, and useful to the audience
4. Materials: accurate and relevant to the intended age group and culture
5. Print size: readable for the intended age group
6. Illustrations: accurate and related to the intended audience

D. Nurse as a tool of teaching: the nursing professional should

1. Show interest, empathy, and enthusiasm
2. Practice expert listening skills; listen between the lines not only to what clients say, but how they say it
3. Note clients' verbal and nonverbal communication that occurs; be aware of your own communication style
4. Take a break when the client indicates a need; vary the schedule
5. Be creative
6. Keep language simple
7. Allow enough time for demonstrations and return demonstrations
8. Summarize at the end with encouragement for any progress, no matter how small

E. Evaluation tips for achievement of education outcomes

1. Evaluation is an ongoing process throughout the entire teaching session
2. If periodic reassessment of learning indicates no progress, try a different approach
3. Ask open-ended questions along with specific questions
4. Ask clients to evaluate themselves

F. Intervention tips for different age groups

1. Pediatrics: the play approach works best with dolls or models; coloring, comic, or storybooks
2. Teenagers and persons in their 20s: use peer speakers, entertainment, and peer groups and keep in mind that body image and independence are a priority for these age groups
3. Persons in their 30s to mid-40s: written materials work well with follow-up time to answer questions or clarify information
4. Persons from mid-40s to early 60s: a few long, single sessions to discuss how the effects of the health problem will interfere with attainment of or plans for lifelong goals
5. Persons over mid-60s: use short, frequent, one-to-one meetings with material in larger print and keep in mind that maintaining functional abilities is a priority

SUMMARY

A working knowledge of the content in Chapter 1, the essential elements for nursing, will enhance the application of the remainder of the content in the review series. Most nursing professionals incorporate the two elements into their practice, which is based on the changing needs of clients who pursue the acquisition of healthcare services and actions to prevent pathological deterioration of the body. The nursing process and client education are intertwined in the areas of primary (preventive), secondary (early diagnosis), and tertiary (restorative, rehabilitative) health promotion.

NANDA-APPROVED NURSING DIAGNOSES

Activity intolerance
Activity intolerance, risk for
Adaptive capacity, decreased: intracranial
Adjustment, impaired
Airway clearance, ineffective
Anxiety
Aspiration, risk for

Body-image disturbance
Body temperature, altered, risk for
Bowel incontinence
Breastfeeding, effective
Breastfeeding, ineffective
Breastfeeding, interrupted
Breathing pattern, ineffective
Cardiac output, decreased
Caregiver role strain
Caregiver role strain, risk for
Communication, impaired verbal
Community coping, ineffective
Community coping, potential for enhanced
Confusion, acute
Confusion, chronic
Constipation
Constipation, colonic
Constipation, perceived
Coping, defensive
Coping, family: potential for growth
Coping, ineffective family: compromised
Coping, ineffective family: disabling
Coping, ineffective individual
Decisional conflict (specify)
Denial, ineffective
Diarrhea
Disuse syndrome, risk for
Diversional activity deficit
Dysreflexia
Energy field disturbance
Environmental interpretation syndrome: impaired
Family processes, altered
Family processes, altered: alcoholism
Fatigue
Fear
Fluid volume deficit
Fluid volume deficit, risk for
Fluid volume excess
Gas exchange, impaired
Grieving, anticipatory
Grieving, dysfunctional
Growth and development, altered

Health maintenance, altered
Health-seeking behaviors (specify)
Home maintenance management, impaired
Hopelessness
Hyperthermia
Hypothermia
Incontinence, functional
Incontinence, reflex
Incontinence, stress
Incontinence, total
Incontinence, urge
Infant behavior, disorganized
Infant behavior, disorganized: risk for
Infant feeding pattern, ineffective
Infection, risk for
Injury, perioperative positioning: risk for
Injury, risk for
Knowledge deficit (specify)
Loneliness, risk for
Management of therapeutic regimen, community: ineffective
Management of therapeutic regimen, families: ineffective
Management of therapeutic regimen, individuals: effective
Management of therapeutic regimen, individuals: ineffective
Memory, impaired
Mobility, impaired physical
Noncompliance (specify)
Nutrition, altered: less than body requirements
Nutrition, altered: more than body requirements
Nutrition, altered: risk for more than body requirements
Oral mucous membrane, altered
Pain
Pain, chronic
Parent/infant/child attachment altered, risk for
Parental role conflict
Parenting, altered
Parenting, altered, risk for
Peripheral neurovascular dysfunction, risk for
Personal identity disturbance
Poisoning, risk for
Posttrauma response
Powerlessness
Protection, altered

Rape-trauma syndrome
Rape-trauma syndrome: compound reaction
Rape-trauma syndrome: silent reaction
Relocation stress syndrome
Role performance, altered
Self-care deficit, bathing/hygiene
Self-care deficit, dressing/grooming
Self-care deficit, feeding
Self-care deficit, toileting
Self-esteem disturbance
Self-esteem, chronic low
Self-esteem, situational low
Self-mutilation, risk for
Sensory/perceptual alterations (specify) (visual, auditory, kinesthetic, gustatory, tactile, olfactory)
Sexual dysfunction
Sexuality patterns, altered
Skin integrity, impaired
Skin integrity, impaired, risk for
Sleep pattern disturbance
Social interaction, impaired
Social isolation
Spiritual distress (distress of the human spirit)
Spiritual well-being, potential for enhanced
Suffocation, risk for
Swallowing, impaired
Thermoregulation, ineffective
Thought processes, altered
Tissue integrity, impaired
Tissue perfusion, altered (specify type) (renal, cerebral, cardiopulmonary, gastrointestinal, peripheral)
Trauma, risk for
Unilateral neglect
Urinary elimination, altered
Urinary retention
Ventilation, inability to sustain spontaneous
Ventilatory weaning process, dysfunctional
Violence, risk for: self-directed or directed at others

CHAPTER 2

Human Conception and Fetal Development

STUDY OUTCOMES

After completing this chapter, the reader will be able to do the following:

- Define the key terms listed.
- Discuss the impact of genetic factors, teratogens, and maternal lifestyle on fetal-newborn health and well being.
- State the importance and content of genetic counseling.
- Describe the process of conception and the initiation of pregnancy.
- Discuss the preembryonic, embryonic, and fetal stages of development.
- Describe the function of structures essential to fetal growth and development

    amniotic membranes and fluid
    placenta
    umbilical cord

KEY TERMS

Amniotic fluid	Clear, slightly yellow alkaline fluid that surrounds the fetus; usually 1000 mL in volume at term of pregnancy.
Amniotic membranes	Amnion and chorion membranes that enclose the fetus in amniotic fluid and protect it from infectious microorganisms that may ascent through the maternal vagina.
Chromosome	Threadlike strands composed of hereditary material known as deoxyribonucleic acid (DNA); many genes, which are small segments of DNA, compose each chromosome.
Conception	The process whereby a sperm fertilizes (unites with) an ovum to create a zygote, the first cell of a new human being.
Embryo	Term used to refer to the fertilized ovum from day 15 until 8 weeks' gestation.
Fetus	Term used to refer to the embryo from 8 weeks' gestation until the pregnancy ends.
Menstrual cycle	Recurring, hormonally regulated process of follicle maturation and endometrial development that results in ovulation and preparation of the uterus for implantation of a fertilized ovum.
Multifactorial inheritance	Pattern of inheritance that reflects the interaction of several genetic and environmental factors creating mild to severe defects depending on the number of factors present.
Placenta	Organ specific to pregnancy that is formed as the chorionic villi (projections from the chorion) imbed into the decidua (endometrium of pregnancy); also called secundines.
Teratogen	Environmental substances-exposures known to be harmful to humans and which can adversely effect fetal-newborn health and well being.
Umbilical cord	Connects the fetus to the placenta, composed of two arteries and one vein.
Unifactorial (single gene) inheritance	Particular trait, health problem, or defect is controlled by one gene as a result of a variety of transmission patterns.

CONTENT REVIEW

I. Overview of genetics and conception

A. A human being's physical characteristics are determined by the genetic material carried in the nucleus of each body cell

B. Abnormalities in chromosomes and defects in genes adversely affect fetal-newborn health and well being in a variety of ways and to varying degrees

C. Defective genes can be transmitted to the offspring of gene carriers whether or not the carriers have the disorder themselves

D. Teratogen can adversely affect fetal-newborn health and well being according to

1. Teratogen's degree of toxicity or ability to harm
2. Amount of substance-exposure
3. Timing of the contact—critical periods of fetal growth and development
4. Degree of fetal susceptibility to the teratogen

E. Congenital disorders present at the time of birth as a result of interference in the process of fetal growth and development; causes include

1. Abnormal chromosomes
2. Defective genes
3. Teratogens
4. Environmental factors

F. Conception resulting in a pregnancy is a process that requires

1. Maturation of gametes—sperm and ovum
2. Menstrual cycle that results in both ovulation and preparation of the uterine endometrium for implantation
3. Intact female and male reproductive systems that allow passage of both sperm and ovum so contact can occur
4. Fertilization of an ovum with a sperm
5. Implantation of the fertilized ovum in the secretory endometrium where further development of supporting structures and the zygote-embryo-fetus can occur

II. Basic principles of human genetics

A. Genetic material is composed of chromosomes and genes, found in the nucleus of each body cell

1. Chromosome—threadlike strands composed of hereditory material known as DNA
2. Genes—small segments of DNA; they compose each chromosome
3. Each body cell is composed of 46 chromosomes
   a. 23 pairs, one from each parent
      (1) 22 pairs of autosomes which control most body traits
      (2) 1 pair of sex chromosomes which determine the sex of the human being along with some other traits
   b. Each pair of chromosomes is homologous, or matched in terms of its composition and traits regulated
4. Each gene occupies a specific location on a chromosome—each individual acquires two genes for every trait: one from the mother and one from the father
   a. Alleles refer to the different variations of a trait. Example: different eye or hair colors.
   b. If the two gene alleles for a trait are the same they are homozygous for that trait. Example: if the two gene alleles for eye color are both blue, the person will have blue eyes.
   c. If the two gene alleles for a trait are different they are heterozygous for that trait. Example: one gene for brown hair and one gene for blond hair.
   d. Genes are dominant or recessive for a trait
      (1) The dominant gene in a pair is expressed even if the other gene is different. Example: the gene for brown eyes is dominant while the gene for blue eyes is recessive; when both are in a gene pair the person will have brown eyes.
      (2) A recessive gene for a trait is only expressed if the other gene in the pair is the same-recessive. Example: two genes for blue eyes are required to express blue eyes.
5. Genotype refers to an individual's entire genetic makeup created when an ovum and sperm unite at fertilization
6. Phenotype refers to an individual's physical appearance that results from the manner in which his genotype is expressed, as influenced by the combination of dominant and recessive genes. Example: a person's genotype includes one blue-eyed gene and one brown-eyed gene while the phenotype is brown eyes.
7. Karyotype is a photograph of an individual's chromosomes arranged in pairs in terms of order, form, and size for the purpose of detecting chromosomal abnormalities

B. Chromosomal abnormalities occur during the process of cellular division-replication as a result of advanced maternal age (>35) and exposure to teratogens; two major types of abnormalities

1. Abnormalities in the number of chromosomes—more than or less than the required 46
   a. Down syndrome (trisomy 21)—the individual has three of chromosome 21 instead of two
   b. Turner's syndrome (monosomy of the X chromosome as XO instead of XX)—the individual has a missing X chromosome and as a result her reproductive system and secondary sexual characteristics are underdeveloped rendering her infertile
   c. Klinefelter's syndrome (trisomy of the sex chromosomes as XXY instead of XY)—resulting in a male with an underdeveloped reproductive system and secondary sexual characteristics rendering him infertile
2. Abnormality in the structure of chromosomes as a result of chromosomal breakage leading to the translocation, addition, or deletion of genetic material
   a. Cri du Chat syndrome—deletion of the short arm of chromosome 5, resulting in an infant born with the characteristics of a typical mewing-like cry, microcephaly, severe mental retardation, and abnormal facial characteristics

C. Transmission of defective genes

1. Unifactorial (single gene) inheritance
   a. Autosomal dominant inheritance—the abnormal gene is dominant, therefore the abnormality is expressed when the gene is present even if the other gene in the pair is normal
      (1) Abnormality may be expressed in varying degrees of severity. Examples: polydactyly (extra digits), Huntington's Chorea, achondroplasia (dwarfism).
      (2) When one parent is affected and one parent is normal, there is a 50% chance in EACH PREGNANCY that the offspring will be affected and a 50% chance that the offspring will not be affected
   b. Autosomal recessive inheritance—the abnormal gene is recessive, therefore the defect is only expressed when the other gene in the pair is the same abnormal recessive gene

(1) If the second gene in the pair is normal the abnormality is not expressed but the person is a carrier of the abnormal gene, which can be transmitted to offspring. Examples: phenylketonuria (PKU), Tay-Sachs disease, sickle-cell anemia, cystic fibrosis.

(2) Two carriers of the recessive gene must each contribute the recessive gene for their offspring to express the abnormality; for EACH PREGNANCY, there is a 25% chance the offspring will be unaffected, a 25% chance the offspring will be affected, and a 50% chance the offspring will be unaffected but a carrier of the abnormal gene

c. X-linked recessive inheritance—defective gene is carried on the X chromosome
   (1) Females are predominately carriers
   (2) Males predominately manifest the disorder when they receive the recessive gene from their mothers since there is no corresponding gene on their Y chromosome; they can transmit the defective gene only to their female offspring
   (3) Females can only express the disorder if they receive a recessive gene from their mother and a recessive gene from their affected father. Examples: hemophilia, color blindness, and Duchenne's muscular dystrophy.

d. X-linked dominant inheritance—defective gene is carried on the X chromosome but since it is dominant it is expressed in both the male and the female offspring who inherit the defective gene carrying X chromosome; females are less severely affected than males since they also carry a normal gene in their second X chromosome. Example: vitamin D-resistent rickets.

e. Inborn errors of metabolism—health problems related to absence of or defect in enzymes responsible for metabolism of protein, fat, or carbohydrate leading to an accumulation of harmful substances (phenylalanine) or absence of a substance (thyroxine) needed for growth and development
   (1) Follows an autosomal recessive pattern of inheritance
   (2) Physical growth and mental development are often adversely affected as the infant gets older; death can be an outcome. Examples: phenylketonuria (PKU), Tay-Sachs disease, and cystic fibrosis.

2. Multifactorial inheritance
   a. Expression of the health problem can occur if
      (1) Required number of defective genes are transmitted
      (2) Less than required defective genes are transmitted but required environmental factors are also present
   b. Family history of the disorder is often present. Examples: cleft lip-palate, neural tube defects, pyloric stenosis, congenital heart disease.

D. Genetic counseling

1. Counseling should be provided when
   a. Parents give birth to a child with a health problem related to inheritance
   b. Family history of genetic problems exists
2. Counselors must be capable of utilizing therapeutic communication techniques that will facilitate the development of a trusting relationship with clients in order to provide education, guidance, and support
3. Counseling should consist of
   a. Determining for each pregnancy probability of having a child that is either normal, affected by the disorder, or a carrier of the disorder
   b. Discussing the implication of the health problems created including
      (1) Effect on fetal-neonatal health and well being
      (2) Treatment approaches available
      (3) Impact on family processes by providing an opportunity to talk to parents who have children with the disorder
   c. Describing the diagnostic measures (advantages, risks, costs) specifically designed to determine if the fetus is affected, such as chorionic villi sampling (CVS), amniocentesis, sonography (see Chapter 6)
   d. Assisting with decision making using an unbiased, nonjudgmental approach—confidentiality and privacy are critical
      (1) Determine influencing factors such as religious and cultural beliefs, personal resources
      (2) If planning a pregnancy—should they risk pregnancy or seek alternatives to having their own biological children
      (3) If pregnant—should they continue with the pregnancy, seek an abortion, or allow the child to be adopted

e. Supporting parents in their decision by providing emotional support, facilitating open communication, and making referrals to appropriate support groups

f. Facilitating the grieving process as parents face
   (1) The loss of the "perfect" child with the loss of the fetus in abortion or with the birth of an affected child
   (2) The loss of the ability to have their own biological children

III. Conception—a number of interrelated steps comprise the process of conception and the beginning of pregnancy

A. Gametogenesis—process that incorporates meiosis (cellular division that reduces the chromosome number from 46 to 23) and maturation of gametes (sperm and ovum) to create cells each containing 23 single chromosomes (haploid) that are capable of uniting in fertilization to create a cell containing 46 chromosomes (diploid), characteristic of human cells

1. Spermatogenesis—maturation of one primary spermatocyte of 46 chromosomes into 4 mature gametes (sperm) each containing 23 chromosomes
   a. 22 autosomes
   b. 1 sex chromosome—either an X (female) or Y (male)
2. Oogenesis—maturation of one primary oocyte of 46 chromosomes into one mature ovum containing most of the cellular material and 3 polar bodies, all of which contain 23 chromosomes
   a. 22 autosomes
   b. 1 sex chromosome—an X chromosome
   c. Second meiotic division is completed at the time of fertilization
   d. Ovum degenerates if fertilization does not occur

B. Menstrual cycle

1. Gonadotrophin releasing hormone (GnRH)—secreted by the hypothalamus in response to the decreasing estrogen and progesterone level that occurs at the end of the menstrual cycle; stimulates the pituitary to secrete FSH and LH
2. Follicle stimulating hormone (FSH)—prepares the follicle
3. Luteinizing hormone (LH)—completes follicular maturation and stimulates ovulation, release of the maturing ovum from the ruptured follicle, as well as the development of the corpus luteum
4. Estrogen—secreted from the maturing follicle and then in smaller quantities from the corpus luteum

   a. Stimulates the proliferation of the uterine endometrium to become thicker and more vascular
   b. Increases the motility of the fallopian tubes which allows the capture of the released ovum and propels it through the tube to the site of fertilization in the ampulla (outer third) of the tube
   c. Increases the motility of the uterus, which along with prostaglandin from sperm, facilitates the forward migration of sperm into the tube to the site of fertilization
   d. Stimulates the formation of a copious amount of thin, elastic, alkaline cervical mucus that is receptive to sperm and allows them to pass through the cervix into the uterus
5. Progesterone—the major hormone secreted by the corpus luteum, formed at the site of the ruptured follicle
   a. Continues the development of the endometrium into a secretory layer capable of providing a bed for the implantation and nourishment of the fertilized ovum
   b. Raises body temperature—an objective sign that ovulation has occurred
   c. Reduces the motility of the uterus to allow for implantation and adherence of the fertilized ovum
6. If fertilization occurs
   a. Corpus luteum continues to function as a result of human chorionic gonadotrophin (HCG) which is secreted by the implanted blastocyst
      ▼ Human chorionic gonadotrophin (HCG), found in maternal urine and serum, is the basis for a positive pregnancy test
   b. Corpus luteum maintains the pregnancy by secreting estrogen and progesterone until the placenta is mature enough to produce these hormones at sufficient levels in about 6 to 10 weeks
7. If fertilization does not occur
   a. Corpus luteum degenerates
   b. Levels of estrogen and progesterone fall
      (1) Vasoconstriction occurs causing the endometrium to break down, slough off, and be discarded in the menstrual flow (day 1 of a new cycle)
      (2) Hypothalamus is stimulated to begin the menstrual cycle again

C. Sexual intercourse that takes place during the time of fertility (ovum viability) may result in fertilization and pregnancy

1. Ovum remains fertile for about 24 hours after ovulation with the optimum time of 2 hours
2. Sperm remain viable for about 48 hours after ejaculation into the female reproductive system
   a. Capability to fertilize lasts about 24 hours
   b. An average of 4 to 6 hours are required for sperm to reach the ampulla of the fallopian tube
   c. Ideally, viable sperm should be in the tube at the time of ovulation

D. Fertilization—the union of one ovum and one sperm to create a zygote; takes place in the ampulla of the fallopian tube

1. When gametes each containing an X chromosome unite, a female is created
2. When one gamete containing an X chromosome and one gamete containing a Y chromosome unite, a male is created
3. Once fertilized, the cell membrane of the ovum becomes impenetrable to other sperm
4. Zygote continues to grow and develop through mitosis, the process of cellular replication resulting in two cells with the same genetic composition (46 chromosomes) as the parent cell
5. Progress of development—zygote to morula (16 cells) to blastocyst (first major differentiation as a fluid filled cavity forms in the morula and an inner solid mass of cells develops into the embryo)
6. During its development the zygote continues to travel through the tube to the uterus and is ready for implantation at the blastocyst stage

E. Implantation (nidation)—the developing zygote reaches the uterus in 3 to 4 days where it attaches itself to the endometrium most often in the anterior or posterior segment of the fundus and completely burrows itself into the endometrium within 7 to 10 days of conception

▼ Slight bleeding may be noted as part of the process of implantation and may be mistaken for a menstrual period. This contributes to the inaccuracy of using Naegle's rule to determine the estimated date of birth (EDB).

IV. Fetal growth and development

A. Three periods or stages

1. Preembryonic or ovum
   a. Period from conception until day 14
   b. Zygote develops into the blastocyst and implants itself into the endometrium

2. Embryonic
    a. Period from day 15 until 8 weeks
    b. Referred to as an embryo
    c. Critical stage for organ and external feature development—highly vulnerable to teratogens
3. Fetal
    a. Period from 9 weeks' gestation until pregnancy ends
    b. Characterized by refinement of structure and function developed during the previous two stages
    c. Referred to as a fetus
    d. Less vulnerable to teratogens except for those that can interfere with the development of the brain and central nervous system (CNS)

B. Progress of fetal development (Figure 2-1)

▼ These illustrations can be an effective prenatal teaching tool when working with pregnant women and their families

V. Structures essential to fetal growth and development

A. Amniotic membranes

1. Amnion (inner) and chorion (outer) membranes enclose the fetus in amniotic fluid
2. Protect the fetus from infectious organisms that may ascend through the maternal vagina

B. Amniotic fluid

1. Derived from maternal plasma, cells of the amnion, and fetal fluids from lung, skin, and fetal urine; clear, slightly yellow, alkaline fluid; approximately 1 liter at term
2. Essential functions of the amniotic fluid
    a. Surrounds to cushion the fetus from trauma
    b. Facilitates fetal movement thereby enhancing the development of the musculoskeletal system
    c. Facilitates symmetrical growth by preventing fetal entanglement in the membranes and allowing for unrestricted positioning
    d. Regulates intrauterine temperature
    e. Provides a source of oral fluid
    f. Cushions umbilical cord and prevents its compression
    g. Serves as a receptacle for fetal substances—fluid can be obtained and then analyzed to determine fetal health status by means of an amniocentesis

C. Placenta—an organ specific to pregnancy; also called secundines

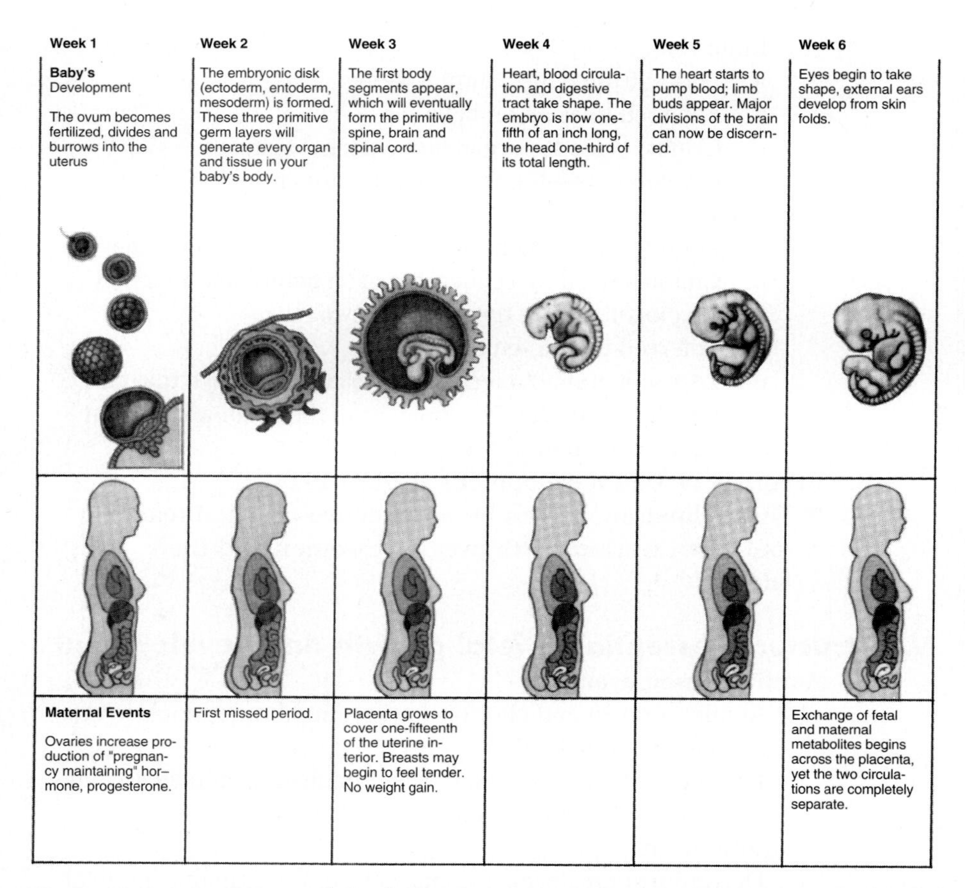

Figure 2-1. Summary of fetal development and maternal events. (From *Safe passage: a woman's guide to a healthier pregnancy,* McNeil Consumer Products Co, Fort Washington, Penn. Bobak IM et al: *Maternity and gynecologic care: the nurse and the family,* ed 5, St Louis, 1993, Mosby.) *(continued)*

1. Fully functional by week 12; it continues to grow larger and thicker as pregnancy progresses; an aging process begins at approximately the 36th week of pregnancy
2. Maternal factors that inhibit circulation (diabetes, hypertension, cardiac disease, smoking) negatively effect the growth and development of the placenta; these placentas tend to be smaller and begin to age prematurely, a fact that compromises the health and well being of the fetus
3. Essential functions of the placenta
   a. Respiration—provides oxygen and removes carbon dioxide
   b. Nutrition—supplies nutrients, fluid, vitamins, and minerals from the mother to sustain fetal growth and development

Week 14	Week 15	Week 16	Week 17	Week 18	Week 19	Week 20
The musculoskeletal system has matured. The nervous system begins to exercise some control over the body; blood vessels rapidly develop.	With hands ready to grasp, the fetus — now weighing about 7 ounces — kicks restlessly against the amniotic sac.	All organs and structures have been formed and a period of simple growth begins.	**Baby's Development**	An oily coating protects the fetus. Fine hair covers the body and keeps the oil on the skin.	Eyebrows, eyelashes and head hair develop.	The fetus is now following a regular scedule of sleeping, turning, sucking and kicking—and has settled upon a favorite position within the uterus.
3–4 lb weight gain. Belly beginning to show.		The fetal heartbeat can now be heard with an amplified stethoscope. Placenta begins producing the estrogen hormone.	**Maternal Events**	3–4 lb weight gain.	Breasts begin secreting colostrum in prepartion for nursing.	The placenta reaches its largest size relative to the fetus, covering one-half of the uterine lining. There is 400 ml of fluid now present in the amniotic sac.

Figure 2-1. *(cont'd)* Summary of fetal development and maternal events. (From *Safe passage: a woman's guide to a healthier pregnancy,* McNeil Consumer Products Co, Fort Washington, Penn. Bobak IM et al: *Maternity and gynecologic care: the nurse and the family,* ed 5, St Louis, 1993, Mosby.) *(continued)*

c. Waste removal—removes the by-products of fetal metabolism
d. Protection
   (1) Creates a barrier that prevents exposure to some but not all harmful substances
   (2) Allows passage of maternal antibodies
e. Endocrine—secretes estrogen, progesterone, human chorionic gonadotrophin (HCG), and human placental lactogen (HPL), all essential for maintenance of the pregnancy

D. Umbilical cord—connects fetus to placenta; composed of the following

1. One vein—carries oxygenated blood and nutrients to the fetus
2. Two arteries—return deoxygenated blood and wastes to the placenta

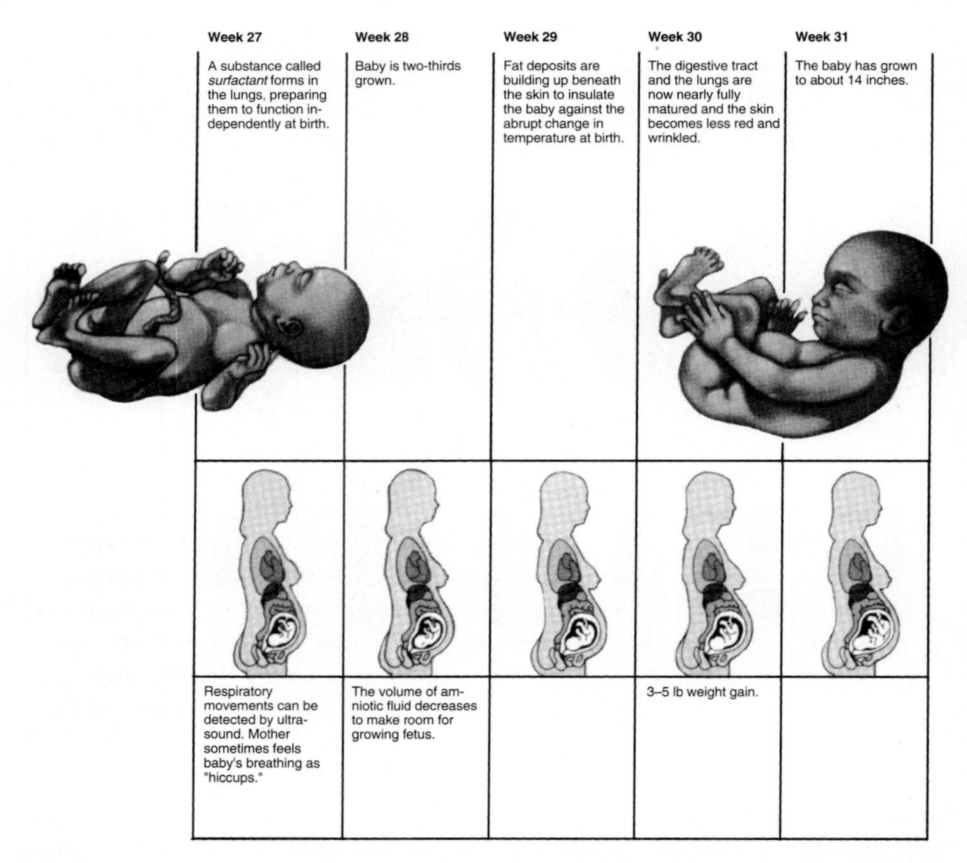

Figure 2-1. *(cont'd)* Summary of fetal development and maternal events. (From *Safe passage: a woman's guide to a healthier pregnancy,* McNeil Consumer Products Co, Fort Washington, Penn. Bobak IM et al: *Maternity and gynecologic care: the nurse and the family,* ed 5, St Louis, 1993, Mosby.)

3. Wharton's jelly—supports and separates the vessels
4. Amnion—membrane that covers the cord

VI. Factors that influence the progress of fetal growth and development—the well being of the fetus-newborn

A. Exposure to teratogens can adversely affect fetal-newborn health, well being, and even survival

1. Nature of the harmful effect is influenced by
   a. Toxicity of the teratogen
   b. Amount and length of exposure compared with the amount required for damage to occur

   c. Timing of the exposure determines the nature of the effect or abnormality
      (1) Preembryonic period—spontaneous abortion
      (2) Embryonic period—structural and anatomic abnormalities as well as spontaneous abortion
      (3) Fetal period—behavioral abnormalities, intrauterine growth retardation, fetal demise
2. Teratogens
   a. Drugs and chemicals such as alcohol, hormones, dilantin, certain antibiotics, cocaine, lead, nicotine
   b. Environmental pollutants
   c. Infectious agents that cause rubella, syphilis, toxoplasmosis, cytomegalovirus, herpes
   d. Radiation
   e. Maternal health problems such as diabetes

B. Maternal health habits and lifestyle can expose the fetus to teratogens or limit the amount of substances (nurtrients) required for optimal growth and development; preconception care and counseling should be used to help women adopt a healthy lifestyle before attempting pregnancy; health and lifestyle practices that can adversely affect the fetus-newborn include

1. Poor nutrition
2. Stressful lifestyle
3. Poor hygiene or unsafe sex practices
4. Environmental pollutants at home and in the workplace
5. Use of tobacco, alcohol, or cocaine (Table 2-1)

C. Paternal health habits and exposure of men to environmental influences are becoming the subject of increasing research

1. Fertility, in terms of sperm (number, viability, motility, morphology), penile erection, and the quality of genetic material transmitted have already been shown to be adversely affected by the same health and lifestyle practices that have been identified for women (see above)
2. Prospective fathers should receive preconception care and counseling to help them adopt a healthier lifestyle

Table 2-1. Effects of Alcohol, Tobacco, and Cocaine on Fetal-Newborn Health and Well Being

Alcohol	Tobacco	Cocaine
Effects of alcohol on the fetus-newborn appears to be related to the amount and timing of exposure ▼ Fetal alcohol syndrome (FAS), more common among women considered to be alcoholics (1 out of 3 alcoholic pregnant women will have infants with FAS), is characterized by retardation, behavioral problems, growth and structural (face-limb) abnormalities ▼ Fetal alcohol effect, which can occur among women who are light to moderate drinkers, is characterized by long-term effects of emotional problems, insomnia, difficulty with decision making or coping with school and/or job ▼ Binge drinking is especially harmful since alcohol crosses the placenta and the fetus is exposed to a large amount at one time	Tobacco has harmful effects on fetus, newborn, and pregnancy according to ▼ Degree that a woman smokes ▼ Age and health status—pregnant women who are older or already at risk from cardiovascular problems such as heart disease, hypertension, and pregnancy induced hypertension experience more harmful effects Stopping or reducing smoking during pregnancy will favorably affect outcome Circulatory effects include ▼ Damaged placenta with smaller vessels and presence of ischemic areas ▼ Double the incidence of stillbirth, LBW ▼ Increased chance for spontaneous abortion, prematurity, and perinatal mortality Nutritional effects ▼ Smoking may interfere with maternal nutrient intake and nutrient absorption ▼ Women may gain less weight	Cocaine has a major effect on pregnancy by causing vasoconstriction ▼ Increased risk of spontaneous abortion, preterm labor and birth ▼ Premature separation of the placenta ▼ Low birth weight and structural defects of the limbs Some women have used cocaine to induce labor and control the time of birth; for example adolescent women may have difficulty coping with a pregnancy that lasts 40 weeks Cocaine has been associated with congenital anomalies especially with regard to brain, CNS, and renal development ▼ Intracranial hemorrhage related to fetal hypertension; seizures ▼ Irregular sleep patterns ▼ Jittery, irritable, hard to console, muscular rigidity ▼ Limited ability to interact, make eye contact, respond to environmental stimuli ▼ Poor feeders

- Alcohol affects events occurring during each stage of development (i.e., during the fetal stage the major effect is on brain-CNS development and growth)

Fetus-newborn is more likely to exhibit intrauterine growth retardation (IUGR) and low birth weight (LBW) as a result of

- Smaller placentas
- Maternal nutritional intake may be adversely affected by alcohol abuse

Women who drink have a higher rate of stillbirth

Stopping or reducing drinking during pregnancy appears to improve outcome

Research has not indicated a safe level or time for alcohol consumption during pregnancy

Alcohol enters breast milk during lactation

No amount of alcohol is considered safe during pregnancy or lactation.

Carcinogenic effect since by-products of smoking reach the fetus, researchers are investigating an apparent increased risk for brain cancer and leukemia among children whose mothers smoked during pregnancy

Research findings into the long-term effects of fetal exposure to tobacco especially neonatal exposure to second hand smoke, are indicating

- Slower growth in height and weight; less adipose tissue
- Language and learning deficits
- Behavioral problems including hyperactivity, anxiety, depression, disobedience

Newborns exposed to parental second hand smoke have exhibited

- Increased incidence of serious infections including respiratory and ear infections
- Increased incidence of asthma and sudden infant death syndrome (SIDS)
- Long-term behavioral and learning problems
- Abnormalities of urinary tract—urethra and meatus

Breathing patterns may be affected especially during sleep—increased risk for SIDS

Coping with a cocaine-affected newborn is especially difficult for a mother who still abuses drugs or is recovering from drug abuse herself

REVIEW QUESTIONS

1. A couple seeking preconception counseling ask the nurse about the effects teratogens can have on future pregnancies. Which statement is *inaccurate* concerning the effects of teratogens?
   a. Teratogens are equally harmful to each fetal system throughout pregnancy
   b. Fetal susceptibility to teratogens varies
   c. Teratogens are not equal in terms of their toxicity or their ability to cause harm
   d. The amount of teratogen and duration of exposure influence the extent of fetal damage that occurs

2. A person's physical appearance as determined by the manner in which their genetic makeup is expressed is termed
   a. Genotype
   b. Phenotype
   c. Karyotype
   d. Dominant inheritance

3. A pregnant woman has been told that her fetus will be born with Down syndrome. Down syndrome is an example of
   a. Unifactorial inheritance
   b. X-linked recessive inheritance
   c. Trisomy of chromosome 21
   d. Chromosomal translocation

4. Based on genetic testing of a newborn, a diagnosis of dwarfism was made. The parents ask the nurse if this could happen to future children. Since this is an example of autosomal dominant inheritance, the nurse would tell the parents
   a. For each pregnancy, there is a 50% chance the child will be affected by dwarfism
   b. This will not happen again since the dwarfism was caused by the harmful genetic effects of the infection you had during pregnancy
   c. For each pregnancy there is a 25% chance the child will be a carrier of the defective gene but unaffected by the disorder
   d. Since you already have had an affected child there is a decreased chance for this to happen in future pregnancies

5. A female carries the gene for hemophilia on one of her X chromosomes. Now that she is pregnant she asks the nurse how this might affect her baby. The nurse should tell her
   a. A female baby has a 50% chance of also being a carrier
   b. A male baby can be a carrier or have hemophilia
   c. Female babies are never affected by this disorder
   d. Hemophilia is always expressed if a male inherits the defective gene

6. A couple planning pregnancy is concerned since the woman has a history of Tay-Sachs, an autosomal recessive disorder, in her family. What should the nurse advise this couple as they begin genetic testing?
   a. If either one of you carry the gene for Tay-Sachs, there will be a 50% chance with each pregnancy that the child will be affected by the disorder and a 50% chance that the child will be unaffected
   b. Both of you must carry the gene for Tay-Sachs in order for one of your children to inherit the disorder
   c. If both of you are carriers there is a 25% chance your future children will also be carriers
   d. A healthy diet and lifestyle can reduce the risk even if both of you are carriers

7. Inborn errors of metabolism such as phenylketonuria (PKU) are an example of
   a. Autosomal dominant inheritance
   b. Autosomal recessive inheritance
   c. X-linked recessive inheritance
   d. Multifactorial inheritance

8. A pregnant woman carries a single gene for cystic fibrosis. The father of her baby does not. Which of the following is true concerning the genetic pattern of cystic fibrosis as it applies to this family?
   a. The pregnant woman has cystic fibrosis herself
   b. There is a 50% chance her baby will have the disorder
   c. There is a 25% chance her baby will be a carrier
   d. There is no chance her baby will be affected by the disorder

9. Which of the following is NOT one of the responsibilities of a nurse working in genetic counseling?
   a. Determine specific diagnostic tests that will be used
   b. Help parents to understand the probability, for each pregnancy, of having a child who is either unaffected, affected, or a carrier of a genetic disorder

c. Assist parents through the grieving process
d. Educate parents so they can make informed decisions

10. If a woman experiences a deficiency in the secretion of luteinizing hormone (LH) from her pituitary gland, the result will be an interference with
a. Initial development of the graafian follicle
b. Proliferation of the endometrium after menstruation
c. Release of the ovum from a ruptured follicle (ovulation)
d. Formation of copious, thin, elastic cervical mucus

ANSWERS, RATIONALES, AND TEST-TAKING TIPS

Rationales	Test-Taking Tips
1. Correct answer: a Fetal effects are influenced by critical periods of development for each organ system.	Cluster responses *b, c,* and *d* under the catagory of "general" or "vague" because of the words "varies," "not equal in toxicity," and "amount duration influence extent." Response *a* has strong specific words: "equally each throughout" and is therefore the most INACCURATE.
2. Correct answer: b Genotype is the entire genetic makeup both expressed and unexpressed. Karyotype is a photograph of an individual's chromosomes. Many patterns of inheritance are responsible for appearance.	Remember *P*henotype—*P*hysical.
3. Correct answer: c Down's syndrome is a chromosomal disorder related to too many chromosomes, in this case three instead of two of chromosome 21. Unifactorial and x-linked recessive inheritance refer to genetic disorders. Translocation relates to structural abnormality of chromosomes associated with breakage.	If you get stumped on this type of question and tell yourself "I'll never be able to remember this," don't worry and be happy! Questions such as this one and the prior question will be minimal on the test. The important test strategy is to STOP the emotional reaction to these types of questions—close your eyes, take a few *slow,* deep breaths, blow the reaction off as you breath. Now, with the emotions gone your best performance is once again ready to answer the remaining questions.

4. Correct answer: a

Autosomal dominant inheritance is unrelated to exposure to teratogens. Each pregnancy has the same potential for expression of the disorder; there is no reduction if one child is already affected. If the gene is inherited, the disorder is always expressed.

Eliminate response *b*, since it introduces information—"infection" is not mentioned in the stem. Key words "inheritance" means disorder is expressed. The best response would have the greatest chance of reoccurrence and this is response *a*.

5. Correct answer: d

There is a 25% chance females will be carriers. If males inherit the defective X chromosome, the disorder will be expressed and they can transmit the gene to female offspring. Females are affected if they receive a gene from both parents.

Cluster responses *a, b,* and *c* with the word "baby" in each and select response *d*—that doesn't have the word "baby." Use this technique if you have no idea of the correct answer.

6. Correct answer: b

Expression of an autosomal recessive disorder requires two recessive genes, one from each parent. For each pregnancy there is a 25% chance offspring will be unaffected, a 25% chance offspring will be affected, and a 50% chance offspring will be unaffected but carriers.

Remember that "recessive" disorders require two. Thus eliminate response *a*. Eliminate response *d* since it is false. Response *b* is a more general statement than response *c* and therefore the better answer since the question is more general.

7. Correct answer: b

PKU is an example of autosomal recessive inheritance, which is a type of unifactorial (single gene) inheritance.

If you have no idea of the correct answer after reading the options, close your eyes, take 3 slow, deep breaths, then reread the question and options, make a selection and go on to the next question. Resist an emotional reaction!

8. Correct answer: d

Cystic fibrosis, as an inborn error of metabolism, follows an autosomal recessive pattern of inheritance. Two defective genes are required for expression of the disorder—she does not have the disorder nor will any of her children but there is a 50% chance they will be carriers.

Repeat the test-taking tip in no. 7. Remember that the majority of questions will be different than these two which are together.

9. Correct answer: a

While *b, c,* and *d* are nursing responsibilities, the ordering of diagnostic testing is a medical responsibility.

Response *a* has a clue from the words "determine specific diagnostic tests;" clearly this is a physician responsibility.

10. Correct answer: c

Follicle stimulating hormone (FSH) is responsible for the initial development of the graafian follicle. Estrogen is responsible for endometrial proliferation and increased production of cervical mucus.

Associate *l*uteinizing hormone *l*ets free the ovum, ovulation. Associate *f*ollicle *s*timulating hormone *f*acilitates *f*ollicle development. Associate *e*strogen affects *e*ndometrial proliferation.

CHAPTER 3

Anatomic and Physiologic Adaptations to Pregnancy

STUDY OUTCOMES

After completing this chapter, the reader will be able to do the following:

- Define the key terms listed.
- Calculate an expected date of birth using Naegele's rule.
- Describe anatomic and physiologic adaptations to pregnancy for
  - the reproductive system
  - oxygenation and circulation
  - nutrition and fluid-electrolytes
  - bowel and urinary elimination
  - physical activity and rest
  - integument
- Identify expected assessment findings during pregnancy.
- Identify the presumptive, probable, and positive changes of pregnancy.
- Identify the warning signs of ineffective anatomic and physiologic adaptation to pregnancy.

KEY TERMS

Antepartal (prenatal, gestation) period	Time of fetal development and maternal adaptation to pregnancy that begins with conception and ends with the onset of labor.
Full term gestation	Birth occurs after the 37th week but before the end of the 42nd week of gestation.
Postterm gestation	Birth occurs after the 42nd week of gestation.
Preterm gestation	Birth occurs prior to the 38th week of gestation but after the age of fetal viability, which is at approximately 20 to 24 weeks' gestation.
Trimester	One of three divisions of pregnancy with the first trimester lasting from week 1 to 13, the second trimester from week 14 to 26, and the third trimester from week 27 until birth.

CONTENT REVIEW

I. General information

A. Antepartal (prenatal, gestation) period of pregnancy

1. Duration of gestation—average of 40 weeks or 280 days from last menstrual period
   a. Full term—after 37th week, before 42nd week
   b. Preterm—before 38th week, after 20th to 24th week
   c. Postterm—after 42nd week
2. Trimester—prenatal period is divided into three segments
   a. First trimester—1 to 13 weeks
   b. Second trimester—14 to 26 weeks
   c. Third trimester—27 to birth
3. Estimation of gestational age and the estimated date of birth (EDB), formerly termed estimated date of confinement (EDC), is determined by using the following methods
   a. Dates—use of Naegele's rule: first day of the last menstrual period (LMP) minus 3 months, plus 7 days and in most cases 1 year

	month	day	year
EXAMPLE: LMP began on	7	14	94
Naegele's rule	– 3	+ 7	+ 1
EDB	4	21	95

   b. Sonogram—use of ultrasonic (sound) waves to visualize the uterus and its contents

(1) Measure gestational sac, fetal crown to rump length, fetal biparietal diameter
(2) Compare to measurements expected for a particular gestational age

c. Date for occurrence of significant events
   (1) Auscultation of fetal heart beat
      (a) 10 to 12 weeks with doppler-ultrasound stethoscope
      (b) 18 to 20 weeks with fetoscope
   (2) Quickening—maternal perception of fetal movement begins by week 16 to 20

d. Fundal height measurement to calculate gestational age in weeks using McDonald's rule—height of fundus (cm) $\times \frac{7}{8} =$ weeks' gestation. Example: 21 cm $\times \frac{7}{8} =$ 24 weeks' gestation.

e. Naegele's rule has limited value if dates are forgotten, menstrual cycles are irregular, or intermittent spotting (vaginal bleeding) occurs during the pregnancy. Therefore, using a combination of the other methods described will enhance the accuracy of the EDB.

B. Pregnancy—healthy state requiring maternal adaptations to support fetal growth and development

1. Is ongoing—occurring throughout the antepartal period as a result of mechanical and hormonal factors
2. Effects nearly every bodily function and structure to some degree
3. Increases the pregnant woman's vulnerability to health problems especially if she is determined to be at high risk
4. Has diagnostic value—presumptive, probable, positive changes of pregnancy (Table 3-1)
5. Is the underlying cause for discomforts experienced during pregnancy (Chapter 5, Table 5-4, p. 99)
6. Requires careful assessment
   a. What is the nature of the adaptation? (assessment findings exhibited, their timing, duration)
   b. Do the adaptations fall within the expected range for pregnancy or are they representative of a pathophysiological process? (such as physiologic anemia vs. pathologic anemia)
   c. Have warning signs representing ineffective adaptation and a change in risk status occurred that require further evaluation and possible intervention?

Table 3-1. Presumptive, Probable, Positive Changes of Pregnancy

Presumptive Changes	Probable Changes	Positive Changes
Definition Subjective findings suggestive, but not diagnostic of pregnancy *Changes* ▼ Breasts: tender, tingling, heaviness ▼ Nausea, vomiting ▼ Fatigue-lassitude ▼ Quickening ▼ Amenorrhea ▼ Urinary frequency	*Definition* Objective findings more suggestive of, but not yet diagnostic of pregnancy *Changes* ▼ Pigmentary changes of integument ▼ Striae gravidarum ▼ Uterine enlargement ▼ Uterine souffle ▼ Braxton-Hick's contractions palpated ▼ Hegar's sign ▼ Goodel's sign ▼ Chadwick's sign ▼ Ballottement ▼ Positive pregnancy test	*Definition* Objective findings diagnostic of pregnancy *Changes* ▼ Fetal heart beat ▼ Fetal outline with ultrasound ▼ Fetal movement detected by examiner

II. Anatomic and physiologic adaptations to pregnancy

A. Reproductive system

1. Breasts
   a. Bilateral changes, stimulated primarily by estrogen, progesterone, and human placental lactogen; begin at approximately 6 weeks' gestation
   b. Gradual increase in size of breasts; glandular and duct tissue develops; alveoli hypertrophy
   c. Precolostrum (thin, clear fluid) is produced at approximately 6 weeks and colostrum (thick, yellowish, precursor to milk) during the third trimester
   d. Circulation-vascularity increases
   e. Lactation is suppressed until estrogen-progesterone level falls after birth and the already elevated level of prolactin begins the lactation cycle

- f. Appearance
  - (1) Second to third trimester—full, heavy, enlarged, striae gravidarum
  - (2) Pigmentation of nipples and areola deepens
  - (3) Montgomery's glands (sebaceous glands found in the areola) enlarge
  - (4) Nipples enlarge, more erectile
  - (5) Nipple leakage of precolostrum and colostrum
- g. Sensitive or tender
- h. Nodular upon palpation

2. Breast self-examination (BSE)—critical to distinguish expected change from pathology; take note of
   - a. New masses especially if fixed and firm
   - b. Recent skin changes—dimpling, erythema, rashes, ulcerations, edema, and nipple retraction
   - c. Breast which has become painful
   - d. Pathologic changes are not usually bilateral in nature
3. Uterus, vagina, perineum
   - a. Changes stimulated primarily by estrogen and progesterone activity and mechanical factor of fetal growth
   - b. Uterus
     - (1) Thin, soft-walled organ enlarges 500 times its prepregnant size
     - (2) Fundus—top muscular portion of the uterus, rises (see Figure 5-1)
       - (a) Above symphysis pubis by 12 to 14 weeks
       - (b) At umbilicus by 20 weeks
       - (c) Just below xiphoid process by 36 weeks
   - c. Uterine softening begins at approximately 7 to 8 weeks and progresses from lower segment to cervix
     - (1) Hegar's sign—lower segment of uterus softens
     - (2) Goodel's sign—cervix softens and becomes more friable (fragile)
   - d. Endometrium (uterine lining) becomes thick, velvety, highly vascular; ideal for implantation; endometrium now termed the decidua
   - e. Uterine vascularity increases resulting in changes beginning at approximately 6 to 8 weeks
     - (1) Chadwick's sign—color of cervix and vagina deepens to a reddish-purple
     - (2) Progressive softening
     - (3) Pelvic congestion and edema

(a) Increase in sexual arousal and orgasms in second trimester
(b) Varicosity formation in third trimester as enlarged uterus increases pelvic pressure and inhibits venous return

f. Cervical and vaginal glands produce more mucus
   (1) Mucous plug (operculum) fills cervical (os) canal creating a barrier to infection
   (2) Leukorrhea, characteristic mucoid discharge of pregnancy occurs
g. Perineum-vulva—softer, more stretchable-vascular
h. Menstrual cycle and menses (amenorrhea) ceases due to suppression of FSH and LH by elevated levels of estrogen and progesterone
i. Fundus rises progressively until lightening (descent of uterus that accompanies movement of fetal presenting part into pelvic inlet) occurs (Figure 3-1)
   (1) Primigravida—2 to 4 weeks before labor onset
   (2) Multigravida—just before labor onset
j. Cervix-vagina change in appearance and consistency—Chadwick's and Goodel's signs

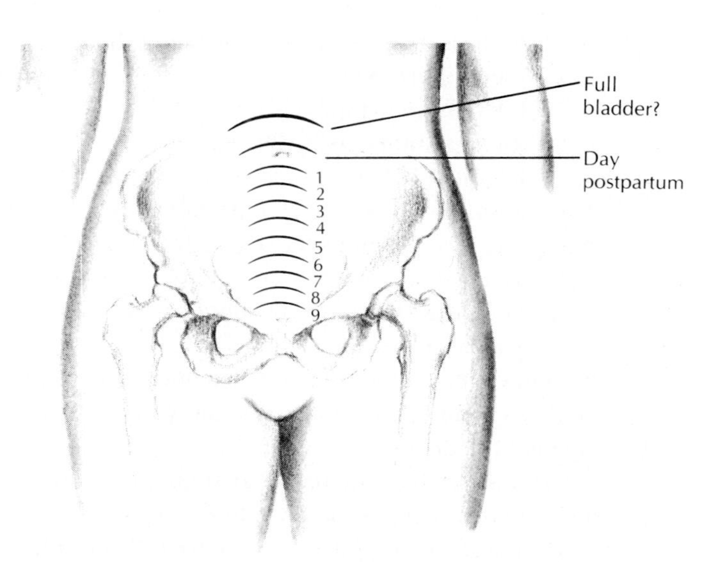

Figure 3-1. Height of the fundus by weeks of normal gestation with a single fetus. Line indicates height after lightening. (From Bobak IM et al: *Maternity nursing,* ed 4, St Louis, 1995, Mosby.)

k. Spotting can occur after examination and intercourse related to increased vascularity and friability of cervix
l. Vulva-labia major are enlarged
m. Ballottement (16 to 18 weeks)—gentle tapping on fetus during vaginal examination causes fetus to rise and then bounce back and tap finger
n. Varicosities are noted on vulva, perineum, around anus (hemorrhoids)
o. Leukorrhea appearance—white-gray, thick, less acidic (Ph 6.5) than usual vaginal discharge, faint musty odor
p. Increased risk for vaginal infections especially yeast, candidiasis, as a result of the less acidic discharge
q. Braxton-Hicks contractions—irregular, painless uterine tightening as it stretches-enlarges; begins at about 6 weeks' gestation and can be palpated after 16 weeks; become more noticeable by 28 weeks' gestation
r. Premonitory signs of labor—signs that the onset of labor is approaching
s. Vaginal bleeding to any degree must be evaluated to determine cause
t. External genitalia changes indicative of reproductive tract infections
   (1) Lesions, pruritus, erythema
   (2) Vaginal secretion changes color, amount, odor, consistency
u. Signs of preterm labor (see Chapter 11)

B. Oxygenation-circulation

1. Oxygenation
   a. Diaphragm is moved upward 4 cm (1.5") by rising fundus (see Figure 2-1)
   b. Ribs flare and expand
   c. Oxygen demand increases from increased maternal basal metabolic rate (BMR), development of reproductive structures, and fetal growth and development
   d. Vascularity of upper airway and respiratory system increases from higher estrogen levels
   e. Respirations
      (1) Slight increase in baseline respiratory rate (2 respirations per minute)
      (2) Volume deeper (hyperventilation of pregnancy)
      (3) Thoracic breathing pattern

(4) Increased awareness of need to breathe with some shortness of breath and slight dyspnea even at rest—diminishes after lightening occurs

f. Chest circumference expands by 5 to 7 cm (2" to 3")
g. Nasal mucosa—swollen, moist, reddened
h. Nasal-sinus stuffiness, clear, watery discharge
i. Inflammatory response to upper respiratory infections (colds) is more severe
j. Episodes of epistaxis (nosebleeds)
k. Sense of fullness in ears with slight impairment of hearing and earaches
l. Voice deepens
m. Slight respiratory alkalosis, compensated by mild metabolic acidosis—decrease in P_aCO_2 of 5 mm Hg at about week 10
n. Signs and symptoms indicative of cardiac decompensation and pulmonary edema in the high risk client, especially those with cardiac, hypertensive, or renal health problems
   (1) Anxiety
   (2) Moderate to severe dyspnea with tightness in chest
   (3) Orthopnea (unable to breathe lying down)
   (4) Crackles/rales
   (5) Cough, frothy sputum

2. Circulation
   a. Blood volume increases beginning at about week 10 to 12 and peaking at about week 20 to 26
      (1) 30 to 50% or 1500 ml increase in a single pregnancy
      (2) Increase of another 500 ml or more in a multiple gestation
   b. Vascular network relaxes-dilates to accommodate volume
   c. Purpose of increase in volume
      (1) Fill expanded vascular network—placenta, enlarged uterus, increased vascularity of body organs
      (2) Protect maternal-fetal unit from hypotension related to impaired venous return
      (3) Safeguard against blood loss during birth
   d. Hemodilution—most noticeable in the second trimester
      (1) Initially plasma increases faster than red blood cells
      (2) Red blood cell production catches up by the third trimester as plasma volume expansion peaks or levels off

e. Cardiac output increases by 30 to 50%—peaks at 32 weeks and then declines
f. Cardiac workload increases
g. Heart enlarges slightly
h. Heart and apex moves upward and to the left—left axis deviation on the 12 lead ECG
i. Inferior vena cava and pelvic blood vessels are compressed to varying degrees by enlarging uterus and maternal position (supine, upright); results in
    (1) Impaired venous return
    (2) Decreased cardiac output from decreased preload
    (3) Increased venous pressure in the lower extremities
j. Circulation and cardiac output is enhanced in the lateral position (right or left)
k. Hypercoagulability (increase in fibrin-fibrinogen, decrease in fibrolytic activity)
    (1) Protects against hemorrhage
    (2) Hypercoagulability combined with sluggish circulation in lower extremities increases risk of thrombophlebitis
l. Blood pressure
    (1) Decreases 5 to 10 mm Hg systolic and diastolic during first and second trimester
    (2) Returns to prepregnant baseline during third trimester
    (3) Supine hypotension, vena caval syndrome—pressure of enlarging uterus on inferior vena cava when in the supine position
    (4) Postural hypotension—fall in BP with sudden change from supine to upright position
    (5) Hypotension results in dizziness, lightheadedness, pallor, diaphoresis, anxiety
m. Heart rate and pattern
    (1) Point of maximal intensity (PMI) shifts ½" (1.5 cm) to left
    (2) Rate increases by 10 to 15 beats per minute by approximately 14 to 20 weeks, persisting until term
    (3) Transitory systolic murmurs, benign dysrhythmias, palpitations
n. Edema and varicose vein formation in lower extremities, around anus, and vulva-perineum

o. Physiologic anemia related to hemodilution
   (1) Hematocrit (Hct) should fall no lower than 33% (first, third trimesters) and no lower than 32% (second trimester)
   (2) Hemoglobin (Hgh) should fall no lower than 11 g/dL (first, third trimesters) and no lower than 10.5 (second trimester)
   (3) Stabilizes by midpregnancy with gradual return to prepregnant range
p. Signs of pregnancy induced hypertension (PIH)
   (1) Hypertension
      (a) BP increases more that 30 mm Hg systolic and 15 mm Hg diastolic over baseline
      (b) BP is ≥140/90 after 20 weeks if woman's baseline is not known
      (c) Elevation present on at least two separate assessments 6 hours apart
   (2) Edema
      (a) Upper body edema—face, hands, fingers
      (b) Sudden sharp increase in weight (i.e., >2 pounds in one week)
   (3) Headaches, visual disturbances such as double vision, spots before eyes, blurring
   (4) Epigastric pain
   (5) CNS irritability, brisk deep tendon reflexes
   (6) Proteinuria ≥1+
q. Signs of pathologic anemia
   (1) Hct and Hgh levels fall below accepted minimums
   (2) Often related to poor nutrition especially a low intake of iron (see Chapter 5, Table 5-3)
r. Signs of thrombophlebitis (more common third trimester)—primarily noted unilaterally in lower extremity, especially calf
   (1) Discomfort, feeling of heaviness in leg
   (2) Heat, erythema; found over inflamed vein if superficial vein is affected
   (3) Edema, increase in calf size
   (4) Positive Homan's sign—sharp pain in calf upon dorsiflexion of the foot
   (5) Once a positive Homan's sign is established, do not recheck since clots may be dislodged.

C. Nutrition and fluid-electrolytes

1. Basal metabolic rate (BMR) increases by approximately 20%
2. Increased activity of the thyroid gland with slight enlargement and elevated T_3 and T_4 levels
3. Nutrient needs increase and metabolism is altered to supply demands of increased BMR, maternal adaptations and fetal growth and development
   a. Increased nitrogen (protein) retention
   b. Moderate increase in iron absorption
   c. Increase in calcium absorption, enhanced parathyroid activity
   d. More complete fat absorption with deposition in subcutaneous tissue in preparation for lactation
   e. Carbohydrate metabolism-glucose level regulated by a changing production of insulin—the diabetogenic effect of pregnancy preserves glucose to meet fetal demands through the placental production of insulin antagonists
4. Weight increases (average pounds)
   a. Fetal growth (7.5+)
   b. Placenta and amniotic fluid (3)
   c. Expansion of maternal fluid volume, including blood (4)
   d. Maternal fat deposition (4 to 8)
   e. Breast and uterine development (5.5)
5. Motility of upper gastrointestinal tract decreases from an increasing progesterone level; results in
   a. Relaxation of cardiac sphincter causing a reflux of gastric contents into esophagus leading to pyrosis or heartburn
   b. Slower gastric emptying time for maximum nutrient absorption
   c. Slower emptying time of gallbladder creates potential for gallstone formation
6. Nausea and vomiting can occur as a result of slower emptying time of stomach, elevated level of human chorionic gonadotrophin (HCG), fetal demands for glucose, emotions
7. Vascularity of oral cavity increases from higher estrogen level
8. Emotional factors such as stress, anxiety, fear, ambivalence can result in GI symptoms as noted above
9. Weight gain recommendations for the entire pregnancy and the weekly pattern during second and third trimesters are based on the woman's body mass index (BMI) which is calculated using height and weight measurements (standardized tables are available)

a. First trimester weight gain—2 to 5 pounds for all BMI classifications
b. Normal weight (BMI 19.8 to 26)—25 to 35 pounds; 1 pound/week
c. Underweight (BMI <19.8)—28 to 40 pounds; 1.1 pound/week
d. Overweight or obese (BMI > 26)—15 to 25 pounds; 0.6 pound/week

10. Twin gestation weight gain recommendation—35 to 45 pounds
11. Morning sickness—nausea and/or vomiting
    a. Can occur at anytime of day
    b. Should subside by second trimester
    c. Should not result in nutritional and fluid deficits
12. Increased appetite; cravings for or aversion to certain foods
13. Pyrosis—heartburn
14. Changes in oral cavity occur by week 9 to 12
    a. Softened, tender, vascular gums that bleed more easily
    b. Epulis—localized vascular lesion present on gums
15. Laboratory values
    a. Lower fasting blood sugar (FSB)—65 mg/dL
    b. Higher cholesterol levels—243 to 305 mg/dL
16. Weight gain pattern that does not follow expected norms
    a. Too much or too little related to excessive or inadequate nutrient intake
    b. Sudden, sharp increase related to fluid retention of pregnancy induced hypertension
17. Hyperemesis gravidarum—severe vomiting leading to fluid-electrolyte imbalance, malnutrition, ketosis
18. Pica—craving for and ingestion of nonnutritive substances (i.e., laundry starch, dirt, chalk) leading to anemia and malnutrition
19. Signs of cholecystitis-cholelithiasis

D. Elimination

1. Bowel elimination
    a. Intestinal displacement and increased pressure on anal blood vessels from enlarging uterus
    b. Intestinal motility-peristalsis decreases from higher progesterone levels
    c. Increased fluid absorption from feces related to slower movement through intestine
    d. Diminished bowel sounds
    e. Flatulence

f. Constipation
g. Hemorrhoids
   (1) Combination of pelvic pressure and straining to pass constipated stool
   (2) Aggravated after lightening occurs
h. Abdominal cramping or pain—evaluate for cause; could indicate presence of appendicitis, separation of placenta, abortion, etc.
i. Diarrhea—frequent watery stools could indicate presence of intestinal tract infection, influenza, etc.

2. Urinary elimination
   a. Increase in the amount of metabolic wastes for excretion
   b. Increase in renal blood flow and glomerular filtration rate
   c. Interference in renal blood flow as a result of uterine pressure when supine or upright leads to fluid retention and edema
   d. Enhanced renal blood flow occurs when in the lateral position (left or right)
   e. Decrease in bladder capacity as a result of displacement and compression by enlarging uterus
   f. Decrease of renal tone and peristalsis in pelves, ureters, bladder and peristalsis from higher progesterone level leads to stasis-back flow of urine
   g. Urinary frequency-urgency, stress incontinence during first trimester and after lightening
   h. Increased urine production when in lateral position
      (1) Decrease in edema
      (2) Nocturia—increased urination at night
   i. Alteration in urine characteristics
      (1) Glycosuria (trace, +1)
      (2) Proteinuria (trace especially if urine is concentrated)
      (3) Higher nutrient content
   j. Positive pregnancy test as a result of presence of human chorionic gonadotrophin (HCG)
   k. Asymptomatic bacturia
      (1) Positive urine culture with no clinical signs of UTI
      (2) Associated with pregnancy and fetal complications
   l. Signs of pyelonephritis or urinary tract infection (UTI)
      (1) Flank pain
      (2) Fever
      (3) Frequency-urgency accompanied by dysuria (painful urination)

(4) Change in characteristics of urine (cloudy, hematuria, odor)

E. Physical activity and rest

1. Decrease in abdominal muscle tone and stretching from enlarging uterus
2. Nerve pressure and postural changes from enlarged, heavier breasts; change in center of gravity associated with enlarged uterus, and increased joint-ligament mobility (relaxin)
3. Increased fetal demand for calcium coupled with low intake may lead to hypocalcemia
4. Postural changes in blood pressure and cardiac output
5. Stressors related to pregnancy may interfere with rest and sleep
6. Alteration in appearance
   a. Lordosis—accentuated lumbar curve
   b. Waddling gait, awkward movement
7. Discomfort
   a. Neck and shoulder strain, numbness or tingling of hands
   b. Low back pain
   c. Muscle cramps-tetany especially of lower extremities
8. Faintness, dizziness
9. Fatigue, lassitude, decreased energy level especially in the first and third trimester
10. Diastasis recti—separation of recti muscles of abdomen
11. Tension headache
12. Signs of carpal tunnel syndrome—sustained tenderness, weakness of thumb muscles radiating to the elbow
13. Signs of pregnancy induced hypertension
    a. Severe persistent headache
    b. Irritability, restlessness, insomnia
    c. Brisk deep tendon reflexes (DTR), ankle clonus

F. Integument

1. Increased production of melanotrophin, melanocyte stimulating hormone (MSH) results in a deepening of body pigmentation
2. Increased activity of sweat and sebaceous glands from elevated levels of estrogen
3. Increased fragility and elasticity of connective tissue from increased adrenocortical activity
4. Increase in basal body temperature from increased BMR and higher progesterone level requires heat dissipation though sweat gland activity and peripheral vasodilation

5. Pigmentary changes
   a. Melasma (chloasma, mask of pregnancy)—blotchy brownish discoloration of face usually over cheeks, forehead, and nose beginning about week 16
   b. Linea nigra—darkening of vertical line along middle of abdomen beginning about week 12 and rising as fundal height increases
   c. Darkening of nipples, areola, vulva, moles, freckles, and birth marks
   d. Increased sensitivity to sunlight, sunburns more easily
6. Diaphoresis, acne, oily skin
7. Striae gravidarum—reddish-purple stretch marks on breasts, abdomen, buttocks, thighs beginning in second half of pregnancy
8. Changes related to peripheral vasodilation
   a. Hair—lustrous, fuller; hirsutism
   b. Fingernails—thinner, softer, fragile
   c. Palmar erythema
   d. Vascular spiders (spider angiomas-telangiectasis)—tiny red circular elevations with several thin branching arms; found on neck, thorax, arms of fair-skinned women about the second to fifth month of pregnancy
9. Signs of physical abuse—bruises, abrasions, fractures, and other injuries

REVIEW QUESTIONS

1. The first day of a woman's last menstrual period (LMP) was May 3, 1994, and it ended on May 7. Using Naegele's rule, this woman's estimated date of birth (EDB) would be
a. February 10, 1995
b. February 14, 1995
c. July 31, 1995
d. August 6, 1995

2. After measuring a woman's fundus, a nurse used McDonald's rule to estimate the gestational age of the pregnancy in weeks. Since the woman's fundal height was 24 cm, the gestational age of the pregnancy would be approximately how many weeks?
a. 16
b. 18
c. 21
d. 27

3. During a physical examination of a woman who suspects she is pregnant, the nurse records the following findings: darkening of nipples and areola; Hegar's, Goodel's, and Chadwick's signs present. These findings would be considered what kind of pregnancy changes?
a. Presumptive
b. Probable
c. Positive
d. Subjective-Objective

4. The external genitalia of a pregnant woman are examined during a routine prenatal visit. The nurse notes a whitish-gray, thick vaginal discharge with a faint, musty odor. The nurse should
a. Notify the physician
b. Obtain a specimen of the discharge for culture
c. Treat the woman for a yeast infection
d. Record the finding as leukorrhea

5. Upon examination of a pregnant woman at 10 weeks' gestation, the nurse notes that her vagina and cervix is a deep reddish-purple color. The nurse would record this as
a. Chadwick's sign
b. Hegar's sign
c. Goodel's sign
d. Hyperpigmentation of the genitalia

6. A pregnant woman at 14 weeks' gestation arrives for her prenatal visit and tearfully tells the nurse that she noticed a few drops of blood from her vagina when she urinated this morning. "My husband and I had intercourse last night. We thought it was safe now that I am in my second trimester. Am I losing my baby?" The nurse's best response would be
   a. "I will schedule a sonogram this afternoon so we can find out"
   b. "This is warning sign that intercourse may no longer be safe during your pregnancy"
   c. "The spotting you experienced occurs because your cervix is more fragile during pregnancy and some spotting is normal after intercourse or even vaginal exams"
   d. "Try not to have an orgasm the next time"

7. A pregnant woman in her third trimester tells the nurse that if she gets out of bed too fast she feels dizzy and lightheaded. This client is most likely experiencing
   a. Orthopnea
   b. Postural hypotension
   c. Supine hypotension
   d. A warning sign of cardiac decompensation

8. While her fundal height is being measured, a pregnant woman at 20 weeks' gestation begins to complain of dizziness and lightheadedness. The nurse notes that the woman's skin has become pale and diaphoretic. This woman is most likely experiencing
   a. Supine hypotension
   b. Anxiety reaction to pregnancy
   c. Postural hypotension
   d. Circulatory collapse

9. Which hematocrit (Hct) and hemoglobin (Hgb) result represents the lowest acceptable values for a woman in the third trimester of pregnancy?
   a. 38% Hct; 14 g/dl Hgb
   b. 35% Hct; 13 g/dl Hgb
   c. 33% Hct; 11 g/dl Hgb
   d. 32% Hct; 10.5 g/dl Hgb

10. A pregnant woman's prepregnant weight is 125 pounds and her BMI is 24. By the end of her pregnancy, her weight should fall between what range of pounds?
   a. 140 to 150
   b. 150 to 160
   c. 153 to 165
   d. 160 to 180

ANSWERS, RATIONALES, AND TEST-TAKING TIPS

Rationales | **Test-Taking Tips**

1. Correct answer: a

Naegele's rule: subtract 3 months and add 7 days and one year to the first day of the last menstrual period.

5	3	1994
–3	+7	+1
2	10	1995

Test-Taking Tip: Remember that with this rule 3 comes before 7 numerically, therefore always subtract 3 from the given month first. So immediately the responses can be narrowed to either *a* or *b*. Now remember that the first day is the starter day so that date is the one to use with the 7 and the correct answer is obvious.

2. Correct answer: c

McDonald's rule: height of fundus (cm) $\times \frac{7}{8}$ = number of weeks' gestation 24 cm $\times \frac{7}{8}$ = 21 weeks.

Test-Taking Tip: Eliminate the highest and lowest numbers, responses *a* and *d.* With the remaining choices 21 is the closest to 21 cm.

3. Correct answer: b

These are all probable changes of pregnancy—objective findings highly suggestive of but not diagnostic pregnancy.

Test-Taking Tip: Note the three levels of findings given: presumptive, probable, and positive. Use the numbers approach and eliminate the top and bottom levels; the one left is presumptive, which is the correct answer.

4. Correct answer: d

Cervical and vaginal glands are more active during pregnancy—the characteristics described reflect the expected characteristics of this mucoid discharge called leukorrhea. No further action is required except to encourage good genital

Test-Taking Tip: Given the data in the stem, it is inappropriate to call the physician; the nurse should do further assessment eg. ask what length of time it was there, get a temperature. Response *b* cannot be done without an order. In response *c,* yeast has a curdled cottage cheese type of consistency and a whitish color.

hygiene since increased risk for reproductive tract infection is present related to the less acidic nature of this discharge.

5. **Correct answer: a**

Color change is related to the increased vascularity of genitalia not increased pigmentation. Hegar's sign is softening of the lower uterine segment and Goodel's sign is softening of the cervix.

Think alphabetically for the signs and from external to internal: Chadwick's = vagina and color Goodel's = cervix and softening Hager's = uterine and softening

6. **Correct answer: c**

The spotting described is expected after intercourse because of the increased vascularity and friability of the cervix. A change in position to decrease penetration may be suggested. Continued bleeding would require further assessment. Orgasm is not responsible for the bleeding.

The longest answer describing the nurse's response is many times the best answer since it gives the most information.

7. **Correct answer: b**

A sudden change in position (posture) caused the drop in blood pressure responsible for the symptoms experienced—it is expected and not a warning sign. Orthopnea refers to difficulty breathing when supine. Supine hypotension occurs when the vena cava is compressed by the uterus when the woman lies on her back.

Match up the event described in the stem, the client changes position—postural hypotension. There is not enough information in the stem to consider response *d* as a correct choice.

8. Correct answer: a

Signs exhibited relate to a drop in blood pressure from uterine compression of the vena cava—it is an expected finding and unrelated to circulatory problems or maternal anxiety. Postural hypotension occurs when rising from a supine to an upright position.

Match up the position of the client in the stem. She would be flat on her back the fundus measured, so select supine hypotension. There is not enough data in the stem to even consider responses *b* and *d.*

9. Correct answer: c

Responses *a* and *b* are within the normal range for a nonpregnant woman. Response *c* represents the lowest acceptable value during the first and third trimester while *d* represents the lowest acceptable value for the second trimester.

Eliminate the highest and lowest numbers, responses *a* and *d.* Reread the question, which is asking for the lowest acceptable value, so select the lower number, response *c.*

10. Correct answer: b

BMI of 24 indicates a normal weight therefore the recommended weight gain would be 25 to 35 pounds.

If you have no idea of a correct answer, eliminate the options with the highest and the lowest number, options *a* and *d.* Reread the question. Go with what you know—an average recommended weight gain is between 25 to 35 pounds. Add the minimum 25 to 125 pounds of prepregnant weight. Select option *b,* 150 to 160 pounds. Or another approach, between options *b* and *c* select the one with the most conservative numbers, option *b.*

CHAPTER 4

Psychosocial Impact of Pregnancy and Impending Parenthood

STUDY OUTCOMES

After completing this chapter, the reader will be able to do the following:

- Define the key terms listed.
- Describe the psychosocial impact of pregnancy on the pregnant woman and her family.
- Discuss the crisis potential of pregnancy and birth.
- Identify factors that influence personal perceptions of pregnancy, birth, and parenting.
- Discuss the developmental tasks involved in preparation for the role of mother and the role of father.
- Describe sibling responses and need for support during pregnancy.
- Discuss the role of grandparent with changes during pregnancy.

KEY TERMS

Couvade	Culturally determined paternal behaviors during pregnancy and birthing.
Maturational crisis	Associated with an expected change related to growth and development, such as transition to the role of parent.
Situational crisis	Associated with a change in circumstances, such as the death of a family member or a preterm birth.

CONTENT REVIEW

I. Family and support system characteristics

A. Definition of family

1. Many different definitions and views of family exist
2. For this text, the definition of family is an open, living system that is composed of two or more persons who support each other; the nature of the support may be physical, economic, emotional; the degree of support may vary among family members and may be influenced by such factors as age, need, geographic location
3. Family types include
    a. Nuclear—parents and their children; becoming less common as the dominant family type in the United States
    b. Single parent—parent and his or her children; becoming more common as the dominant family type in the United States as a result of separation, divorce, death, or never being married
    c. Extended family—expansion of a nuclear or single parent family to include other family members such as grandparents, siblings, aunts, uncles, cousins
    d. Blended or combined families—parent-stepparent and children-stepchildren
4. The nurse must determine through a psychosocial assessment of each pregnant woman various factors
    a. Meaning or definition of family
    b. Composition of the family and the degree of support each family member provides
    c. Father of the baby—considered by many pregnant women to be the most important and influential person in their lives

(1) They may or may not be married to each other
(2) He may or may not be willing to play a role in the pregnancy of his partner or the raising of their child

B. Tasks that should be accomplished by the childbearing-childrearing family include

1. Alteration in career and lifestyle demands to accommodate the responsibilities of meeting the needs of children for physical care, emotional support, nurturing, and developmental guidance
2. Incorporation of children into the family system
   a. Assigning roles and responsibilities that are developmentally appropriate
   b. Developing communication patterns
   c. Providing rules of acceptable behavior (morals, values) and cultural-religious beliefs and traditions
3. Preparation of children for entry into society—the socialization process
   ▼ The reader is encouraged to consult a maternity, child health, or family health textbook for a more in-depth discussion of the concept of family

C. Definition of support system

1. For this text, the definition of support system is a group of individuals deemed by a person to be important to that person's well being
2. Composition of a support system is highly individualized and can include family members, friends, healthcare providers, clergy, other members of the community including social workers, counselors, teachers, supervisors, colleagues
3. The nurse must determine through psychosocial assessment the composition of each pregnant woman's support system and the degree and type of support offered by each individual identified as part of the support system

D. Pregnancy affects the pregnant woman, her family, and in some cases, specific members of her support system; effects include

1. Reaction to the physical and emotional changes experienced by the pregnant woman
2. Changes in roles, responsibilities, and relationships
3. Alteration in family dynamics-processes as a result of the addition of a new family member

II. Pregnancy creates a potential for the development of a maturational crisis and/or a situational crisis. Examples: change in family finances, stability, health status of a family member, complication of pregnancy, preterm birth.

A. **Perception of the event**
   1. Realistic—see pregnancy as a growth experience; recognize that adjustments and increased responsibilities are required
   2. Unrealistic—see pregnancy as stressful, a time of fear; see newborn as someone to love them or as someone who can strengthen a shaky relationship; anticipate that life will go on as usual

B. **Coping mechanisms**
   1. Usual methods of coping with stress and responding to change are called into play
   2. Effective-constructive—healthy lifestyle changes made; seek out and participate in parenting groups, childbirth classes, prenatal care
   3. Ineffective—delay confirming pregnancy or seeking prenatal care; hide pregnancy by limiting weight gain

C. **Situational supports**
   1. Availability and degree of support offered by family-support group
      a. Emotional support especially from partner
      b. Physical support in terms of household tasks, transportation, child care
      c. Role models, source of information-expertise related to pregnancy and parenting
   2. Degree to which pregnant woman accepts support offered
   3. Availability of health care and community support agencies to meet the needs of the pregnant woman and her support group—consider eligibility, quality of services, available transportation, convenience of location, and appointment times

III. Maternal psychosocial adaptations to pregnancy and impending parenthood

A. **Maternal role and responsibilities define**
   1. Activities acceptable and required during pregnancy including self-care measures, nutritional practices, activity-rest cycles, participation in health care
   2. Birthing practices
   3. Parenting activities

B. Perception of maternal role and responsibilities influenced by

1. Family experiences especially relationship with own mother
2. Cultural norms and expectations regarding a woman's behavior when pregnant and as a mother
3. Previous experiences with pregnancy and as a mother or caretaker of children
4. Attitude toward the pregnancy—desired, planned, unplanned, unwanted
5. Society—changing views regarding women and motherhood
   a. Women combining career-work role and parent role
   b. More active involvement of the father and other family members especially grandparents in helping the mother meet her parenting responsibilities
   c. Postponement of childbearing until ready for responsibilities
   d. Increasing numbers of women in the United States and even worldwide are opting for single parenthood

C. Preparation for the maternal role—developmental tasks

1. First trimester—accomplish acceptance of pregnancy: "I am pregnant"
   a. Seek confirmation of pregnancy
   b. Reaction to confirmation influenced by readiness and desire to be pregnant; most experience at least some ambivalence (feeling of "someday but not now")
   c. Adjustment to bodily changes and sensations (morning sickness, fatigue, breast tenderness, frequency); leads to
      (1) Egocentricity—concern centers on self and bodily changes
      (2) Emotional lability (moods swings)—related to hormonal changes and anxiety regarding ability to successfully cope with pregnancy
      (3) Diminished sex drive results from body changes, fear of harming fetus, mood swings
2. Second trimester—reach acceptance of the fetus as distinct from herself: "I am going to have a baby"
   a. Fetus becomes a reality and attachment to the fetus is stimulated by
      (1) Hearing the fetal heart beat
      (2) Feeling fetus move (quickening)
   b. Woman becomes introspective with attention now focused on the fetus

(1) Fantasize about the baby, themselves as mothers
(2) Review relationship with own mother
(3) Observe the mothering activities of others
(4) Family members may feel left out

c. Discomforts of first trimester diminish
d. Sexual drive resumes or increases—pelvic congestion enhances orgasm
e. Body contours begin to change—pregnancy "shows" and body boundaries become less definite

3. Third trimester—reach acceptance of impending birth and the reality of parenthood: "I am going to be a parent"
   a. Concerns center on
      (1) Securing safe passage of the fetus
      (2) Separating self from fetus
      (3) Accepting the newborn
   b. Discomforts increase, which enhances the desire for labor to begin and the fetus to be born
      (1) Fetal activity may interfere with rest
      (2) Enlarging uterus creates a change in the center of gravity increasing awkwardness and clumsiness, making it more difficult to
         (a) Ambulate, move
         (b) Accomplish tasks of living
         (c) Assume a position of comfort
      (3) Lightening leads to
         (a) Urinary frequency
         (b) Varicosities of legs, vulva, rectum-anus
         (c) Edema of legs, ankles, feet
   c. Reality of impending birth stimulates motivation to
      (1) Participate in childbirth and parenting classes
      (2) Prepare a birth plan—both parents work together to create a realistic and mutually acceptable plan to guide their birth experience
   (d) Major alterations in body contours occur—pregnant woman is sensitive to the reaction of significant others, especially the father
   (e) Decrease in sexual drive results from an increase in discomforts, a change of body-image, dyspareunia, and concerns regarding injury to fetus and stimulation of labor

D. Adolescents may experience difficulty accomplishing the tasks of pregnancy

1. Pregnancy is often unexpected; fear of discovery and possible rejection by family and support system can lead to
   a. Denial; delay in acceptance of pregnancy
   b. Avoidance of health care including prenatal care
   c. Attempts to conceal pregnancy by limiting nutrition and changing style of clothing
2. Immaturity in terms of own development may result in
   a. Limited motivation to seek and follow through with prenatal care, healthy lifestyle practices during pregnancy, or childbirth preparation classes
   b. An unrealistic, idealized view of babies and the impact of parenting
3. Successful physical and psychosocial adaptation of the adolescent to pregnancy is dependent upon the support and acceptance provided by her family and support system

E. Warning signs of ineffective maternal psychosocial adaptation to pregnancy

1. Intense denial of pregnancy as evidenced by
   a. Avoidance of or delay in confirmation of pregnancy and participation in prenatal care and expectant parent classes
   b. Concealment of pregnancy by limiting weight gain, refusal to wear maternity clothes
   c. No preparation for the newborn in terms of name, living space, supplies
2. Unrealistic expectations predominate of birth and parenting
3. Intolerance of the physical changes related to pregnancy results in an interference with ability to participate in daily activities of living
4. Refusal to alter lifestyle to ensure healthy outcome of the pregnancy and optimal fetal growth and development

IV. Paternal psychosocial adaptations to pregnancy and impending parenthood

A. Perception of paternal role influenced by

1. Factors similar to that of mother, including
   a. Family experiences and relationship with own father; single parent families with the absence of a father figure as role model may have an impact on the fathering ability of future fathers
   b. Views of his partner regarding paternal role responsibilities

c. Cultural norms and expectations regarding acceptable behaviors of the father during pregnancy and birth and as a parent
d. previous experiences with fatherhood or as a caregiver to children
e. Attitude toward his partner and the pregnancy

2. Societal norm is becoming a more equitable sharing of parenting responsibilities
3. Ideally, responsibilities of the maternal and paternal role are mutually determined and acceptable since conflict regarding role perceptions can lead to family crisis

B. Preparation for the paternal role—developmental tasks

1. Accept reality that partner is pregnant: "I am going to be a father"
   a. Views pregnancy as a confirmation of virility
   b. Experiences uncertainty or doubt regarding ability to support partner, especially during childbirth, and ability to be a father
   c. Experiences concern regarding impact of pregnancy and newborn on finances, lifestyle, sexuality
   d. Influenced by couvade
      (1) Identification with partner's pregnancy—related discomforts by experiencing nausea and vomiting, weight gain, fatigue
      (2) Role responsibilities and practices during childbirth, including degree and nature of participation
   e. Reviews relationship with own father
   f. Develops view of fetus
      (1) Becomes introspective—fantasizes about baby, self as a father
      (2) Develops attachment to fetus as he participates in the pregnancy and is given the opportunity to feel fetal movement and responses, and to hear fetal heart beat
2. Cope in a positive manner with partner's changing body and emotions
   a. Feelings regarding the changes and response to partner
      (1) Expresses pleasure in her changing body
      (2) Views physical and emotional changes of pregnancy as natural
      (3) Records changes with photographs
   b. Alteration in sexual relationship with partner related to partner's changing sex drive, body contours, and his fear of injuring partner and fetus

(1) Communicates concerns
(2) Works with partner to find mutually satisfying ways to express love and affection

3. Participate in the process of pregnancy and birth
   a. Increases involvement in creative activities such as self-improvement, enhancement of living space, job advancement
   b. Determines with his partner the degree and nature of his participation
      (1) Roles can include observer, active caregiver, provider of emotional support
      (2) Negotiate role with partner—develop birth plan together
      (3) Cope with fears regarding safety of mother-fetus and his effectiveness as a participant

C. Paternal feelings and behaviors have an influence on the success and ease of the mother's adaptation to pregnancy and parenting

D. Warning signs of ineffective paternal psychosocial adaptation to pregnancy

1. Unwilling or unable to meet the physical and emotional needs of his pregnant partner and to participate in preparation activities
2. Refusal to discuss fetus-newborn; views or fantasizes about baby as an older child
3. Expressions of anger regarding required changes in lifestyle, sexuality, financial situation may lead to abuse of partner, infidelity, abandonment
4. Expressions of disgust-displeasure with changes in partner's appearance
5. Difficulty with sexual expression with partner, may lead to infidelity or impotence

   ▼ The incidence of physical and psychological abuse of the pregnant woman by her partner is reported to have increased

V. Sibling responses to pregnancy and the newborn

A. Pregnancy and addition of a new family member has a major impact on siblings

1. May be the child's first situational-maturational crisis
2. Anxiety is created when familiar daily patterns-routines of living and relationships change
3. Perceive a loss of position and status in the family; feelings of jealousy may result
4. Stress related to separation from mom during hospitalization

B. Sibling reactions depend on age, developmental status, and life experiences

1. Toddlers—aware of mom's changing appearance; most likely to have difficulty with separation from mother and to exhibit signs of regression
2. Preschoolers and schoolagers—ask increasingly detailed questions regarding the pregnancy and express eagerness to participate in the care of the newborn
3. Adolescents—may express embarrassment regarding apparent sexual activity of parents and change in mother's bodily appearance; may be very sensitive to the needs of their mother at this time

C. Parental views and practices regarding sibling preparation are critical to successful sibling adjustment (Box 4-1)

VI. Grandparent responses to children's pregnancy and parenting

A. Must react to implications that their children are having children

1. They are old enough to be grandparents and their children are adults
2. Society's image of "grandparenthood"
3. Their children's pregnancy, birthing, and parenting practices may conflict with their views and "the way things were done when we had you"
4. Provides an opportunity to do things with their grandchildren they didn't have the time or resources to do with their own children

B. Grandparents can serve as

1. Family historians
2. Sources of support, strength, and nurturing
3. Role models, friends, and teachers

C. Nature of grandparents' role and degree of involvement influenced by

1. Experiences with own parents in the role of grandparents
2. View of the grandparent role
3. View of the grandparent role held by the expectant parents
4. Nature of the relationship between the grandparents and the expectant couple
5. Ability to develop with their children mutually agreed upon role responsibilities and involvement; failure to do so can increase the risk for family conflict and crisis

Box 4-1. Preparing Children for a New Baby

Begin preparations and use methods that are consistent with the developmental level of each child involved

- Toddlers and preschoolers should be told about the pregnancy when changes in the mother become noticeable
- Schoolagers and adolescents should be told about the pregnancy as soon as parents know

Include children in preparations made for the new baby

- Discuss anticipated changes in roles and responsibilities for each family member and the impact the baby will have on family life
- Help with choosing a name, getting the baby's room ready, picking out toys, clothing

Make plans in advance for the care of children during the time of birth

- Seek input from the children involved—who they would want to stay with and where they would want to go—and honor their input as much as possible
- Arrange for introductions, sleepovers to help younger children become familiar with temporary caregiver(s) and to prepare them for separation

Make changes, especially those regarding younger children, early in pregnancy

- Environmental changes—room change, advance from crib to bed
- Developmental changes—toilet training, enrollment in day care
- Preserve the rituals (i.e., mealtime, bedtime) of young children as much as possible

Use developmentally appropriate books, videos, classes to educate children regarding

- Sexuality
- Pregnancy and birth
- Newborns: their characteristics, needs, and care

Enhance the development of a realistic view of newborns

- Provide opportunities for children to interact with families who have newborns
- Allow older children to accompany mother to a prenatal care visit to hear the fetal heart beat and learn the importance of health care during pregnancy
- Encourage children to feel the movements of the fetus and to talk to the fetus
- View family photo albums, showing the children what they looked like as babies
- Enroll children in sibling preparation classes

REVIEW QUESTIONS

1. Which of the following behaviors is least likely to contribute to the crisis potential of pregnancy?
   a. A mother plans to surprise her pregnant daughter by moving in with the daughter after the neonate's birth and show her daughter the right way to take care of a baby
   b. A woman, pregnant for seven months, expresses pride that by limiting her weight gain she can still wear her regular clothes
   c. A pregnant woman has started to modify her work schedule in anticipation of the added responsibilities of parenting after her baby is born
   d. A 19-year-old single woman, pregnant for the first time, decides not to participate in parenting classes since she has experience as a babysitter and therefore knows how to take care of babies

2. The type of crisis represented by the typical role and responsibility changes related to pregnancy and parenting is termed
   a. Maturational
   b. Gestational
   c. Situational
   d. Family

3. During the first trimester, the pregnant woman would be most motivated to learn about
   a. Fetal development
   b. Impact of a new baby on family members
   c. Measures to reduce nausea and fatigue so she can feel better
   d. Location of childbirth preparation and breastfeeding classes

4. An expectant father confides in the nurse that his pregnant wife, 10 weeks' gestation, is driving him crazy. "One minute she seems happy and the next minute she is crying over nothing at all. Is there something wrong with her?" The nurse's best response would be
   a. "This is normal behavior and should begin to subside by the second trimester"
   b. "She may be having difficulty adjusting to pregnancy, I will refer her to a counselor that I know"
   c. "This is called emotional lability and is related to hormone changes and anxiety during pregnancy. The mood swings will eventually subside as she adjusts to being pregnant."
   d. "You seem impatient with her—perhaps this is precipitating her behavior"

5. During the second trimester, the nurse would expect a pregnant woman to exhibit
   a. Excitement when quickening occurs
   b. Egocentricity
   c. Interest in childbirth techniques
   d. Diminished sex drive related to fatigue, nausea, and breast tenderness

6. During the third trimester, the pregnant woman is working toward the accomplishment of which developmental task of pregnancy?
   a. Acceptance of the pregnancy
   b. Identification of the fetus as distinct from herself
   c. Reduction in ambivalent feelings about being pregnant
   d. Acceptance of the reality of impending birth and parenthood

7. A pregnant adolescent may have difficulty accomplishing the developmental tasks of pregnancy. Behaviors reflective of this difficulty would include all *except* which of the following?
   a. Denial of the pregnancy
   b. Participation in early and ongoing prenatal care
   c. Limitation of nutritional intake to conceal pregnancy
   d. Refusal to alter habits that could be harmful to the developing fetus

8. A Chinese-American expectant father tells the nurse he does not view his role during childbirth to be that of a coach. The nurse recognizes that this behavior is most likely a reflection of
   a. Limited interest in the well being of his wife
   b. Embarrassment
   c. Couvade
   d. Ambivalence regarding the pregnancy

9. Which of the following, if exhibited by an expectant father, would be a warning sign of ineffective adaptation to his partner's first pregnancy?
   a. Views pregnancy with pride as a confirmation of his virility
   b. Consistently changes the subject when the topic of the fetus-newborn is raised
   c. Expresses concern that he might faint at the birth of his baby
   d. Experiences nausea and fatigue, along with his partner, during the first trimester

ANSWERS, RATIONALES, AND TEST-TAKING TIPS

Rationales	Test-Taking Tips
1. Correct answer: c Response *c* represents a realistic perception of the impact of parenthood and constructive coping mechanisms; *a* represents a situational support problem; *b* represents ineffective coping to deal with changes in body-image; *d* represents an unrealistic perception of full-time parenting and ineffective coping mechanisms.	Be aware of the important word "least." In reading over the question too quickly and then getting involved with reading through the long responses, this word can be forgotten. It's best on these types of lengthy responses to reread the question after the first read through of the responses.
2. Correct answer: a Situational crisis would occur if there were a change in circumstances or unexpected events such as illness of a family member, loss of a job, or preterm labor. Responses *b* and *d* are not terms used to describe a crisis.	Think of maturational as developmental concerns or markers over the lifetime of a person. For situational think of a situation or event at one given moment.
3. Correct answer: c During the first trimester, a woman is egocentric and concerned about how she feels. Responses *a* and *b* would be of greater interest during the second trimester and response *d* in the third trimester.	Maslow's hierarchy of needs can be applied here in that the physiologic needs take priority over higher needs.

4. Correct answer: c

Response *a* does not provide enough information while responses *b* and *d* ascribe the wrong rationale for the mood swings described.

In response questions typically the longest response is the best response since it gives the most information. Response *c* is better than *a*; reread the father's question to the nurse: "Is there something wrong with her?" Response *c* is a more accurate description for an explanation.

5. Correct answer: a

Egocentricity is typical of the first trimester. Diminished sex drive typically occurs during the first and third trimesters. Interest in childbirth is prominent in the third trimester as the onset of labor approaches.

Remember the three trimesters with this technique, the three *E*'s: first = *e*go for me go; second = *e*xcitement—baby is really there; third = *e*xit—plans and preparation.

6. Correct answer: d

Responses *a* and *c* are tasks of the first trimester related to acceptance of "I am pregnant" while *b* is a task of the second trimester, "I am going to have a baby."

Associate third trimester with terminal phase of pregnancy. Option *d* best describes this—"impending birth."

7. Correct answer: b

Adolescents are more likely to deny pregnancy and as a result they may delay entry into prenatal care and try to conceal or prevent the body changes. Immaturity may limit their ability to follow through on healthy lifestyle practices.

Cluster the three responses *a, c,* and *d* under the umbrella of a negative approach from the words "denial," "limitation," and "refusal." The correct response is a positive approach.

8. Correct answer: c

Couvade refers to the culturally determined paternal behaviors during pregnancy and birth.

There is not enough data in the stem to support options *a, b,* and *d* as they are stated. Select option *c* even if you don't know what it is.

9. Correct answer: b

Responses *a, c,* and *d* are all expected behaviors of an expectant father especially in a first pregnancy. Persistent refusal to talk about the fetus-newborn may be a sign of a problem and should be assessed further.

Cluster responses *a, c,* and *d* with identification that the given information is positive and points to some type of relationship with the pregnancy. Response *b* relates negativeness toward the pregnancy and is the different and correct response.

CHAPTER 5

Application of the Nursing Process during Pregnancy

STUDY OUTCOMES

After completing this chapter, the reader will be able to do the following:

- Define the key terms listed.
- Discuss the role of prenatal care in facilitating an optimum outcome to pregnancy.
- Identify the components of a prenatal health history and physical assessment.
- Identify the laboratory tests most commonly used in a low risk pregnancy.
- Identify the common discomforts of pregnancy.
- Describe measures found to be effective for the relief of the common discomforts of pregnancy.
- Utilize the nursing process to address the most common health problems experienced by pregnant women and their support system.

KEY TERMS

Gravida	Refers to the total number of times the woman has been pregnant.
Para	Number of pregnancies delivered after the age of fetal viability has been reached, irregardless of outcome.
Preconception counseling-care	Health assessment and guidance within the year prior to becoming pregnant to ensure optimal physical and psychosocial condition for pregnancy.
Prenatal care	Early, comprehensive health care during pregnancy.

CONTENT REVIEW

I. General information for prenatal care

A. Prenatal care—only about 76% of women in the United States receive prenatal care

1. Benefits of prenatal care appear to be
   a. Reduced incidence of low birth weight (LBW) and preterm birth
   b. Increased likelihood of a positive outcome to pregnancy
2. Major factors which interfere with participation in prenatal care
   a. Demographic
      (1) Age—<20, >40
      (2) Education level—<12 years
      (3) Parity—>3
      (4) Marital status—single
      (5) Minority status
   b. Financial
      (1) Unemployed
      (2) Poverty
      (3) Inadequate or no health insurance
   c. Healthcare system
      (1) Limited capacity
      (2) Cultural insensitivity
      (3) Unwelcoming clinic atmosphere
      (4) Inconvenient hours open and limited choice for appointment times
   d. Client
      (1) Personal-cultural views with regard to healthcare during pregnancy

(2) Knowledge deficit regarding pregnancy, importance of prenatal care, and where to go for care
(3) Concurrent stressful life experiences
(4) Fear, embarrassment
(5) Attitude toward the pregnancy

3. Major services of prenatal healthcare providers
   a. Ongoing assessment of health and risk status (see Chapters 4, 7)
   b. Guidance in health promotion activities
   c. Prompt medical and psychosocial intervention
   d. Follow-up when warning signs-health problems occur
   e. Involvement with multidisciplinary health team approach and community agencies
4. Recommended prenatal care schedule—based on woman's risk status (see Table 5-1 for laboratory test for low risk clients)
   a. Preconception counseling-care—prospective father of the baby should also be included
   b. Postconception care—most common schedule
      (1) First 28 weeks—once per month
      (2) Week 28 to 36—every 2 weeks
      (3) Week 36 to birth—every week
      (4) Postterm—twice a week
5. Content of prenatal care—first visit and subsequent visits are outlined in Box 5-1, p. 83

B. The nursing process should be utilized when planning care for the pregnant woman and her family

1. Assessment of the pregnant woman and her family should
   a. Consider pregnant woman-family health history and pregnant woman's health problems-medications-treatment
   b. Involve pregnant woman and her family in the assessment process and teach them how to recognize the expected changes and warning signs of pregnancy
   c. Determine reaction to pregnancy and the adaptations it entails
   d. Focus on progress in the physical and psychosocial adaption to pregnancy taking note of expected assessment findings and warning signs (see Chapters 3, 4)
   e. Address discomforts of pregnancy—may represent a developing health problem and/or increase anxiety which may interfere with adjustment to pregnancy (Table 5-2, p. 84)
   f. Utilize consistent-accurate techniques to facilitate comparison of changes over time. Examples: BP technique, weight, fundal height measurement.

Table 5-1. Common Laboratory Tests for Low-Risk Pregnancies

Laboratory Tests	Purposes and Scheduling	Expected Results
Blood Tests		
Hematocrit, hemoglobin	Detect anemia, first visit and at 28 to 32 weeks	32 to 42%, 10.5 to 14 g/dL
White blood cells	Detect infection, first visit and as required	5000 to 15,000/mm^3
Platelets	Evaluate blood clotting mechanism, first visit and as required	150,000 to 350,000/mm^3
Blood type, Rh, coombs	Determine Rh status of mother; if mother is Rh negative and father is Rh positive a coombs (indirect) is done to detect if antibodies against Rh positive blood cells have been formed; first visit and as required	Coombs negative indicating sensitization has not occurred and Rhogam can be given during third trimester
Sickle-cell anemia screen	Detect sickle-cell hemoglobin in African American women; first visit	Negative is the desired result; if positive, further testing is required to differentiate between carrier and disease status
Rubella titer, also called Rubella antibody test	Determine immunity to rubella; first visit	>1:10 ratio indicates immunity to rubella (German measles)
VDRL/RPR/FTA-ABS	Screen for exposure to syphilis; first visit, 32 weeks	Negative, nonreactive
Hepatitis B surface antigen (HBsAG)	Screen for hepatitis B infection; first visit and as required	Negative

Glucose—1 hour	Screen for gestational diabetes: administer 50 gm of glucose by mouth and draw blood one hour later; 24 to 28 weeks	<140 mg/dL 1 hour after administration of the 50 g of glucose; if >140, a 3-hr glucose tolerance test (GTT) is done; some authorities believe that a GTT should be done if the glucose value is >130 mg/dL
Maternal serum alpha-fetoprotein (MsAFP)	Screen for open neural tube defects; spina bifida (elevated) or Down's syndrome (decreased); 16 to 18 weeks	Desired result is within the normal range; consult with laboratory performing the test for the normal range
Urine Tests—use clean catch, midstream specimen if possible		
Analysis	Detect cells, casts, pH, specific gravity to determine presence of health problems related to renal function; first visit and as needed	No differences in usual values are expected during pregnancy
Human chorionic gonadotrophin (HCG)	Basis of pregnancy test; first visit and when pregnancy is suspected	Positive test indicates presence of (HCG)
Microscopic-culture	Screen for asymptomatic bacteria; first visit and as needed (i.e., signs of urinary tract infection)	Negative
Glucose, acetone, protein	Screen for signs of diabetes, ketosis, pregnancy induced hypertension; every visit using the dipstick method	Trace for glucose and protein, negative for acetone

Continued.

Table 5-1. Common Laboratory Tests for Low-Risk Pregnancies—cont'd

Laboratory Tests	Purposes and Scheduling	Expected Results
Other		
Tuberculin skin test	Screen for tuberculosis, first visit	Nonreactive; if reactive, chest x-ray after 20 weeks' gestation, screen family members, discuss findings with client and family
Pap smear	Screen for atypical cells that can indicate cancer of cervix or certain types of reproductive tract infections; first visit	Negative
Testing of cervical and vaginal secretions	Screen for reproductive tract infections such as gonorrhea, group B streptoccus, chlamydia; first visit, at 28 weeks, and as needed	Negative

Box 5-1. Recommended Content of Prenatal Visits

First Visit

Assessment: Determine Baseline Health Status

Health history
Psychosocial status
Physical examination
- ▼ Vital signs
- ▼ General assessment of body systems with emphasis on changes associated with pregnancy
- ▼ Height and weight with determination of body mass index (BMI)
- ▼ Reproductive assessment (see Chapter 2)
  - — Breasts
  - — External and internal examination
  - — Determine pelvic adequacy now or near term (see Chapter 6)

Laboratory testing (see Table 5-1, p. 80)

Health Guidance

Emphasize importance of regular prenatal health care to promote and maintain health of the mother and her baby
Discuss the components of prenatal care—schedule of visits, what to expect, and why
Begin health teaching regarding pregnancy, self-assessment regarding expected findings and warning signs, self-care measures and health-lifestyle habits
Make appointment for next visit

Subsequent Visits

Assessment: Monitor Changes in Baseline Data and Progress of Adaptations

Update health history
Psychosocial status
Physical examination
- ▼ Vital signs
- ▼ Physical adaptations to pregnancy—expected assessment findings, presence of warning signs
- ▼ Weight
- ▼ Reproductive assessment
  - — Breasts
  - — Fundal height
  - — External genitalia; repeat internal examination near term to determine cervical changes or as required (i.e., signs of preterm labor, reproductive tract infection)
- ▼ Fetal status—fetal heart rate (FHR), fetal movements, presentation

Laboratory testing (see Table 5-1, p. 80)

Health Guidance

Discuss areas of concern such as common discomforts of pregnancy, health-lifestyle habits
Provide health teaching consistent with developmental tasks of pregnancy (see Chapter 4)

Table 5-2. Common Discomforts Associated with Pregnancy and Relief Measures

Discomforts	Recommended Relief Measures
Reproductive System Breasts ▼ Tenderness, pain, tingling (1st)* ▼ Leakage (2nd, 3rd)* (r/o mastitis)	▼ Wear supportive maternity bra ▼ Use absorbent pads, change frequently ▼ Keep nipples-areola clean and dry, avoid soap
Leukorrhea (2nd, 3rd)* (r/o infection)	▼ Perform daily perineal care, washing from front to back with soap and water then rinse with water ▼ Use pantyliners, change frequently ▼ Wear loose cotton underwear ▼ Avoid pantyhose and tight pants ▼ *Never douche*
Braxton-Hick's contractions (3rd)* (r/o labor)	▼ Change position ▼ Ambulate for short periods ▼ Practice childbirth breathing and relaxation techniques ▼ Increase fluid intake ▼ Keep bladder empty
Oxygenation-Circulation	
Nasal stuffiness, epistaxis (1st, 2nd, 3rd)*	▼ Use humidifier, cool air vaporizer ▼ Apply normal saline nasal spray or drops
Dyspnea, shortness of breath (3rd)* (r/o pulmonary edema)	▼ Maintain good posture ▼ Raise arms and stretch above head ▼ Use extra pillows at night ▼ Avoid large meals ▼ Stop smoking ▼ Balance activity and rest
Hypotension related faintness-dizziness (2nd, 3rd as uterus enlarges)*	▼ Assume side-lying position when in bed ▼ Place small pad under one hip when supine ▼ Avoid sudden position changes; move slowly and carefully

*Trimester(s) in which discomfort is most likely to occur.

Table 5-2. Common Discomforts Associated with Pregnancy and Relief Measures—cont'd

Discomforts	Recommended Relief Measures
	▼ Avoid warm and crowded areas ▼ Wear support stocking ▼ Exercise moderately to enhance venous return, increase preload ▼ Avoid hypoglycemia by eating small, frequent meals
Varicose veins, edema of lower extremities (3rd)*	▼ Avoid long periods of uninterrupted standing or sitting ▼ Do not wear constrictive clothing ▼ Avoid crossing legs ▼ Perform moderate exercise, leg and foot exercises; ambulate frequently ▼ Rest with legs and hips elevated ▼ Wear support stockings ▼ Assume lateral position when in bed to enhance renal blood flow and urine formation
Nutrition, Fluid and Electrolytes Nausea and vomiting (1st)* (r/o hyperemesis)	▼ Avoid empty or overdistended stomach by eating small, frequent meals (5 to 6/day with snacks or every 2 to 3 hours); eat foods that are liked or craved, high in potassium and magnesium, easily digested ▼ Do not brush teeth immediately after meals ▼ Eat dry carbohydrates such as unsalted crackers, dry popcorn or toast in AM before getting out of bed slowly ▼ Eat bedtime snack of slowly digested protein food such as yogurt, milk, cheese, boiled egg, lean meat

*Trimester(s) in which discomfort is most likely to occur.

Continued.

Table 5-2. Common Discomforts Associated with Pregnancy and Relief Measures—cont'd

Discomforts	Recommended Relief Measures
	▼ Avoid spicy, fried, gas-forming foods ▼ Plan relaxed mealtimes and rest periods ▼ Sit upright after meals ▼ Drink fluids between meals not with them; herbal teas are helpful ▼ Use acupressure—put pressure on wrist point with fingers at midpoint between ulnar and radial sides about ¼" from distal wrist line or wrist bands ▼ Reduce stress by using relaxation techniques and verbalizing feelings ▼ Avoid strong, unpleasant odors; lemon scent and fresh air are helpful
Bleeding, tender gums; epulis (3rd)* (r/o gum disease)	▼ Perform gentle, frequent oral care especially after episodes of vomiting ▼ Perform dental care ▼ Maintain good nutrition
Pyrosis (2nd, 3rd)*	▼ Avoid overdistended stomach by eating smaller, more frequent meals ▼ Do not eat gas-forming, fatty, spicy foods ▼ Remain upright for at least one hour after meals ▼ Maintain good posture ▼ Try sips of milk, hot tea, chewing gum, low sodium antacids (Maalox)
Elimination	
Urinary frequency, urgency, stress incontinence (1st, 3rd)* (r/o UTI)	▼ Perform kegel exercises to strengthen pelvic muscles

*Trimester(s) in which discomfort is most likely to occur.

Table 5-2. Common Discomforts Associated with Pregnancy and Relief Measures—cont'd

Discomforts	Recommended Relief Measures
	▼ Drink fluids during the day but limit fluids before bedtime; limit caffeine ▼ Establish regular elimination patterns ▼ Wear pantyliners
Constipation (2nd, 3rd)*	▼ Maintain adequate intake of fluid (6 to 8 glasses) and roughage daily ▼ Exercise moderately ▼ Establish regular elimination patterns ▼ Avoid over-the-counter remedies unless approved by healthcare provider ▼ *Never use mineral oil, since it increases elimination of fat-soluble vitamins*
Flatulence, bloating, belching (2nd, 3rd)*	▼ Chew foods slowly ▼ Avoid gas-forming foods, fatty foods, and large meals ▼ Exercise moderately ▼ Establish regular elimination patterns to prevent constipation
Hemorrhoids (3rd)*	▼ Avoid constipation—straining at stool ▼ Use sitz baths, medicated pads (Tucks) ▼ Assume Sims position to elevate buttocks
Physical Activity, Rest	
Fatigue, diminished energy level, insomnia (1st, 3rd)* (r/o anemia, depression, inadequate nutrition)	▼ Schedule rest periods (home, workplace) ▼ Perform relaxation exercises ▼ Exercise moderately on a regular basis

*Trimester(s) in which discomfort is most likely to occur.

Continued.

Table 5-2. Common Discomforts Associated with Pregnancy and Relief Measures—cont'd

Discomforts	Recommended Relief Measures
	▼ Follow a balanced diet with iron supplementation ▼ Enlist help of support system ▼ Support body parts when at rest or sleep ▼ Use safe measures to induce sleep such as warm milk, warm relaxing shower or bath ▼ *Avoid saunas, hot tubs since they can elevate body temperature leading to fetal damage*
Low back pain (2nd, 3rd)* (r/o preterm labor)	▼ Perform exercises: pelvic rock (Figure 5-1), Tailor sit position, squatting ▼ Wear maternity girdle, low heeled shoes ▼ Maintain good posture and use good body mechanics ▼ Rest on firm mattress ▼ Use local measures such as heat and massage ▼ Avoid lifting heavy objects or climbing ladders or step stools
Leg cramps (2nd, 3rd)* (r/o thrombophlebitis)	▼ Extend leg and dorsiflex foot or stand and lean forward on effected leg ▼ Apply heat, massage over effected area ▼ Include calcium rich foods in the diet or take approved calcium supplement

*Trimester(s) in which discomfort is most likely to occur.

2. Nursing diagnoses most often arise from
   a. Ineffective anatomic-physiologic adaptation to pregnancy
   b. Difficulty coping with the required alterations in lifestyle-behaviors required to ensure health of the maternal-fetal unit

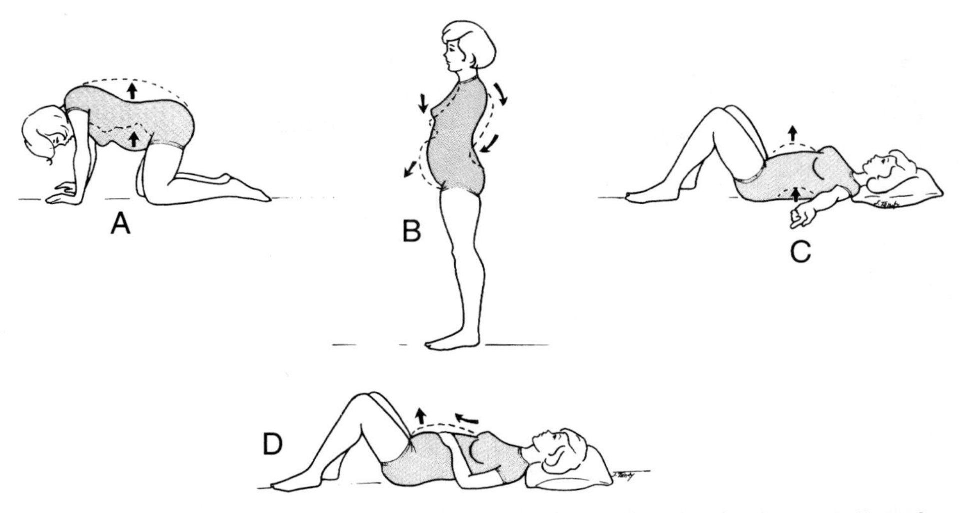

Figure 5-1. Exercises. **A-C,** Pelvic rocking relieves low backache (excellent for relief of menstrual cramps as well). **D,** Abdominal breathing aids relaxation and lifts abdominal wall off uterus. (From Bobak IM et al: *Maternity and gynecologic care: the nurse and the family,* ed 5, St Louis, 1993, Mosby.)

c. Discomforts that accompany the adaptations to pregnancy (see Table 5-2)
d. Knowledge deficits in terms of pregnancy, childbirth, parenting
e. Anxiety and stress in response to pregnancy and prospective parenting
f. Deficits in family and support system

3. Plans of care for common nursing diagnoses are described in Table 5-3

II. Assessment: physical and psychosocial adaptations of the pregnant woman and her family

A. Assess reproductive adaptations

1. Health history
   a. Gynecologic history
      (1) Menstrual pattern
      (2) Reproductive problems such as infections, benign-malignant conditions, infertility, surgeries
      (3) Birth control practices
   b. Obstetrical history
      (1) Gravida
         (a) Nulligravida—never pregnant

Table 5-3. Common Nursing Diagnoses Encountered During the Antepartal Period

Client Outcomes	Nursing Interventions	Evaluation Criteria
A. Risk for alteration in nutrition, less than or more than body requirements related to lack of knowledge regarding nutrient requirements during pregnancy, inadequate intake associated with nausea and vomiting		
Client Will Identify nutrient requirements during pregnancy Consume a diet that reflects the nutrients required during pregnancy Report a decrease in nausea and vomiting Will gain approximately one pound per week during the second and third trimester	Teach client about the nutrient needs of the pregnant woman (Table 5-4, p. 99) Discuss the relationship of nutrition to her own health, the outcome of pregnancy, and the growth of her fetus ▼ Good nutrition is a major factor in preventing low birth weight Teach client about the recommended weight gain for a pregnant woman based on her BMI; explain distribution of weight gained (see Chapter 3) Develop a diet WITH the client that reflects data from nutrition assessment, food diary, cultural preferences, activity level, nutrient requirements during pregnancy (see Table 5-4, p. 99) Serving suggestions ▼ Milk, yogurt, cheese group: 3 servings, 4 for teenager ▼ Meat, poultry, fish, dry beans, eggs, nuts group: 2 to 3 servings ▼ Vegetable group: 3 to 5 servings ▼ Fruit group: 2 to 4 servings ▼ Bread, cereal, rice, pasta group: 6 to 11 servings Discuss food preparation methods to preserve nutrient content	*Client* Accurately identified nutrient requirements Kept a 24-hour diary that reflected appropriate nutrient intake Reported fewer episodes of nausea, vomiting along with an increased tolerance for food and fluids Exhibited expected weight gain pattern

Caution client that

- ▼ Vitamin supplementation with prenatal vitamins is not a substitute for a balanced, nutritious diet
- ▼ Megadoses of vitamins especially fat soluble vitamins, A, D, E, K, can be toxic and result in fetal damage
- ▼ Fat and simple carbohydrate intake should be limited
- ▼ Alcohol should not be ingested during pregnancy

Instruct client to take iron supplement on an empty stomach if tolerated to enhance absorption; gastroninstestinal upset and constipation can occur; try a change in preparation, (i.e., ferrous sulfate to ferrous fumarate)

Teach client measures that are helpful in diminishing nausea and vomiting (see Table 5-2, p. 85)

Continued.

Table 5-3. Common Nursing Diagnoses Encountered During the Antepartal Period—cont'd

Client Outcomes	Nursing Interventions	Evaluation Criteria
B. Constipation related to decreased peristalsis associated with elevated progesterone levels and inadequate intake of fluid and roughage		
Client Will Report regular elimination of soft, formed feces Follow a diet that reflects sufficient intake of roughage and fluids	Review client's diet for sources of roughage and amount of fluid included each day Determine usual bowel elimination patterns and measures client already uses to facilitate elimination Discuss physiologic and anatomic basis for the occurrence of constipation during pregnancy and importance of roughage, fluids, and activity as safe and natural prevention measures Teach client to ▼ Drink 6 to 8 glasses of fluid each day ▼ Include sources of roughage (fiber) in the diet such as whole grains, fresh fruits and vegetables, nuts ▼ Participate in moderate level of activity each day such as walking ▼ Caution to check with healthcare provider before using stool softeners, laxatives, mineral oil, enemas	*Client* Reported having a bowel movement of a moderate amount of soft, brown stool every day or every other day Described her diet which included 8 glasses of water and fruits, vegetables, bran cereal, whole wheat bread daily

C. Altered sexuality patterns related to physiologic and anatomic changes that occur during pregnancy

Expectant Couple Will Openly discuss concerns regarding effects of pregnancy on their sexuality Identify a variety of mutually acceptable ways to express their sexuality	Describe effects of pregnancy on sexuality and sexual expression Emphasize importance of open communication of feelings and concerns regarding changes related to pregnancy and their effects on sexuality Reassure couple that in a normally progressing pregnancy there is no evidence that intercourse is harmful although some vaginal spotting (fragility of cervix and vagina) and mild uterine cramping may normally occur after intercourse Emphasize the importance of safer sex techniques to prevent infection Discuss the expectant couples current sexual practices as required Provide information concerning alternative means of sexual expression ▼ More comfortable positions ▼ Massage, oral sex, masturbation ▼ Touch to feel bodily changes ▼ Relaxation techniques Identify maternal problems that may limit the manner of sexual expression such as bleeding, premature rupture of membranes, history of spontaneous abortions or preterm labor; intercourse and orgasm may be contraindicated Counsel couple together and separately as appropriate Make referrals such as for sexual counseling if needed	*Couple* Sought guidance from nurse regarding their concerns about their sex life and openly discussed the problems they were having Participated in problem solving to find mutually acceptable ways of expressing their sexual feelings Reported satisfaction with massage and using different positions for intercourse Stated they felt more comfortable talking about sex with each other

Continued.

Table 5-3. Common Nursing Diagnoses Encountered During the Antepartal Period—cont'd

Client Outcomes	Nursing Interventions	Evaluation Criteria
D. Anxiety related to a lack of knowledge concerning the expected anatomic and physiologic changes of pregnancy		
Client Will Identify the anatomic and physiologic adaptations for each trimester of pregnancy Identify effective measures to relieve the discomforts of pregnancy Follow a lifestyle that reflects health habits conducive to a positive pregnancy outcome Express feeling more prepared to cope with changes of pregnancy Utilize appropriate measures to facilitate family adjustment to pregnancy	Use teaching approaches that take into consideration the change in concerns as pregnancy progresses ▼ First trimester, egocentric, accepting pregnancy—ready to learn about adaptations of pregnancy as they are effecting her and measures to facilitate her well being and comfort ▼ Second trimester, focusing on fetus, introspective—ready to learn about fetal growth and development, role changes, measures to facilitate fetal well being ▼ Third trimester, separation from fetus in childbirth—ready to learn about baby care, what will be needed, childbirth classes, and measures to cope with the process of labor at informal instruction or formal Use a variety of methodologies ▼ Lectures ▼ Group discussions, role playing ▼ Films ▼ Demonstration, redemonstration ▼ Written literature—pamphlets, prepared handouts, books ▼ Tour of agency where birthing will occur	Participated in prenatal education and childbirth classes Explained basis of body changes noted and identified signs that could indicate a problem requiring evaluation by her healthcare provider Enrolled in a smoking cessation program Reported use of appropriate measures for constipation and nausea and experienced relief Enrolled four-year-old child in a sibling preparation class

Essential topics should include

- Anatomic-physiologic adaptations expected during pregnancy, why they occur and how they are exhibited; warning signs of pregnancy and signs of approaching labor
- Effect of pregnancy on each member of the family including siblings and grandparents; preparation methods for siblings
- Measures to enhance well being and optimal pregnancy outcome, such as appropriate nutrition, appropriate physical activity, sufficient rest and relaxation, stress reduction, lifestyle changes—absence of smoking, alcohol, drugs
- Discomforts of pregnancy—why and when they occur, appropriate relief measures (see Table 5-2)
- Preparation for childbirth
- What to expect during the postpartum period
- Preparation for parenting and care of newborn

        (b) Primigravida—first pregnancy
        (c) Multigravida—two or more pregnancies
      (2) Para—(viability is reached at approximately 20 to 24 weeks' gestation; some authorities say at least 22 weeks)
        (a) Nullipara—no pregnancy completed to viability
        (b) Primipara—completion of one pregnancy to viability
        (c) Multipara—completion of two or more pregnancies to viability
      (3) 5-digit system to describe pregnancies-outcomes
        (a) G—gravida
        (b) T—number of term birth(s)
        (c) P—number of preterm birth(s)
        (d) A—number of abortion(s), termination of pregnancy before age of viability
        (e) L—number of living children. Example: 6-4-0-2-4.
      (4) Past obstetrical outcomes related to
        (a) Pregnancy, birth, or postpartum events
        (b) Fetus-newborn status
      (5) Current pregnancy experiences
        (a) Adaptations made
        (b) Progress noted
        (c) Warning signs observed
        (d) Fetal movement patterns experienced

2. Physical assessment
   a. Breasts
      (1) Observe appearance, leakage
      (2) Palpate for consistency, tenderness
      (3) Review BSE technique
   b. Fundal height measurement—use consistent technique
      (1) Use pliable, nonstretchable tape
      (2) Assist woman into supine position with head and shoulders elevated with small pillow for comfort
      (3) Measure along midline of abdomen from notch of symphysis pubis to top of fundus
   c. Uterus—palpate for
      (1) Braxton-Hick's contractions
      (2) Fetal movement
      (3) Fetal presentation-position following the systematic abdominal palpation of Leopold's maneuvers
   d. Lower uterine segment, cervix, vagina

(1) Palpate softening of lower uterine segment (Hegar's sign)
(2) Palpate softening of cervix (Goodel's sign)
(3) Observe change in color of cervix-vagina to deep reddish-purple from increased vascularity (Chadwick's sign)
(4) Perform pelvic examination at first visit and again near term

e. Observe-palpate external genitalia and vaginal discharge for evidence of reproductive tract infection
f. Observe vulva, perineum for varicosities, lesions, rashes

B. Assess oxygenation and circulation adaptations

1. Health history
   a. Health problems
      (1) Asthma, respiratory infections (bronchitis, sinusitis)
      (2) Cardiovascular disease
      (3) Hypertension
      (4) Thrombophlebitis
   b. Harmful lifestyle practices-situations
      (1) Tobacco, drug abuse, alcohol use
      (2) Exposure to environmental pollutants
      (3) Inadequate or unbalanced nutritional intake
   c. Presence of changes in respiratory tract and breathing patterns
      (1) Dyspnea, shortness of breath (SOB), orthopnea
      (2) Cough, sputum-discharge
      (3) Epistaxis
   d. Changes in hearing, earaches
   e. Presence of dizziness-faintness, fatigue, difficulty performing activities of daily living
   f. Presence of cardiovascular changes
      (1) Palpitations
      (2) Signs of pregnancy induced hypertension (see Chapter 7)
2. Physical assessment
   a. Determine maternal vital signs—BP, temperature, pulse (apical, radial), respirations
   b. Assess fetal heart rate (see Chapter 6)
   c. Auscultate chest—heart and breath sounds
   d. Observe and palpate extremities
      (1) Circulatory status—color, temperature, peripheral pulses, capillary refill <3 sec

(2) Edema—degree, over what period of time did it develop

(3) Signs of thrombophlebitis or deep vein thrombosis

C. Assess nutritional and fluid-electrolyte adaptation

1. Health history
   a. Useful tools—nutritional self-assessments, nutrition diaries for 24-hour or 3-day nutritional recalls; facilitate individualized approach to nutrition counseling-teaching
   b. Nutritional habits and resourses
      (1) Typical food and fluid intake; food preferences
      (2) Food preparation methods
      (3) Facilities for food preparation and storage
      (4) Availability of and ability to obtain food
      (5) Knowledge of nutritional requirements for pregnancy (see Table 5-4)
      (6) Cultural-religious influences; vegetarianism
   c. History of nutritional problems
      (1) Inappropriate intake—dietary imbalance
      (2) Underweight, overweight
      (3) Bulimia, anorexia
      (4) Cholecystitis, ulcers
      (5) Food allergies
   d. History of endocrine problems
      (1) Pregestational or gestational diabetes mellitus
      (2) Hyperthyroidism, hypothyroidism
      (3) Adrenal insufficiency; steroid use with health problems such as lupus, arthritis
   e. Gastrointestinal health with this pregnancy
      (1) Appetite
      (2) Pyrosis—heartburn
      (3) Cravings-pica; altered food tolerances. Examples: pain after fatty meals, aversions
      (4) Nausea, vomiting—onset, duration, pattern, severity, precipitating factors, actions that relieve or minimize
2. Physical assessment
   a. Determine
      (1) Prepregnant weight, height
      (2) Body mass index (BMI)
      (3) Pattern of weight gain
      (4) Weight assessment must follow a consistent approach for accurate determination of pattern

Table 5-4. Recommended Nutrient Requirement Increases during Pregnancy

Nutrient	Requirement*	Food Sources
Calories Essential to supply energy for ▼ Increased metabolic rate ▼ Utilization of nutrients ▼ Protein sparing so it can be used for — Growth of fetus — Development of structures required for pregnancy including placenta, amniotic fluid, tissue growth	300 calories/day above the prepregnancy daily requirement to maintain ideal body weight and meet energy requirements of activity level ▼ Begin increase in second trimester ▼ Use weight-gain pattern as an indication of adequacy of calorie intake ▼ Failure to meet caloric requirements can lead to ketosis as fat and protein are used for energy; ketosis has been associated with fetal damage	Caloric increase should reflect ▼ Foods of high nutrient value such as protein, complex carbohydrates (whole grains, vegetables, fruits) ▼ Variety of foods representing food sources for the nutrients required during pregnancy ▼ No more than 30% fat
Protein Essential for ▼ Fetal tissue growth ▼ Maternal tissue growth including uterus and breasts ▼ Development of essential pregnancy structures ▼ Formation of red blood cells and plasma proteins ▼ Inadequate protein intake has been associated with onset of pregnancy induced hypertension (PIH)	60 mg/day or an increase of 10% above daily requirements for age group Adolescents have a higher protein requirement than mature women since adolescents must supply protein for their own growth as well as protein to meet the pregnancy requirement	Protein increase should reflect ▼ Lean meat, poultry, fish ▼ Eggs, cheese, milk ▼ Dried beans, lentils, nuts ▼ Whole grains ▼ Vegetarians must take note of the amino acid content of protein foods consumed to ensure ingestion of sufficient quantities of all amino acids

Continued.

Table 5-4. Recommended Nutrient Requirement Increases during Pregnancy—cont'd

Nutrient	Requirement*	Food Sources
Calcium-Phosphorous Essential for ▼ Growth and development of fetal skeleton and tooth buds ▼ Maintenance of mineralization of maternal bones and teeth ▼ Current research is demonstrating an association between adequate calcium intake and the prevention of pregnancy induced hypertension	**Calcium** Calcium increases of ▼ 1200 mg/day representing an increase of 50% above prepregnancy daily requirement ▼ 1600 mg/day is recommended for the adolescent 10 mcg/day of vitamin D is required since it enhances absorption of both calcium and phosphorous	Calcium increase should reflect ▼ Dairy products: milk, yogurt, ice cream, cheese, egg yolk ▼ Whole grains, tofu ▼ Green leafy vegetables ▼ Canned salmon and sardines with bones ▼ Calcium fortified foods such as orange juice ▼ Vitamin D sources: fortified milk, margarine, egg yolk, butter, liver, seafood

Iron Essential for ▼ Expansion of blood volume and red blood cell formation ▼ Establishment of fetal iron stores for first few months of life	30 mg/day representing a doubling of the prepregnant daily requirement ▼ Begin supplementation at 30 mg/day in second trimester, since diet alone is unable to meet pregnancy requirement ▼ 60 to 120 mg/day along with copper and zinc supplementation for women who have low hemoglobin values prior to pregnancy or who have iron deficiency anemia ▼ 70 mg/day of vitamin C which enhances iron absorption ▼ Inadequate iron intake results in — Maternal effects—anemia, depletion of iron stores, decreased energy and appetite, cardiac stress especially during labor and birth — Fetal effects—decreased availability of oxygen thereby affecting fetal growth ▼ Iron deficiency anemia is the most common nutritional disorder of pregnancy	Iron increases should reflect ▼ Liver, red meat, fish, poultry, eggs ▼ Enriched, whole grain cereals and breads ▼ Dark green leafy vegetables, legumes ▼ Nuts, dried fruits ▼ Vitamin C sources: citrus fruits and juices, strawberries, cantalope, tomatoes, green peppers, broccoli or cabbage, potatoes ▼ Iron from food sources is more readily absorbed when served with foods high in vitamin C

Continued.

Table 5-4. Recommended Nutrient Requirement Increases during Pregnancy—cont'd

Nutrient	Requirement*	Food Sources
Zinc		
Essential for the formation of enzymes May be important in the prevention of congenital malformations of the fetus	15 mg/day representing an increase of 3 mg/day over prepregnant daily requirements	Zinc increases should reflect ▼ Liver, meats ▼ Shell fish ▼ Eggs, milk, cheese ▼ Whole grains, legumes, nuts
Folic Acid, Folacin, Folate		
Essential for ▼ Formation of red blood cells and prevention of anemia ▼ DNA synthesis and cell formation; may play a role in the prevention of neural tube defects (spina bifida), abortion, abruptio placenta	400 mcg/day representing an increase of more than 2 times the daily prepregnant requirement 300 mcg/day supplement for women with low folate levels or dietary deficiency	Increases should reflect ▼ Liver, kidney, lean beef, veal ▼ Dark green leafy vegetables, broccoli, asparagus, artichokes, legumes ▼ Whole grains, peanuts ▼ Oranges
Additional Requirements		
Minerals		
▼ Iodine	175 mcg/day	Increased requirements of pregnancy can easily be met with a balanced diet that meets the requirement for calories and includes food sources high in the other nutrients needed during pregnancy
▼ Magnesium	320 mg/day	
▼ Selenium	65 mcg/day	
Vitamins		
E	10 mg/day	
Thiamine	1.5 mg/day	
Riboflavin	1.6 mg/day	
Pyridoxine (B_6)	2.2 mg/day	
B_{12}	2.2 mcg/day	
Niacin	17 mg/day	

*Represents requirements for a healthy, well-nourished woman with a singleton pregnancy. Additional requirements, including supplementation, are

(a) Reduce stress involved in the "weigh in"
(b) Balance scale before use
(c) Wear same amount of clothing (examination gown, no shoes)

b. Evaluate hydration status—turgor, diaphoresis, edema, concentration and amount of urine
c. Observe condition of oral cavity—integrity of gums and teeth, vascular lesions, bleeding
d. Palpate thyroid gland

D. Assess elimination adaptations

1. Health history
   a. History of health problems. Examples: urinary tract infections (UTIs), pyelonephritis, colitis, chronic constipation, hemorrhoids.
   b. Usual pattern of bowel-bladder elimination—recent changes such as pain, decreased or increased frequency
   c. Usual characteristics of feces and urine—any recent changes noted in consistency, color, odor, clarity, and amount with potential contributing factors
   d. Measures used to facilitate bowel elimination such as specific foods, fluids, medications
2. Physical assessment
   a. Auscultate bowel sounds
   b. Observe urethral meatus for redness-edema and anus for hemorrhoids

E. Assess physical activity and rest adaptations

1. Health history
   a. Usual activity patterns
      (1) Type and frequency of activity
      (2) Participation in exercise programs
      (3) Any changes in activity patterns-tolerance since pregnant
   b. Usual rest-sleep patterns
      (1) Change in amount of rest-sleep
      (2) Sufficiency of rest-sleep for feeling of well being
      (3) Interference in rest-sleep since pregnant
   c. Measures used to facilitate rest-sleep
   d. Knowledge of safety measures, body mechanics related to changing body contours, center of gravity
2. Physical assessment—observe
   a. Muscle tone—overall, abdominal

b. Range of motion
c. Ambulation, gait, balance
d. Posture
e. Signs of fatigue
f. Appropriateness of dress. Examples: nonrestrictive clothing, low heeled shoes.

F. Assess integument adaptations

1. Health history
   a. History of integumental problems such as rashes, birth marks, acne, excess dryness or oiliness
   b. Hygiene and grooming practices; products used for care
2. Physical assessment; observe and palpate
   a. Appearance in terms of hygiene and grooming
   b. Condition of skin-mucous membranes
      (1) Color
      (2) Integrity, texture, moisture
      (3) Signs indicative of physical abuse
   c. Condition of hair and nails—integrity, growth
   d. Expected pregnancy changes
      (1) Pigmentary
      (2) Acne or oiliness
      (3) Striae gravidarum
      (4) Palmar erythema, spider nevi

G. Laboratory-diagnostic testing

1. Pregnancy tests—determine level of human chorionic gonadotropin (HCG) in urine or serum
   a. Urine most commonly used specimen—first voided, morning specimen obtained before eating or drinking using a clean catch method facilitates accuracy
   b. Radioimmunoassay (RIA) test—uses serum to detect the beta subunit of HCG as early as 8 days after conception; laboratory test
   c. Enzyme-linked immunosorbent assay (ELISA) test uses serum or urine to detect the beta subunit of HCG as early as 7 to 10 days after conception; may be a home or office test
   d. Home pregnancy tests are accurate-sensitive if instructions are carefully followed; most are ELISA
      ▼ Early diagnosis of pregnancy facilitates prompt initiation of prenatal care
2. Common laboratory tests to monitor adaptation to pregnancy and facilitate early detection of health problems (see Table 5-1)

▼ Test findings during pregnancy should always be evaluated utilizing expected ranges for a pregnant woman since in many cases these ranges differ from the ranges for a nonpregnant woman

H. Psychosocial assessment

1. Self-concept
   a. Perceptions of physical self
      (1) Description of current health status
      (2) Feelings expressed about changing body-image and sensations
      (3) Measures taken to enhance health during pregnancy; these include views about health guidance during pregnancy (prenatal care)
   b. Perceptions of personal self
      (1) Reaction to and feelings about pregnancy
      (2) Perception of pregnancy and parenting—realistic, unrealistic
      (3) Coping mechanisms used to respond to stress; measures used to cope with the demands of pregnancy and parenting—effective, ineffective
      (4) Cultural beliefs regarding pregnancy, parenting
      (5) Progress in meeting the developmental tasks of pregnancy and age related developmental tasks (see Chapter 4)
      (6) Moral-ethical-spiritual values, beliefs, standards of behavior
   c. Level of knowledge concerning pregnancy
      (1) Adaptations
      (2) Self-assessment and self-care measures
   d. Father—consider self-concept and perceptions, meeting of developmental tasks, coping mechanisms (refer to items above under *b. Perceptions of personal self*)
2. Role function
   a. Description of
      (1) Current roles
      (2) Role responsibilities and expectations as defined by self, family, and support system
      (3) Role performance as determined by self, family, and support system
      (4) Presence of role conflicts
   b. Potential for role conflict with the addition of the pregnant woman role and then the parent role

   c. Awareness of high risk for role conflicts and preparations made
   d. Perceptions regarding the role of mother
   e. Present knowledge and skill regarding the mother role and measures taken to prepare for the mother role
   f. Assess the father and the paternal role
3. Interdependence
   a. Family and support system
      (1) Who are they?
      (2) Capability of giving support
      (3) Degree of support offered during pregnancy and after the baby is born
   b. Relationship of expectant mother and father with each other and with family and support system
      (1) Willingness to accept support
      (2) Strength to appropriately refuse or limit support
   c. Responses of family and support system to pregnancy—partner, siblings, grandparents, friends, coworkers
   d. Sibling preparation measures
   e. Stability-safety of the home-work environment
   f. Financial security
   g. Community agency support required—accepted, rejected, available

REVIEW QUESTIONS

1. A woman is pregnant for the second time. Her first pregnancy ended in a spontaneous abortion at 12 weeks. The correct terms to use to describe this woman's obstetrical history would be
   a. Primigravida, nullipara
   b. Multigravida, primipara
   c. Primigravida, primipara
   d. Multigravida, nullipara

2. A woman is pregnant for the second time. Her first pregnancy resulted in the birth of twin boys at 35 weeks' gestation. The boys are now three years old. Using the 5-digit system to describe this woman's current obstetrical history, the nurse would record
   a. 1-0-2-0-2
   b. 1-1-0-0-2
   c. 2-0-1-0-2
   d. 2-2-0-0-1

3. When examining a pregnant woman's cervix, the nurse notes a softening of the cervix's consistency. The nurse would record that which sign was present?
   a. Chadwick's
   b. Hegar's
   c. Goodel's
   d. Homan's

4. A home pregnancy test based on the ELISA testing method can detect human chorionic gonadotrophin (HCG) in the urine as early as
   a. 7 to 10 days after conception
   b. 1 week after the first menstrual period is missed
   c. 2 to 3 weeks after conception
   d. 3 weeks after the first menstrual period is missed

5. Which of the following laboratory results would be a cause for concern if exhibited by a woman at her first prenatal visit during the second month of her pregnancy?
   a. Hematocrit 38%, hemoglobin 13 g/dL
   b. White blood cell count 6000/mm^3
   c. Platelets 300,000/mm^3
   d. Rubella titre 1:6

6. A woman must collect her urine and bring it to the laboratory of the prenatal clinic so a pregnancy test can be performed. To ensure accuracy the woman should

a. Collect the urine during her last voiding of the day and refrigerate the specimen
b. Void immediately upon arising in the morning, drink two glasses of water, and collect urine from her next voiding
c. Before eating or drinking, collect the urine of her first voiding in the morning using a clean catch technique
d. Collect urine after eating breakfast in the morning and just before coming to the clinic

7. At 24 to 28 weeks' gestation, a 1 hour glucose test is usually performed as a screening test for gestational diabetes. A finding above what mg/dL level would require the performance of a three-hour glucose tolerance test?

a. 110
b. 115
c. 125
d. 135

8. A maternal serum alpha-fetoprotein (MsAFP) test is performed at 16 to 18 weeks' gestation. An elevated level has been associated with

a. Down syndrome
b. Sickle-cell anemia
c. Cardiac defects
d. Open neural tube defects (spina bifida)

9. When planning a diet with a pregnant woman, the nurse's first action would be to

a. Review the woman's current dietary intake
b. Teach the woman about the food pyramid
c. Caution the woman to avoid large doses of vitamins
d. Instruct the woman to limit the intake of fatty foods

10. Which of the following serving suggestions would be appropriate for a pregnant woman?

a. Milk, yogurt, cheese group: 6 servings
b. Meat, poultry, fish, beans, eggs, nuts group: 5 to 7 servings
c. Vegetable group: 3 to 5 servings
d. Fruit group: 6 servings

ANSWERS, RATIONALES, AND TEST-TAKING TIPS

Rationales	Test-Taking Tips
1. Correct answer: d Multigravida represents two or more pregnancies, irregardless of the outcome. Nullipara indicates that no pregnancy has been completed to the age of viability. Primigravida refers to the first pregnancy while primipara indicates that one pregnancy has been completed to the age of viability.	Remember: gravida = pregnancies; para = births. Narrow your choices to responses *b* and *c* since two pregnancies are "multiple" and with no births select response *d*: "nulli" = none.
2. Correct answer: c Gravida (the first number) = 2 since this woman has been pregnant twice Para (next four numbers) T = 0 term births P = 1 preterm birth at 35 weeks A = 0 abortions L = 2 living children (twins).	The number of pregnancies are two; thus the responses are immediately narrowed to either *c* or *d*. Next the number of term births is none so the correct response is *c*. Term pregnancy is on the average 38 to 42 weeks.
3. Correct answer: c Chadwick's sign is a deep purplish-red color of the vagina and cervix from increased vascularity; Hegar's sign is softening of the lower uterine segment; Homan's sign, used to detect thrombophlebitis, is sharp pain in the calf upon dorsiflexion of the foot.	To remember the signs easily think of them alphabetically and think external to internal anatomically: Chadwick—vagina Goodel—cervix Hegar—lower uterine.

4. Correct answer: a

Home pregnancy tests are highly accurate if directions are followed carefully.

Use common sense to realize that home tests are done to find out if the woman is pregnant as soon as possible. Therefore responses *c* and *d* are unlikely. In reference to response *b*, think that if one waits until one week after a missed period the woman could likely be already 3 to 4 weeks pregnant. The most logical answer is response *a*.

5. Correct answer: d

Responses *a, b,* and *c* are within expected ranges. Rubella titres of less than 1:10 indicate a lack of immunity to rubella, an infection that has the potential for teratogenic effects on the fetus.

Cluster responses *a, b,* and *c* under normal components in the blood. Select *d* since titres are checked to evaluate the degree of immunity to an exposure of a pathological condition such as hepatitis and rubella.

6. Correct answer: c

Using the first voided specimen in the morning before eating and drinking will result in a concentrated urine specimen and an increased amount of HCG. Clean catch technique will enhance accuracy since debris in urine could interfere with results. Responses *a, b,* and *d* will not yield the most concentrated specimen of urine.

Cluster responses *a, b,* and *d* since the collection method has no specifics. Note that response *c* has the specific method of a clean catch.

7. Correct answer: d

The results of the 3-hour glucose test should be below 130 mg/dL, the more sensitive value. If above this level, a 3-hour glucose tolerance test should be performed.

Remember three—do a three-hour glucose tolerance test if glucose is greater than 135 mg/dL. The other given glucose numbers are within the normal range for glucose.

8. Correct answer: d

Response *a* is associated with decreased levels; *b* and *c* are not detected with MsAFP testing.

Remember that *D* in Down syndrome is a clue that the serum level is *D*ecreased and that the other defect, spina bifida, is the opposite. Tip: remember one and then that the other is the opposite.

9. Correct answer: a

While *b, c,* and *d* are correct actions on the part of the nurse, the *first* action should be to assess the client's current dietary pattern, since instruction should be geared to what she already knows and does.

Use the nursing process—further assessment is usually the best response before intervening especially if assessment data is not stated in the stem. Cluster responses *b, c,* and *d* under the focus of interventions and this leaves response *a*, to do additional assessment.

10. Correct answer: c

Correct servings per responses: response *a* = 3 to 4 servings milk group; response *b* = 2 to 3 servings meat group; and response *d* = 2 to 4 servings fruit group.

If you have no idea of the correct answer, cluster options *a, b,* and *d* since they have 6 servings. Select option *c* that falls outside the clustered group.

CHAPTER 6

Assessment of Fetal Health during Pregnancy

STUDY OUTCOMES

After completing this chapter, the reader will be able to do the following:

- Define the key terms listed.
- Describe the methods used to assess fetal health in a low risk pregnancy.
- Identify signs indicative of fetal health.
- Identify signs indicative of fetal compromise.
- Describe the purpose, indicators, preparation method, and interpretation of results for each of the following antepartal tests
  - ultrasound
  - nonstress test
  - biophysical profile
  - contraction stress test
  - amniocentesis
  - chorionic villi sampling

KEY TERMS

Amniocentesis — Insertion of a needle transabdominally into the uterus in order to obtain a sample of amniotic fluid for the purpose of genetic screening and determination of fetal well being and maturity.

Biophysical profile — Test using external fetal monitoring and ultrasound to assess fetal status by evaluating fetal heart rate (FHR) following movement, nonstress test (NST), fetal breathing movements, fetal body movements, fetal muscle tone, and amniotic fluid volume.

Chorionic villius sampling — Removal of a tissue sample from the fetal portion of the developing placenta, chorionic villi, for the purpose of genetic testing.

Contraction stress test — Performed to assess the response of the FHR to uterine contractions to determine fetal risk for hypoxia during labor as a result of uteroplacental insufficiency.

Nonstress test — Performed to assess the response of the FHR to periods of fetal movement.

Ultrasound — Diagnostic test which uses sound waves to reflect off of tissue; allows for visualization of the contents of the uterine cavity including the fetus, fetal movement, placenta, amniotic fluid, and blood flow through the umbilical cord.

CONTENT REVIEW

I. Risk status in pregnancy

A. Assessment methods used to determine fetal health status vary according to the risk status of the pregnancy

1. Low-risk pregnancy—mother exhibits good health status at the start of pregnancy and the maternal-fetal unit adapts to the changes of pregnancy and parturition in an effective manner; risk factors known to jeopardize the maternal-fetal unit are absent
2. High-risk pregnancy—risk factors which place the maternal-fetal unit in jeopardy are present before pregnancy or develop as the maternal-fetal unit adapts to the changes of pregnancy and parturition

B. The mother and her family must be prepared for diagnostic testing that is required during pregnancy

II. Assessment methods to determine fetal health status: low-risk pregnancy

A. Fetal heart rate (FHR)—assessed at every prenatal visit once it is first detected

1. Instruments used
   a. Doppler or ultrasound stethoscope
      (1) Instrument that uses sound waves to detect blood flow by producing an audible sound that can be counted and evaluated
      (2) Contact gel must be placed on the skin to facilitate transmission of sound waves
      (3) Fetal heart sounds can be detected by the 10th to 12th week gestation
   b. Fetoscope
      (1) Special stethoscope designed to auscultate FHR but is less sensitive than Doppler
      (2) Detects fetal heart sounds by 18th to 20th week gestation
2. Assessment method
   a. Identify sounds
      (1) Fetal heart beat
      (2) Uterine souffle—beatlike sound of blood flowing through enlarged uterine blood vessels; rate corresponds to mother's heart beat
      (3) Funic souffle—beatlike sound of blood flowing through umbilical cord; rate corresponds to fetal heart beat
   b. Count fetal heart beat for one full minute
   c. Expected rate 120 to 160 beats per minute, regular rhythm
   d. If a low FHR (<100 beats per minute) is obtained, count the maternal pulse since the beat of the uterine souffle may have been counted inadvertently; if not, report finding to physician immediately
   e. Provide parents, siblings with the opportunity to hear the fetal heart beat—provides reassurance and facilitates attachment by making fetus a reality

B. Measurement of fundal height (see Chapter 5)—enlargement of uterus indirectly implies fetal growth

C. Leopold's maneuvers—systematic palpation of the abdomen to determine fetal presentation-position, degree of fetal descent into pelvis, uterine contours

D. Daily fetal movement count (DFMC)

1. Assessment of fetal movement based on principle that
   a. Vigorous fetal activity = fetal well being
   b. Alteration in pattern of fetal movement (FM), for example decreased frequency, weakening, cessation = possible fetal compromise related to hypoxia
2. Effective, easy, convenient, noninvasive, inexpensive screening tool recommended with increasing frequency for all pregnant women whether low or high risk; assessment is performed at home, results are recorded, and then reviewed at prenatal visits
3. Determining pattern of fetal movements can facilitate maternal attachment to fetus as she recognizes the unique responses of her fetus to such stimuli as sounds (voices, music), emotions, food
4. Protocol
   a. Begin at 27th week when 90% of fetal movements can be perceived
   b. Counting times should take into consideration
      (1) Fetal sleep-wake cycles
      (2) Maternal food intake—increase FM
      (3) Drug-nicotine use—decrease FM
      (4) Environmental stimuli, such as music
      (5) Maternal position—supine position causes uterus to compress vena cava, which causes maternal cardiac output to decrease, placental perfusion to then diminish, and fetal gas exchange to be inhibited, resulting in hypoxia
   c. Explain to the patient
      (1) Timing and position—count in a comfortable, side-lying position after a meal
      (2) Counting method to be used—a variety of methods are currently available
      (3) Expected findings
      (4) Warning signs and importance of reporting them to healthcare provider
   d. Cardiff count to 10 method—one method currently available
      (1) Begin at the same time each day (usually in the morning, after breakfast) and count each fetal movement, noting how long it takes to count 10 fetal movements (FMs)
      (2) Expected findings—10 movements in 1 hour or less
      (3) Warning signs

(a) More than 1 hour to reach 10 movements
(b) Less than 10 movements in 12 hours
(c) Longer time to reach 10 FMs than on previous days
(d) Movements are becoming weaker, less vigorous
▼ Movement alarm signal—<3 FMs in 12 hours

(4) Warning signs should be reported to healthcare provider immediately; often require further testing. Examples: nonstress test (NST), biophysical profile (BPP).

III. Assessment methods to determine fetal health status: high-risk pregnancy

A. More frequent prenatal visits

1. Assess status of maternal-fetal unit on a more frequent basis since appearance of warning signs can occur at any time. NOTE: include assessment of emotional status since stress can adversely influence fetal health.
2. Instruct client-family regarding self-assessment measures, warning signs, and importance of participation in health guidance and treatment regime

B. Daily fetal movement count (DFMC) refer to prior explanation pp. 115-116 under low-risk pregnancy, II, D

C. Specialized testing may be required

1. Purpose
   a. Facilitate early detection of fetal warning signs and prompt intervention to prevent fetal morbidity and death
   b. Identify fetal anomalies
   c. Avoid premature intervention
   d. Determine timing and method of delivery that is of lowest risk to maternal-fetal unit
2. Guidelines
   a. Use with discretion—advantages must outweigh risk, cost, and maternal discomfort
   b. One test may not be definitive—often a combination of tests is required moving from simple to more complex testing. Example: daily fetal movement count (DFMC), then nonstress test (NST), then biophysical profile (BPP), then contraction stress test (CST).
   c. Tests may be repeated to monitor changes in status and to confirm abnormal results
      (1) Serial ultrasounds to monitor fetal growth

(2) Weekly NST to monitor fetal health in a postterm pregnancy
(3) Repeat a positive CST in 24 hours

d. Client-support group preparation is critical
(1) Frightening issues to cope with—baby in jeopardy, pregnancy different from expected
(2) Testing procedures—tiring, uncomfortable, time consuming, costly, embarrassing
(3) Stress response can affect results, such as FHR pattern

e. Role of nurse as an educator, advocate, provider of emotional support
(1) Reassure woman and family with a calm, competent, knowledgeable approach
(2) Explain testing method and procedure
(a) Why it is done
(b) When it is done, including frequency
(c) What will happen
(d) What the results mean
(e) How it will affect the mother and her baby
(f) How the mother and family can participate
(3) Provide time for expression of feelings
(4) Identify need for referrals

D. Ultrasound

1. Purpose
a. Diagnose pregnancy by visualizing gestational sac as early as week 4
b. Date pregnancy by evaluating size or volume of gestational sac and crown to rump length (CRL)
c. Detect multiple gestation
d. Monitor fetal growth by making serial measurements of crown to rump length, biparietal diameter, femur length, abdomen, and head to abdomen ratio

▼ An accurate gestational age facilitates the use of growth charts when evaluating fetal growth; be alert for flattening of the growth curve; this suggests no or minimal fetal growth

e. Evaluate fetal structure and function
(1) Fetal movement
(2) Presence of structural anomalies
(3) Blood flow through the umbilical cord—umbilical velocimetry

f. Estimate amniotic fluid volume

g. Evaluate placental location and efficiency of function—degree of aging, presence of ischemic-calcified areas
h. Facilitate safe performance of other antepartal tests by locating essential structures—placenta, chorion villi, fetus

2. Approaches—transabdominal, transvaginal
3. Specific preparation and support measures
   a. Full bladder for transabdominal approach when woman is ≤20 weeks' gestation
      (1) Facilitates identification of pelvic organs and positioning of uterus for visualization
      (2) Drink 1 to 1½ liters of water approximately 1 to 2 hours before the examination
      (3) Full bladder produces discomfort
   b. Test lasts 20 to 30 minutes—time may be used to point out fetal structures which enhance reality of fetus and facilitate attachment; support woman if abnormalities are noted or if she does not want to look
   c. Position woman—supine with transabdominal or lithotomy with transvaginal
      ▼ Be alert for signs of supine hypotension during test and postural hypotension when arising at the end of the test

E. Nonstress test (NST)

1. Purpose—assess the response of the FHR to periods of fetal movement
   a. Testing begins after the 27th to 30th week when the fetal autonomic nervous system is mature enough to respond effectively
   b. Performed either weekly, twice a week, or daily depending on condition of maternal-fetal unit
2. Indications—pregnancies at risk for placental insufficiency
   a. Postmaturity
   b. Pregnancy induced hypertension (PIH), diabetes
   c. Warning signs noted during DFMC
   d. Maternal history of smoking, inadequate nutrition
3. Protocol
   a. Take into account typical sleep-wake cycle for this fetus (ask mom)
   b. Perform test during a time of activity (mornings are usually good)
   c. Maternal preparation
      (1) Refrain from smoking (2 hours before) or using sedatives before the test

(2) Eat about 2 hours before test to raise glucose level
(3) Position—semifowlers with small pillow under one hip or lateral position

d. Assess maternal vital signs especially BP, before and during test

e. Attach external noninvasive fetal monitors
(1) Tocotransducer over fundus to detect uterine contractions and fetal movements (FMs)
(2) Ultrasound transducer over abdominal site where most distinct fetal heart sounds are detected

f. Monitor until at least 2 FMs are detected in 20 minutes
(1) If no FM after 40 minutes provide woman with a light snack or gently stimulate fetus through abdomen
(2) If no FM after 1 hour further testing may be indicated, such as a CST

4. Interpretation of results
   a. Reactive result
   (1) Baseline FHR between 120 and 160 beats per minute
   (2) At least two accelerations of the FHR of at least 15 beats per minute, lasting at least 15 seconds in a 10 to 20 minute period as a result of FM
   (3) Good variability—normal irregularity of cardiac rhythm representing a balanced interaction between the parasympathetic (decreases FHR) and sympathetic (increases FHR) nervous systems; noted as an uneven line on the rhythm strip (see Chapter 10)
   (4) Result indicates a healthy fetus with an intact nervous system
   b. Nonreactive result
   (1) Stated criteria for a reactive result are not met
   (2) Could be indicative of a compromised fetus
   (3) Requires further evaluation with another NST, biophysical profile, (BPP) or contraction stress test (CST)

F. Biophysical profile

1. Purpose—assess fetal status (healthy, compromised, or at risk) by evaluating several factors
   a. Nonstress test (NST)
   b. Fetal breathing movements—number and duration; first to be effected by early stress and may be predictive of preterm labor since prostaglandins that stimulate labor also decrease breathing movements

c. Fetal body movements—gross-discrete movements of the fetal body and limbs
d. Fetal muscle tone—presence of active extension with a return to flexion of limb, trunk (spine), hand; least sensitive to hypoxia and last sign to be effected
e. Amniotic fluid volume—presence and size of fluid pockets; oligohydramnios (diminished fluid volume) may indicate an extended episode of fetal stress with reduced formation of urine; certain fetal anomalies also affect amount of amniotic fluid
f. Placental grading—evaluation of placental efficiency and degree of maturity-aging is included in some BPP assessments; check testing agency policy; scoring is adjusted appropriately

2. Protocol—follow guidelines for ultrasound and for NST; approximately 40 to 60 minutes are required to perform test in order to accommodate to the fetal sleep-wake cycle
3. Indications—as for NST and CST; often used to follow up on a nonreactive NST or warning signs found with DFMC
4. Interpretation of results
   a. Each sign receives a score of 0 (abnormal) or 2 (normal)—some testing procedures use a 0, 1, 2 scoring system with 2 being the most favorable score for each sign and a total score of 10 as perfect
   b. Total score of ≥8 is considered reflective of a healthy fetus
   c. Low scores may indicate compromise
      (1) Require follow-up by repeating BPP or performing another test, such as a CST
      (2) Score of ≤6 requires determination of need for delivery of fetus—consideration must be given to maturity of fetal lungs
   d. Low incidence of false positives—more accurate than NST or CST alone in detecting fetal compromise and risk

G. Contraction stress test

1. Purpose—use of external noninvasive fetal monitoring and stimulation of uterine contractions to assess fetal risk for hypoxia related to uteroplacental insufficiency since inadequate circulation impairs gas exchange with the fetus especially during contractions
2. Indications—assess pregnancies at risk for placental insufficiency that could compromise the fetus especially during labor (see Nonstress test, discussed earlier in this chapter)

3. Contraindications—history or danger of preterm labor, third trimester bleeding as with placenta previa
4. Protocol
   a. Begin testing at 32 to 34 weeks' gestation
   b. Repeat at weekly intervals
   c. Maternal preparation
      (1) Empty bladder
      (2) Restrict solid food during testing since labor could be stimulated; liquids are permitted
      (3) Position—as for NST
      (4) Encourage mother to use childbirth breathing techniques with contractions
   d. Assess maternal vital signs before and during test
   e. Attach external monitor as for NST and run a baseline strip for 15 minutes; look for accelerations with FM and spontaneous occurrence of uterine contractions
   f. Obtain a pattern of three uterine contractions lasting at least 40 seconds each in a 10-minute period; stimulation is usually required
      (1) Administration of Pitocin IV piggyback to a primary infusion, gradually increasing dosage to desired contraction pattern; takes about 60 to 90 minutes
      (2) Nipple stimulation to facilitate release of endogenous oxytocin from the posterior pituitary gland
         (a) Stimulate only one nipple—2- to 3-minute stimulation with a 2-minute rest interval between stimulation
         (b) Repeat until desired contraction pattern is obtained—takes about 15 to 45 minutes
   g. Be alert for hyperstimulation of the uterus
      (1) Uterine contractions lasting 90 seconds or longer AND/OR
      (2) Contractions that occur at a frequency of every 2 minutes or less
   h. Measures related to hyperstimulation
      (1) Discontinue uterine stimulus immediately
      (2) Continue IV fluids
      (3) Turn mother on her side
      (4) Administer oxygen via tight mask at 8 to 10 L/min
      (5) Monitor maternal VS and FHR
      (6) Suppression of uterine contractions with tocolytics such as Terbutaline 0.25 mg subcutaneously may be needed

i. After test is completed client must wait until uterine activity subsides (<4 contractions in 30 minutes) and vital signs and FHR are stable, returning to baseline levels

5. Interpretation of results
   a. Negative result
      (1) No late deceleration patterns, decrease in FHR after the peak of a contraction related to uteroplacental insufficiency (see Chapter 10)
      (2) Baseline FHR between 120 to 160
      (3) Good variability
      (4) FHR accelerations with FM
      (5) Indicates good functioning of the fetal-placental unit; repeat in one week
   b. Positive result
      (1) Repetitive, persistent late deceleration patterns with more than 50% of the uterine contractions
      (2) More ominous if accompanied by a decrease in variability and an absence of acceleration of the FHR with FM
      (3) May indicate inadequate placental function and fetal risk
      (4) Action taken may be further testing or immediate delivery
   c. Equivocal result—late decelerations occur but with less than 50% of the contractions; further testing required

H. Amniocentesis

1. Purpose—obtain a sample of amniotic fluid by inserting a needle through the abdomen into the amniotic sac; fluid is tested for
   a. Genetic screening
      (1) Early testing time—12th to 14th week with results available in 10 to 14 days
      (2) Traditional testing time—14th to 16th week, with results available in 2 to 4 weeks
      (3) Performed to determine presence of such problems as
         (a) Chromosomal abnormalities. Example: Down syndrome with decreased alpha-fetoprotein (AFP) levels.
         (b) Inborn errors of metabolism. Example: Tay-Sachs disease.
         (c) Other genetic disorders known to have marker genes

            (d) Open neural tube defects indicated by elevated AFP levels in the fluid
    b. Determination of fetal maturity primarily by evaluating factors indicative of lung maturity
        (1) Testing time—during third trimester around 36 weeks' gestation (a little before, at, or just after) when lung maturation is likely to have occurred
        (2) Factors—both should be present at approximately 36 weeks' gestation
            (a) L/S ratio (lecithin/sphingomyelin) greater than 2:1
            (b) Presence of phosphatidylglycerol (PG), termed PG positive
2. Indications
    a. Family history of genetic problems
    b. Women of advanced age, >35 years of age
    c. Assurance of lung maturity prior to inducing labor or performing an elective cesarian section
3. Overall complication rate is <1% primarily related to the invasiveness of the procedure—infection, maternal-fetal damage, bleeding, preterm labor
4. Protocol
    a. Ultrasound—identify placental and fetal location to avoid damage and pinpoint amniotic fluid pockets
    b. Preparation
        (1) Provide emotional support and assistance with relaxation techniques since woman may be restless and frightened
        (2) Verify informed consent forms are complete
        (3) Assist woman to empty bladder
        (4) Position—supine, be alert for supine hypotensive syndrome during and postural hypotension after the test
    c. Assessment of maternal vital signs and FHR before, during, and after the procedure
    d. Preparation of site with betadine; surgical asepsis is critical
    e. After procedure
        (1) Encourage woman to rest on her side
        (2) Monitor maternal vital signs
        (3) Use external monitor to assess for uterine contractions and FHR patterns
        (4) Administer Rhogam to the Rh-negative mother

f. Discharge instructions
    (1) Report
        (a) Changes in FM
        (b) Vaginal discharge—clear fluid, blood, thick purulent malodorous discharge
        (c) Presence of pain
        (d) Signs and symptoms of infection. Examples: fever (>100° F), malodorous discharge, pain, malaise
    (2) Rest for remainder of day
    (3) Avoid heavy lifting, bending, strenuous exercise for several days
g. Discuss results
    (1) When they will be available and who to call
    (2) Provide emotional support during the period of waiting and if results indicate fetal problems

I. Chorionic villi sampling (CVS)—removal of tissue sample from the fetal portion of the developing placenta

1. Purpose—to determine the presence of genetic abnormalities; a transabdominal or transcervical approach may be used
2. Indications—as for amniocentesis but CVS can be performed earlier (9 to 12 weeks' gestation) and results obtained sooner (1 to 2 weeks)
3. Complication rate is slightly higher than for amniocentesis primarily related to bleeding, spontaneous abortion, rupture of membranes, infection, preterm birth, fetal limb defects such as missing fingers or toes
4. Protocol
    a. Ultrasound—used throughout to guide the procedure
    b. Client preparation—similar to that of an amniocentesis except full bladder may be needed to position the uterus for easier catheter insertion
    c. Position depends on approach—transabdominal (supine) or transcervical (lithotomy)
    d. Vital signs are monitored
    e. Care after the procedure and discharge instructions are similar to those for an amniocentesis

REVIEW QUESTIONS

1. A pregnant woman, at 4 weeks' gestation, asks the nurse when she will be able to hear the baby's heart beat. The nurse can tell her that with a special ultrasound stethoscope, which amplifies sounds, the baby's heart beat can be heard in approximately how many more weeks?
   a. 2 to 4
   b. 6 to 8
   c. 10 to 12
   d. 14 to 16

2. When assessing the fetal heart rate (FHR) of a woman at 30 weeks' gestation, the nurse counts a rate of 82 beats per minute. Initially, the nurse should
   a. Recognize that the rate is within normal limits and record it
   b. Assess the woman's radial pulse
   c. Notify the physician
   d. Allow the woman to hear the heart beat

3. A pregnant woman is taught how to assess fetal status using a daily fetal movement count (DFMC) that follows the Cardiff protocol. The woman exhibits need for further instruction if she
   a. Begins DFMCs at the 27th week of pregnancy
   b. Performs the count in a comfortable side-lying position
   c. Begins counting before getting out of bed in the morning
   d. Recognizes that 10 movements in 1 hour or less is a reassuring sign of fetal well being

4. The fetal movement alarm signal (MAS) is defined as
   a. More than 1 hour to reach 10 movements
   b. Less than 10 movements in 12 hours
   c. Less than 3 movements in 12 hours
   d. Weakened, less vigorous movements

5. A pregnant woman at 15 weeks' gestation is scheduled for a transabdominal ultrasound to assess fetal size and confirm the estimated date of birth. Which of the following is an appropriate nursing measure for this test?
   a. Obtain a written, informed consent from the woman
   b. Instruct woman to drink 1 to 1½ liters of water within 2 hours of the test
   c. Place the woman in a lithotomy position in preparation for the test
   d. Instruct the woman not to eat or drink for 6 hours prior to the test

6. Which of the following preparation measures is NOT required prior to a nonstress test?
   a. Avoid eating for at least 2 hours before the test
   b. Attach both a tocotransducer and an ultrasound transducer to the woman's abdomen
   c. Use the woman's description of the typical sleep-wake cycle of her fetus to schedule the test
   d. Refrain from smoking for 2 hours before the test

7. Which of the following would be defined as hyperstimulation of the uterus and require that the uterine stimulation of a contraction stress test (CST) be discontinued?
   a. Uterine contractions of 3 in 10 minutes, each lasting 40 seconds
   b. Uterine contractions occurring every 3 minutes, each lasting 60 seconds
   c. Uterine contractions occurring every 2 minutes or less, each lasting 90 seconds or longer
   d. Uterine contractions of 3 in 15 minutes lasting 50 seconds each

8. A pregnant woman is having a contraction stress test (CST) performed. Which of the following is NOT a criteria for a negative test result?
   a. Absence of FHR accelerations with FM
   b. Absence of late deceleration patterns
   c. Baseline FHR of 120 to 160 beats per minute
   d. Good variability

9. Which of the following amniocentesis results reflects adequate fetal lung maturity?
   a. L/S ratio 1:1 and phosphatidylglycerol (PG) negative
   b. Alpha-fetoprotein level within the normal range
   c. L/S ratio 2:1 and phosphatidylglycerol (PG) positive
   d. Creatinine present

10. Which of the following is true regarding chorionic villi sampling (CVS)?
   a. It is usually performed at approximately 16 weeks' gestation
   b. Results are obtained in 3 to 4 weeks
   c. Fetal limb defects, such as missing digits, can occur
   d. One purpose of the test is to determine fetal lung maturity

ANSWERS, RATIONALES, AND TEST-TAKING TIPS

Rationales	Test-Taking Tips
1. Correct answer: b Fetal heart sounds can be detected using an ultrasound stethoscope/Doppler by week 10 to 12 of pregnancy. Since this woman is already 4 weeks pregnant, the fetal heart beat should be heard in 6 to 8 more weeks. Fetal heart sounds can be auscultated with a fetoscope by week 18 to 20 of pregnancy or in 14 to 16 more weeks.	Be very cautious in reading the question. It is worded in terms of how "many more weeks" from her 4 weeks, not in terms of at what number of weeks. The type of equipment is essential to note in the stem. An ultrasound-Doppler, being more specialized, can pick up sounds earlier than a fetoscope which is similar to a regular stethoscope.
2. Correct answer: b The expected FHR is 120 to 160 beats per minute. The nurse may have inadvertently counted the uterine souffle, the beatlike sound of blood flowing through uterine blood vessels, which corresponds to the mother's heart beat. The physician should be notified if the FHR is confirmed to be 82 beats per minute. Allow the woman to hear the heart beat as soon as a full assessment is made.	Use the nursing process—do further assessment before interventions when findings are presented.
3. Correct answer: c Fetal movements should be counted after meals since fetal movements are increased and more vigorous at this time as a result of increased glucose levels.	The key to selection of the correct answer is to read the question slowly and carefully to note "need for further instruction." You will select a wrong item. Then use common sense that the fetus will probably be least active prior to the mother getting out of bed.

4. Correct answer: c

Responses *a*, *b*, and *d* are warning signs related to fetal movement. Both the MAS and the warning signs should be reported to the healthcare provider immediately.

Key words in the stem are "alarm signal" which are different than "warning signals." Of the given responses, response *c* is the most drastic finding and therefore probably the best choice.

5. Correct answer: b

This is a noninvasive test which does not require a written consent. No GI preparation is needed. Woman should be placed in a supine position. The lithotomy position is used for the transvaginal approach.

Key word in the stem is "transabdominal" and thus, response *c* can be eliminated. With abdominal ultrasounds the bladder needs to be full to act as a landmark for evaluation of other internal structures. The actions in response *b* meet the need to fill the bladder.

6. Correct answer: a

A woman should eat within 2 hours of the test since maternal glucose levels affect fetal movement; *b*, *c*, and *d* are all required for the test.

Since the test does not involve the gastrointestinal structures, eating is not restricted. Read slowly and correctly to avoid missing the key word "not" in the question.

7. Correct answer: c

Response *a* reflects the uterine contraction pattern required for the test; *b* and *d* do not reach the criteria for uterine hyperstimulation.

Key words in the stem are "hyperstimulation" and "test to be continued." Select the most irritable pattern, which is response *c*.

8. Correct answer: a

Acceleration of FHR with fetal movement is a sign of a healthy fetus. Absence of this acceleration with movement is one of the criteria for a positive test.

The wording of these types of questions—"not criteria for a negative" require close reading. One approach is to rephrase the question to what is criteria for a negative test or normal result. Select three of the responses and the one left would not be criteria and indicate an abnormal response.

9. Correct answer: c

Both an L/S ratio of 2:1 and PG present-positive are required to be assured of fetal lung maturity especially if the mother is a diabetic. Alpha-fetoprotein and creatinine are not related to lung maturity.

Recall tip: Lungs are 2 in number; associate *L*/S, *L* with *l*ung and ratio of *2*:1, *2* lungs. Also, read the question carefully; it is asking about adequate maturity.

10. Correct answer: c

CVS is performed between 9 to 12 weeks' gestation with results obtained in 1 to 2 weeks. Since the test is done only in early pregnancy, it is not used to determine lung maturity.

"Go with what you know." Eliminate option *d*; L/S ratio determines lung maturity. Associate that the sampling is taking of tissue; therefore defects may occur.

CHAPTER 7

High Risk Pregnancy

STUDY OUTCOMES

After completing this chapter, the reader will be able to do the following:

- Define the key terms listed.
- Identify major risk factors which place the maternal-fetal unit in jeopardy.
- Identify nursing diagnoses typical of high risk pregnant women and their families.
- Discuss the physiologic basis, impact on maternal-fetal unit and family, and treatment approaches for
  - spontaneous abortion
  - ectopic pregnancy
  - placenta previa-abruptio placenta
  - pregnancy induced hypertension (PIH)
  - hyperemesis gravidarum
  - gestational diabetes
- Describe the manner in which pregnancy is influenced by
  - pregestational diabetes
  - cardiac disease
  - infection

KEY TERMS

Abortion — Termination of pregnancy prior to the age of fetal viability.

Abruptio placenta — Premature separation of a normally implanted placenta (fundal implantation).

Ectopic pregnancy — Implantation of the fertilized ovum occurs at a site other than the body of the uterus, most often in the fallopian tube.

Gestational diabetes — Diabetic state that develops in some nondiabetic women during the second half of their pregnancies, usually the third trimester.

High risk pregnancy — Pregnancy in which the life or health of the maternal-fetal unit is in jeopardy.

Hyperemesis gravidarum — Excessive, intractable vomiting during pregnancy, most often during the first 16 weeks; it results in fluid, electrolyte, metabolic, and nutritional imbalance.

Placenta previa — Placenta is implanted in the lower uterine segment rather than in the fundus.

Pregnancy induced hypertension (PIH) — Syndrome associated with pregnancy that begins after the 20th week of pregnancy through the early postpartum period; it is characterized by hypertension alone (gestational hypertension) or in combination with varying degrees of edema and proteinuria (preeclampsia, eclampsia).

CONTENT REVIEW

I. Application of the nursing process to high risk pregnancy

A. **High risk pregnancy—has a resultant impact on the pregnant woman's family; encompasses the period from conception through the postpartum period**

B. **The greatest risk for perinatal morbidity and mortality of mother, fetus, and newborn occurs in a high risk pregnancy**

C. **Early, ongoing health care is critical to assess the degree and the nature of risk and to intervene in a timely manner to enhance the likelihood for a positive outcome of the pregnancy**

1. Preconception care and counseling must be made available to women and men to help them achieve the best possible health

state and reduce the impact of risk factors prior to pregnancy. Examples: stop smoking, reverse nutritional deficits, stabilize chronic health problems.

2. Comprehensive prenatal care must be accessible to all pregnant women and include ongoing assessment of risk status since risk factors can appear or worsen at any time during pregnancy
3. Health assessment and care must utilize a holistic approach that focuses on all aspects of a pregnant woman's life since risk can arise from many sources including psychosocial

D. Nursing diagnoses need to be identified and then utilized to organize an individualized plan of care; they can include

1. Alteration in nutrition—less than body requirements related to
   a. Insufficient oral food and fluid intake associated with persistent vomiting
   b. Loss of appetite associated with activity restriction
2. Risk for fluid volume deficit related to
   a. Excessive blood loss associated with placenta previa, abruptio placenta, spontaneous abortion, or ectopic pregnancy
   b. Persistent vomiting
   c. Shift of fluid to interstitial space associated with pregnancy induced hypertension
3. Risk for maternal injury related to
   a. Increased CNS irritability associated with pregnancy induced hypertension
   b. Muscle atrophy and orthostatic hypotension associated with prolonged activity restriction
4. Impaired gas exchange related to fluid accumulation in the lungs (pulmonary edema) associated with cardiac decompensation
5. Risk for fetal injury related to
   a. Increased maternal core temperature associated with infection
   b. Alteration in placental perfusion associated with pregnancy induced hypertension, abruptio placenta, or decreased cardiac output
6. Anxiety related to unexpected need for medical intervention during pregnancy and concern for the safety of the pregnant woman and her fetus
7. Alteration in family processes related to limitation on the pregnant woman's activity level

E. Nursing measures should facilitate the healthy coping of high risk pregnant women and their families as well as the safe and effective implementation of the treatment plan. Nurses should

1. Provide time for meeting the needs of high risk pregnant women and their families
   a. Meet with family members together and separately with a provision of adequate time for discussion of feelings, frustrations, concerns, fears
   b. Educate pregnant women and their families regarding the health problem and the components of the treatment plan. Prepare them for the possibility of increasingly complex interventions such as hospitalization, antepartal monitoring, and cesarean section.
   c. Encourage participation in the plan of care and provide positive reinforcement for this participation
2. Reduce stress associated with medical treatment requirements
   a. Arrange for home care if possible since the home environment with support from family members is generally more conducive to healing than is the hospital
   b. Organize client groups on high risk pregnancy units so clients can share experiences and feelings and support each other; liberal visiting hours, diversional activities, and health teaching sessions may further reduce the stress of hospitalization
   c. Coordinate efforts of interdisciplinary team to facilitate continuity of care and the formation of therapeutic relationships with the clients—primary nursing or a nurse case manager is especially helpful in meeting the individualized needs of high risk pregnant women and their families in a consistent manner
   d. Identify stressors related to such factors as finances, child care, home maintenance; make appropriate referrals
3. Provide time for family interaction after the delivery to facilitate the attachment process; use creative approaches if separation occurs as a result of treatment requirements
4. Assist family through the grieving process if the outcome of pregnancy is not a positive one, such as death of mother, fetus, or newborn or the development of serious, long-term health problems in the mother or newborn
5. Facilitate recovery by providing health teaching and arranging for needed support in the home since recovery is often a longer process that requires follow-up care

6. Help women and their families to view the high risk experience in realistic terms—What happened? Why did it happen? What are the implications for future pregnancies?

F. Evaluation criteria—the woman and/or family have exhibited

1. An adaptation to the treatment plan with acceptance of assistance from healthcare providers and family members
2. A positive outcome for the maternal-fetal unit
3. Successful progress through the grieving process reaching acceptance of maternal and/or fetal-newborn demise or morbidity
4. An integration of the high risk pregnancy into self-concept

II. Risk factors which place the maternal-fetal unit in jeopardy

A. Factors arising from the woman's characteristics and lifestyle

1. Age—<15 years of age or >35 years of age
2. Nutritional habits and status
    a. Less than or greater than desired weight
    b. Inadequate intake of appropriate nutrients
3. Stature—5 feet or under
4. Abuse of tobacco, alcohol, drugs
5. Hostile environment at home or at work, with exposure to teratogens

B. Factors arising from the health status and lifestyle of the father of the baby

1. Abuse of drugs, alcohol, tobacco
2. Harmful sexual practices including bisexuality
3. Exposure to environmental hazards

C. Preexisting health problems

1. Health problems present prior to the onset of pregnancy include
    a. Cardiovascular and renal dysfunction
    b. Diabetes
    c. Anemia
    d. Neurological dysfunction such as epilepsy
    e. Infections such as herpes, HIV
2. Pregnancy effects the health problem and the health problem effects the pregnancy. Examples: medication needed to treat epilepsy can cause congenital defects to develop in the fetus and insulin requirements change during the pregnancy of a pregestational diabetic.
3. Preconception care and counseling is critical

D. Health problems that arise during pregnancy

1. Include
   a. Pregnancy induced hypertension (PIH)
   b. Anemia
   c. Hyperemesis gravidarum
   d. Hemorrhage
   e. Gestational diabetes
2. Occur as a result of ineffective adaptation to the changes that occur with pregnancy
3. More likely to occur among women who are already at risk. Examples: a woman with pregestational diabetic, a very young or an older pregnant woman, a woman with hypertension.

E. Obstetrical-gynecological factors

1. Number of pregnancies (gravida) and births (para)—for example the primigravida or the grand multiparous woman (≥5 births)
2. Pelvic and uterine malformations and abnormalities
3. History of STDs and pelvic inflammatory disease (PID)
4. History of complications with previous pregnancies. Examples: spontaneous abortions, hemorrhage, preterm labor, birth.
5. History of infertility
6. Exposure to diethylstilbesterol (DES) as a fetus

F. Psychosocial risk factors

1. Instability of family relationships
   a. Separation or divorce
   b. Abusive relationship with partner-father of the baby
   c. Paternal lack of interest or participation in the pregnancy
   d. Single status of mother especially if family has a negative, nonsupportive reaction to the pregnancy
2. Inadequate economic resources
   a. No health insurance
   b. Need to depend on public assistance for health care
   c. Struggle to meet needs of daily living may lower priority given to seeking and participating in prenatal care
   d. Limited means of transportation
3. Limited access to nearby culturally sensitive prenatal care or a high risk pregnancy center
4. Minority status in terms of race-ethnicity—experience higher rates of maternal-infant morbidity and mortality as well as low birth weight (LBW)
5. History of mental health disorders including depression and psychoses

III. Approach to risk factors

A. **Risk factors vary as to the degree of danger they present and the degree of intervention required. Examples: moderate obesity compared to pregestational diabetes and PIH with this pregnancy compared to a history of PIH with a previous pregnancy.**

B. **Risk factors can occur at any time during the pregnancy or postpartum period since pregnancy is a dynamic, ever-changing state**

C. **More than one risk factor can be present. Example: a 15-year-old single parent smokes and uses marijuana, is underweight, and has a history of STDs.**

D. **One risk factor can precipitate the occurrence of another. Example: the diabetic woman is at increased risk for PIH, infection, and abruptio placenta.**

E. **A variety of high risk assessment tools (Goodwin's scale, prenatal risk indicator form) are available that list risk factors and rate them according to the danger that they present—use of such tools**
   1. Facilitates ongoing, systematic assessment for the presence of risk factors in all women, throughout their pregnancies
   2. Allows degree-severity of risk to be determined
   3. Identifies specific areas for intervention

IV. Psychosocial impact of a high risk pregnancy on the pregnant woman and her family

A. **Stressors are often magnified and increased in high risk pregnancies. These stressors must be recognized and addressed since they can contribute to the worsening of an already difficult situation and diminish the energy needed to cope with the pregnancy. Stressors arise from**
   1. A change in lifestyle and normal living patterns
      a. Family processes are altered to the degree that the pregnant woman is unable to fulfill her role responsibilities and is separated from her family
      b. Family members may have difficulty accepting the severity of the pregnant woman's health problem and the need for treatment since she may not look sick
      c. Added healthcare expenses and the loss of a second income can place a strain on family finances
      d. Frequent prenatal visits, antepartal testing, treatment regimes, and possible hospitalization

(1) Increase discomfort, fear, and anxiety
(2) Alter usual lifestyle habits including activity patterns or diet
(3) Separate pregnant woman from her family and home environment
(4) Change the focus of pregnancy from a natural or a normal experience hoped for to one that is medically oriented

2. An interference with the ability to fulfill the developmental tasks of pregnancy (Rubin) including
   a. Securing safe passage for self and fetus
      (1) Having to follow a strict treatment regime which may be difficult and uncomfortable—"Is it worth it?"
      (2) May fear further deviation from the norm
      (3) Feelings of failure and decreased self-esteem can result—"Other women can do it. Why can't I?"
   b. Ensuring acceptance of newborn by significant others including family members and friends
      (1) Fear baby will not survive or will not be normal if it does
      (2) Family and friends may avoid pregnant woman because they do not know what to say or how to help
      (3) Ambivalent feelings or resentment toward fetus-newborn can occur if it is viewed as the cause for maternal risk-discomfort and disruption of family processes
   c. Binding to her child
      (1) Fear an emotional investment in a fetus that may not survive
      (2) Often separated from newborn after birth as a result of needed treatment for self and/or baby
   d. Learning to give of herself
      (1) Energy and time are used to cope with the pregnancy
      (2) Little is left over to care for others

B. Psychological reactions—experienced by all who are involved in the pregnancy

1. Denial and disbelief
   a. "How can this be happening? It has never happened to us before or to anyone we know."
   b. May interfere with full participation in the treatment regime

2. Blame and guilt
    a. Pregnant woman—"What did I do wrong?"; "Maybe if I led a healthier lifestyle or was a better person"; "I am putting my baby in jeopardy"
    b. Father—responsible for impregnating his partner
    c. Blame each other, leading to long-term detrimental effects on their relationship
3. Fear—life and health of mother and fetus-newborn is in jeopardy
4. Grief and mourning
    a. Anticipatory grief
        (1) Preparation for a potential fetal-newborn loss
        (2) If fetus survives then transition must be made to relate to the newborn and its care needs
        (3) "Vulnerable child syndrome" may result—parents are overprotective and may even expect the child to die during childhood
    b. Grieve the loss of the expected "normal" child or grieve the death of the fetus-newborn

V. Bleeding during pregnancy

▼ **Any bleeding during pregnancy should be considered serious until assessment of the pregnant woman proves otherwise**

A. As pregnancy progresses and the uterus becomes more vascular, increases the danger of hemorrhage with massive blood loss and hypovolemic shock

B. The cause of bleeding during pregnancy changes as the pregnancy progresses

C. Early pregnancy—common causes of bleeding include

1. Abortion—authorities believe age of fetal viability is reached somewhere between the 20th and the 24th gestational week or after fetal weight is >500 g
    a. Findings manifested vary according to the type of abortion being experienced as well as the pregnancy's gestational age which influences fetal size, and the size and adherence of the placenta (Table 7-1)
    b. Sonography may be used to assess the integrity of the gestational sac to determine if the bleeding is related to an abortion process and if so what type
    c. Treatment approach utilized is determined by the type of abortion being experienced and ranges from bedrest to dilatation and curettage (D&C) (see Table 7-1)

Table 7-1. Spontaneous Abortion—Manifestations and Management

Type of Abortion*	Manifestations	Management
Threatened: manifestations may persist for several days or weeks, then subside with continuation of the pregnancy or progress to loss of the pregnancy; approximately 50% progress to loss	Slight bleeding Mild uterine cramping, backache Cervix closed—no effacement and dilatation	Confirm status as a threatened abortion ▼ Determine extent of bleeding, presence of uterine contractions, and condition of cervix ▼ Use sonography to determine cause of bleeding and to assess integrity of gestational sac Watchful waiting, expectant management ▼ Bedrest for 48 hours ▼ Avoid stress and intercourse Evaluate response to management Provide emotional support
Inevitable/imminent: pregnancy cannot be saved, abortion is going to occur	Moderate bleeding Moderate uterine cramping, backache Membranes may rupture Cervix open—dilated and soft	Confirm status as an inevitable abortion Wait for expulsion of uterine contents and examine for completeness OR Terminate pregnancy by ▼ Dilatation and curettage (see Chapter 1) or uterine aspiration when ≤12 weeks ▼ Dilatation and evacuation after 12 weeks Provide emotional support and assist through the grieving process

Incomplete: only a portion of the products of conception are expelled; usually it is the placenta that is retained especially after the 10th week	Heavy bleeding associated with the retained placenta Moderate to severe uterine cramping Tissue is passed with the bleeding Cervix is open and dilated	Manage as for inevitable abortion in terms of evacuating uterine contents Contents of uterus must be completely removed ▼ Bleeding and cramping will continue if placenta is retained since adequate, sustained contraction of the uterus cannot occur ▼ Risk of infection increases Provide emotional support and assistance through the grieving process
Complete: all products of conception are expelled; uterus is fully emptied spontaneously and tissue passed is complete and intact	Slight bleeding Mild uterine cramping Tissue is passed–complete products of conception Cervix closed	No medical intervention is required if ▼ Bleeding and cramping subside after passage ▼ Tissue passed is evaluated to be complete and intact ▼ Infection does not occur Provide emotional support and assistance through the grieving process

*Most spontaneous abortions occur prior to the 16th week of gestation.

Continued.

Table 7-1. Spontaneous Abortion—Manifestations and Management—cont'd

Type of Abortion*	Manifestations	Management
Missed: fetus dies but products of conception are not passed or aborted	Slight bleeding, brownish discharge No uterine cramping No tissue passed Cervix closed Signs of pregnancy subside; pregnancy test becomes negative	Wait for approximately one month to allow for spontaneous emptying of uterus Terminate pregnancy using methods described for inevitable abortion (induction of labor in second trimester may also be used) since retention of decomposing fetus can ▼ Affect maternal clotting integrity leading to disseminated intravascular coagulation (DIC), a severe, life-threatening clotting disorder resulting in massive hemorrhage ▼ Increase risk for infection Provide emotional support and assist through the grieving process

*Most spontaneous abortions occur prior to the 16th week of gestation.

2. Ectopic pregnancy
   a. Incidence is increasing with pelvic inflammatory disease (PID) and intrauterine devices (IUDs) as major risk factors
   b. Sites include the fallopian tube, ovary, abdomen, cervix
   c. Findings appear at approximately 6 to 12 weeks' gestation with the rupture of the fallopian tube
      (1) Severe unilateral pelvic-abdominal pain, often referred to the shoulder
      (2) Tender abdominal mass
      (3) Nausea, faintness
      (4) Bleeding which can lead to excessive blood loss and shock
         ▼ Blood may accumulate in the abdominal cavity with only spotting or irregular bleeding may be apparent externally from vagina
   d. Clinical manifestations may be similar to other health problems including appendicitis and ruptured ovarian cyst; a pregnancy test facilitates diagnosis
   e. Treatment primarily involves abdominal surgery to remove tube and products of conception (fetus, placenta, membranes)

D. Late pregnancy—common causes of bleeding include

1. Placenta previa
   a. Varies as to degree—marginal to complete
   b. Findings occur when the placenta is loosened as the lower uterine segment changes and the cervix ripens, toward the end of pregnancy, in preparation for the labor process
      (1) Bright red, *painless* bleeding
      (2) Bleeding increases as the placenta continues to separate
         ▼ Vaginal examination of a woman experiencing fresh bleeding must never be done unless immediate delivery of the fetus can be accomplished, since further separation of the placenta may occur
   c. Management varies based on the degree of bleeding, placental location in terms of the cervix, and gestational age
      (1) Watchful waiting—bedrest with close observation if pregnancy has not reached term, fetal lungs are immature, and separation-bleeding is limited
      (2) Immediate delivery if bleeding is excessive with continuing separation since fetal viability is endangered, along with maternal well being

(3) Vaginal delivery is possible if placenta does not cover cervical os and impede fetal descent

d. Major postpartum complications associated with placenta previa

(1) Hemorrhage related to limited contractility of the lower uterine segment

(2) Infection related to location of healing placental site

2. Abruptio placenta

a. Separation can occur spontaneously or as a result of such factors as trauma or a convulsion

b. Findings vary according to degree of separation and its location

(1) Bleeding—scant to massive depending on the degree of separation

(a) Concealed hemorrhage results if separation occurs from the center rather than the margins; blood is forced into the uterine myometrium (couvelaire uterus)

(b) Overt-apparent hemorrhage of dark red blood results if separation occurs at the margins

(2) Pain-discomfort and abdominal tenderness occurs as the placenta separates and increases in severity with concealed hemorrhage

c. Management is determined by the degree of separation and severity of blood loss and can range from watchful waiting to emergency cesarean delivery

d. Hemorrhage is a major postpartum complication as a result of

(1) Diminished contractility of the uterine fundus if couvelaire uterus occurs

(2) Exhaustion of clotting factors with bleeding associated with premature separation

VI. Pregnancy induced hypertension (PIH)—a major cause of maternal-fetal morbidity and mortality

A. Risk factors for the development of PIH

1. Chronic health problems that may effect the vascular system such as diabetes, renal disease, chronic hypertension
2. Family or personal history of PIH
3. First pregnancy (primigravida) perhaps related to first exposure to chorionic villi (immunologic reaction)—a similar association has been noted with

a. First pregnancy with a new partner
b. Multiple gestation, hydatidiform mole, large fetus with a large placenta, increased number of chorionic villi

4. Age—<20 or >35 years of age
5. Poor nutrition especially in terms of inadequate protein and calcium

B. Classification of PIH is determined by severity of the clinical findings

1. Gestational hypertension—development of hypertension after 20 weeks of pregnancy in a woman who was not hypertensive prior to pregnancy; edema and proteinuria do not occur
2. Preeclampsia—mild, moderate, or severe as determined by degree of hypertension, edema, and proteinuria
3. Preeclampsia can occur in women who are hypertensive prior to pregnancy (chronic hypertension)—pregnancy adversely effects chronic hypertension, necessitating careful monitoring throughout pregnancy and continued treatment of chronic hypertension
4. Eclampsia—seizure(s) occurs
5. HELLP syndrome—severe form of PIH that involves hemolysis (H), liver dysfunction (EL: elevated liver enzymes), and a low platelet count (LP), along with multisystem organ failure that places the life of the maternal-fetal unit in serious jeopardy

▼ All cases of PIH should be considered severe and taken seriously since PIH is unpredictable and can progress rapidly. Baseline data gathered during prenatal care is a critical factor in the early detection of signs indicative of PIH.

C. Pathophysiological basis for the clinical manifestations of PIH

1. Vascular network does not dilate to accommodate the increasing blood volume that occurs with pregnancy
   a. Typical second trimester diastolic pressure decrease does not occur
   b. Systolic and diastolic BP increases
   c. Intravascular fluid is forced into the interstitial spaces as a compensatory mechanism resulting in
      (1) Edema—peripheral and organ
      (2) Hypovolemia with hemoconcentration—Hct increases and tissue perfusion is decreased further
2. Venospasm occurs increasing peripheral vascular resistance

a. BP increases
b. Perfusion of organs including the placenta becomes impaired

D. Clinical manifestations of PIH

1. Elevated BP
    - a. Early indicator-predictor—second trimester
        - (1) Upward rather than downward trend in diastolic BP
        - (2) Mean arterial pressure (MAP)—vascular resistance against which the heart must work calculated by using the formula: diastolic pressure $+\frac{1}{3}$ of the pulse pressure; sustained MAP >90 mm Hg
    - b. Definitive BP elevation—third trimester
        - (1) BP 140/90 or an increase of ≥30 mm Hg systolic and/or ≥15 mm Hg diastolic on two occasions, at least 6 hours apart (mild)
        - (2) BP ≥160/90 on two occasions, at least 6 hours apart with pregnant woman on bedrest (moderate to severe)
2. Generalized and upper body edema
    - a. Puffy eyelids, face, fingers, hands, legs, feet, and sacrum
    - b. Severity of edema can be determined by assessing
        - (1) Weight gain which is excessive and rapid—often precedes visible edema. Example: a weight gain $>\frac{1}{2}$ to 1 kg/wk in the third trimester.
        - (2) Pitting—depth of depression remaining or the time the depression remains after pressing finger into edematous tissue located over a bone
3. CNS changes related to cerebral edema and venospasm
    - a. Irritability, insomnia, altered level of consciousness
    - b. Headache ranging from transient to severe and constant
    - c. Changes in vision—blurring, spots before eyes, severe photophobia
    - d. Brisk deep tendon reflexes ≥3+ (hyperreflexia) with ankle clonus noted in severe preeclampsia
    - e. Convulsion (grand mal type) occurs in 5% of women with PIH
        - (1) Any stimulus can precipitate a convulsion. Examples: sudden activity in or near client's room, a telephone ring, turning on the light or the televison.
        - (2) 50% occur before labor, 25% during labor, and 25% occur within 48 hours of birth
4. Pulmonary edema

5. Hepatic dysfunction related to venospasm and edema of the liver
   a. Epigastric, upper right quadrant pain related to liver enlargement
   b. Nausea and vomiting
   c. Jaundice
   d. Elevated liver enzymes (ALT and AST)
   e. Liver necrosis with bleeding—liver rupture is a possibility
6. Renal involvement related to diminished perfusion and increased permeability of the glomerular membrane
   a. Proteinuria—a later appearing sign present in two clean catch specimens taken at least 6 hours apart
      (1) 1+ to 2+ (mild)
      (2) 3+ to 4+ (severe)
   b. Increased specific gravity
   c. Oliguria—<25 to 30 ml/hr or <100 ml/4 hours
   d. Increase in serum creatinine and BUN levels
7. Hemolysis and decrease in number of available platelets
   a. Red blood cells change in form and become easily destroyed as they are forced through narrow, contracted blood vessels from the venospasm
   b. Platelets adhere to endothelial lesions in blood vessels resulting from venospasm—clotting may be effected resulting in
      (1) Bruising, epistaxis
      (2) Postpartum hemorrhage
8. Diminished placental perfusion related to hypovolemia and venospasm
   a. Decreased placental size and earlier aging—high risk for abruptio placenta exists
   b. Fetal effects include
      (1) Intrauterine growth retardation (IUGR)
      (2) Preterm birth may be required related to the severity of PIH and its effects on the maternal-fetal unit since the only definitive cure is termination of the pregnancy
      (3) Increased danger of fetal distress during parturition—labor and birth

E. Home care of the woman with mild preeclampsia

1. Monitor progress of PIH and fetal status
   a. Teach pregnant woman and her family how to assess health status including BP, weight, urine (protein level), DFMCs, and signs of worsening condition including headache, vision changes, epigastric pain

b. Encourage woman to keep a record of findings or concerns for review during prenatal visits or during home visits of a healthcare provider
c. Stress importance of keeping prenatal appointments and participating in antepartal monitoring techniques

2. Encourage cooperation with treatment regime
   a. Limitation on activity level—can range from frequent rest periods with an emphasis on sedentary activities to bedrest with bathroom privileges
      (1) Maintain lateral position (alternate between right and left side) when in bed to enhance renal (fluid loss) and placental perfusion
      (2) Utilize relaxation techniques, diversional activities, and gentle range of motion exercises to the extremities to increase tolerance for bedrest or limited activity
      (3) Involve family, friends, and homecare agencies to assist with home maintenance activities
   b. Nutrition
      (1) Maintain a balanced diet appropriate for pregnancy (see Chapter 3)
      (2) Increase protein intake to replace losses and to keep fluid within vascular bed—1.5 g/kg/day
      (3) Maintain a fluid intake of 2000 to 3000 ml/day
      (4) Include roughage to facilitate bowel elimination especially since activity level is reduced
      (5) Avoid highly salted foods, alcohol, and tobacco
         ▼ A low salt diet or calorie restrictions are not recommended as part of the treatment approach for a woman with PIH

F. Hospital care of the woman with moderate to severe preeclampsia

1. Systematic, ongoing assessment of the maternal-fetal unit to detect changes indicative of an improving or worsening condition
2. Bedrest alternating between a left and right lateral position
3. Seizure-precautions care
   a. Reduce environmental stimuli with regard to noise, light, activity; consider room assignment avoiding rooms near high activity areas such as the nurse's station or visitor's lounge
   b. Seizure readiness—pad siderails, keep bed in low position, have client wear loose clothing, keep oxygen and suction equipment nearby or in room

   c. Implement appropriate care should a seizure occur
   d. Following a seizure—observe for onset of labor, signs of fetal distress, and abruptio placenta
4. Medications
   a. Sedatives—combined with bedrest and reduced environmental stimuli can facilitate rest and reduce CNS irritability
   b. Magnesium sulfate
      (1) Primarily used as a CNS depressant; goal of treatment is to prevent a convulsion
      (2) Vasodilation effect produces a slight, temporary decrease in BP
      (3) Smooth muscle relaxation effect reduces uterine contractions thereby potentially interfering with labor process and postpartum contraction of the uterus
      (4) Administered IV piggyback using an IV controller
         (a) Loading dose of 4 to 6 g/250 ml of IV fluid over 20 minutes
         (b) Maintenance dose of 1 to 2 g/hour
      (5) See Chapter 9 for nursing measures required during administration of magnesium sulfate
   c. Antihypertensive medications, such as hydralazine (Apresoline) 10 to 40 mg IV, to reduce BP
      (1) Given according to diastolic pressure, such as when pressure is ≥110 mm Hg
      (2) Monitor BP before and after administration
      (3) Since hypovolemia is present, there is danger of severe reduction in placental perfusion if diastolic pressure is reduced to below 90 mm Hg
5. Vaginal delivery, at term, is the goal—labor induction-augmentation (see Chapter 9) may be required since magnesium sulfate suppresses uterine contractions
6. Postpartal care
   a. Continue PIH treatment until condition stabilizes, with a decrease in BP, edema (diuresis-diaphoresis), and proteinuria
   b. Utilize Pitocin as the oxytocic of choice to enhance fundal contraction since Methergine-Ergotrate can further elevate BP
   c. Observe for signs of hemorrhage
   d. Provide time for interaction with newborn

e. Caution woman to avoid another pregnancy for approximately 2 years to facilitate full recovery

VII. Hyperemesis gravidarum

A. Approximately 1 in 1000 pregnant women have hyperemesis severe enough to require hospitalization

B. Causative factors

1. Hormonal factors
   a. High levels of estrogen, thyroid hormone
   b. Increasing level of HCG associated with early pregnancy
2. Gastrointestinal factors
   a. Decrease in level of HCL acid
   b. Reduction in gastrointestinal motility related to progesterone
3. Psychological-emotional factors
   a. Continuing ambivalence-conflict related to pregnancy and impending motherhood—especially common when pregnancies are unplanned or unwanted
   b. Negative family responses to pregnancy, especially from the father of the baby
   c. Typical response to stressors involves gastrointestinal disturbances

C. Major concern relates to the impact of imbalances on the health status of the maternal-fetal unit

1. Maternal effects include
   a. Weight loss
   b. Fluid volume deficit—dehydration-hypovolemia with resultant alteration in vital signs including tachycardia and hypotension
   c. Acid-base imbalance—metabolic alkalosis progressing to metabolic acidosis
   d. Nutritional deficit
   e. Electrolyte deficit—hypokalemia, hyponatremia
   f. Activity intolerance, fatigue, weakness
   g. Fear regarding welfare of self and fetus
2. Fetal effects include
   a. Hypoxia and intrauterine growth retardation related to diminished placental perfusion and limited nutrient availability from the mother
   b. Anomalies related to exposure to ketosis

D. Major or immediate goal of treatment—restore fluid, electrolyte, and acid-base balances

1. Administer fluids, electrolytes, and nutrients
    a. IV hydration—5% glucose in lactated ringers solution with added multivitamins (MVC9+3, MVI-12), pyridoxine (vitamin B_6), and magnesium sulfate
    b. Provide nutrients with total parenteral nutrition (TPN)
2. Reduce fluid losses by using sedatives and antiemetics (vitamin B_6, compazine, phenergan)
3. Monitor effectiveness of treatment by assessing
    a. Vital signs
    b. Signs of fluid balance including weight, turgor, specific gravity of urine, I&O
    c. Serum electrolyte and glucose levels

E. Additional goals of treatment

1. Rest gastrointestinal tract by maintaining NPO status for 48 hours once vomiting ceases; then gradually introduce oral fluids and foods
2. Restore ability to take and retain oral fluids and food
    a. Gradual introduction and advancement of diet beginning with small amounts of clear fluids such as ice chips, tea alternated with dry carbohydrates such as saltine crackers every 2 to 3 hours
    b. Follow fluid and food preferences
    c. Use measures effective for morning sickness (see Chapter 3)
3. Maintain integrity of oral cavity with frequent oral care to keep mouth clean and moist—especially important after an episode of vomiting, since emesis is acidic
4. Promote rest and relaxation
    a. Create a quiet, restful environment
    b. Provide emotional support
    c. Facilitate expression of feelings and concerns
    d. Teach stress management and relaxation techniques
5. Prepare for discharge
    a. Educate pregnant woman and family regarding her condition, signs of improvement or deterioration, and treatment measures
    b. Make referrals, as appropriate, to monitor or supervise treatments such as TPN
    c. Arrange for follow-up prenatal visits

VIII. Diabetes during pregnancy

A. Pregestational diabetes—diabetes mellitus present prior to pregnancy is effected by pregnancy's influence on glucose

metabolism—a diabetogenic effect designed to supply fetus with the glucose needed for optimal growth and development

1. Alteration in insulin requirements during pregnancy
   a. First trimester—insulin requirement is REDUCED by as much as 33% as a result of
      (1) Fetal utilization of glucose
      (2) Decreased maternal nutritional intake related to nausea and vomiting—"morning sickness"
      (3) Increased tissue response to insulin
   b. Second and third trimester—insulin requirement is INCREASED by as much as 65 to 75% as a result of
      (1) Higher level of cortisol that increases serum glucose level
      (2) Insulin antagonists secreted by the placenta
      (3) Increased tissue resistance to insulin
         ▼ Danger of diabetic ketoacidosis is high during this phase of pregnancy if insulin is not increased to the level required
   c. Parturition—energy demands of labor and birth require a delicate balance of glucose and insulin
   d. Postpartum period—insulin requirement is REDUCED by as much as 25 to 50% as placental insulin antagonists are decreased
      (1) Up to 3 to 4 weeks are required to return to usual pregestational insulin requirements
      (2) Lactating women need to continue careful regulation of glucose levels and insulin requirements
2. Maternal complications related to pregestational diabetes
   a. Polyhydramnios (excessive amniotic fluid)—increases risk for premature rupture of membranes, cord prolapse, preterm labor-birth, postpartum hemorrhage
   b. Acceleration in the progress of vascular changes associated with diabetes increases risk for PIH, placental insufficiency, abruptio placenta
   c. Dystocia (difficult labor) and increased potential for cesarian delivery related to fetal macrosomia, an abnormally large body
   d. Increased risk for infection including monilial vaginitis, urinary tract infection
   e. Increased risk for diabetic ketoacidosis which also endangers fetal well being by effecting growth and development

3. Fetal-newborn complications
   ▼ There is a significant risk for morbidity and mortality unless preconception glucose-insulin balance is attained and pregnant blood glucose levels are maintained at 70 to 120 mg/dL
   a. Alteration in size
      (1) Large for gestational age or macrosomia due to
         (a) Exposure to high glucose levels when maternal control is poor
         (b) Increase in fetal insulin secretion as a response to high glucose levels—insulin accelerates growth rate
      (2) Intrauterine growth retardation if vascular changes associated with diabetes are advanced and affect placental circulation
   b. Congenital anomalies—cardiac, CNS, neural tube and skeletal defects, especially if a woman becomes pregnant in a poorly controlled state
   c. Preterm birth with a higher risk for respiratory distress since surfactant production is inhibited by increased fetal insulin levels
   d. Fetal hypoxia related to
      (1) Placental insufficiency
      (2) Limitation on oxygen availability related to increased level of glycosalated hemoglobin (glucose molecule attaches to hemoglobin altering its oxygen carrying capacity) in poorly controlled diabetic women; fetus compensates by increasing red blood cell production resulting in polycythemia
   e. Neonatal hypoglycemia since newborn continues to secrete high levels of insulin that is no longer balanced by maternal glucose
   f. Neonatal hyperbilirubinemia related to destruction of increased number of red blood cells produced during pregnancy

B. Gestational diabetes

1. Diagnosis
   a. Screening
      (1) All pregnant women should be tested using a 50 g 1-hour glucose test at 24 to 28 weeks' gestation
      (2) Test results >140 mg/dL (some say >130 mg/dL), 1 hour after oral intake of 50 g of glucose requires further testing

b. 3-hour glucose tolerance test (GTT) is used to diagnose gestational diabetes in women with a positive glucose screen or who are at high risk for developing gestational diabetes. Examples: obesity, family history of diabetes, personal history of gestational diabetes.
c. Diagnosis of gestational diabetes is made on the basis of ≥2 abnormal values on the 3-hour GTT

2. Degree of involvement may range from mild with glucose control maintained with diet alone or moderate to severe requiring both diet and insulin to maintain glucose control; ▼ Oral hypoglycemics are teratogenic!
3. Maternal-fetal-newborn complications are the same as those for pregestational diabetes; congenital anomalies are less likely since the onset of gestational diabetes is in the third trimester

C. Management of pregestational and gestational diabetes—goal of a vaginal birth at term will be met if treatment regime is fulfilled and euglycemia (normal glucose between 70 to 120 mg/dL) is maintained

1. Ongoing assessment of the health status of the maternal-fetal unit includes
   a. More frequent prenatal visits
   b. Hospitalization as required to stabilize insulin-glucose balance
   c. Antepartal fetal monitoring
   d. Maternal testing
      (1) Blood glucose levels
         (a) Laboratory testing of fasting (FBS) and 2-hour postprandial (after meals) blood glucose levels
         (b) Home monitoring before meals, 2 hours after meals, and at bedtime
      (2) Glycosalated hemoglobin levels—value of 2.5 to 5.9% indicates effective glucose control over the previous 4 to 12 weeks
      (3) Urine for ketones—negative is desired
2. Dietary management must take into consideration requirements of pregnancy and lactation as well as need to maintain glucose control
   a. First trimester—30 to 35 cal/kg, ideal weight without causing hypoglycemia or ketoacidosis
   b. Second and third trimester—35 to 40 cal/kg, ideal weight without causing hypoglycemia or ketoacidosis
   c. Diet should reflect a balance of 45% carbohydrates with fiber, 20 to 30% protein, and 25 to 30% fat

d. Diet should be distributed over 3 meals (25%, 30%, 30%) and 3 snacks (5% each) or 2 snacks (5% daytime snack and 10% bedtime snack) to maintain stable blood glucose level and prevent hypoglycemia or ketoacidosis
e. Bedtime snack of complex carbohydrate and protein is especially important to cover fasting during sleep

3. Administration of insulin
   a. Daily insulin dosage is based on serum glucose levels with the goal of maintaining a euglycemic state of 70 to 120 mg/dL
   b. NPH and regular insulin is utilized
   c. Frequency of administration is usually twice a day, with ⅔ of the dosage before breakfast and ⅓ of the dosage before supper
   d. Some authorities caution against using the legs as an administration site related to the circulatory changes that occur as pregnancy advances
4. Health teaching and emotional support
   a. Full explanation of diabetes during pregnancy, findings of hypoglycemia and ketoacidosis, need for frequent prenatal visits, antepartal fetal monitoring, a need to follow both a healthy lifestyle during pregnancy and the required therapeutic regime to maintain glucose control
   b. Demonstration, practice, and redemonstration is required for the psychomotor skills of home blood glucose monitoring, urine testing, and insulin administration
   c. Emotional support to reduce the anxiety and fear experienced when changes occur in usual living patterns
      (1) Dietary changes
      (2) Changes in usual insulin doses
      (3) Need to perform invasive procedures including administration of insulin, monitoring blood glucose levels
5. Care during labor and birth commonly includes an IV infusion containing glucose to meet energy needs and administration of insulin (IV/SQ) according to blood glucose levels
6. Postpartum follow-up includes
   a. Observation of the newborn and care if required for
      (1) Hypoglycemia
      (2) Hyperbilirubinemia
      (3) Respiratory distress especially if preterm
   b. Care for the pregestational diabetic woman
      (1) Continue to monitor blood glucose levels as during pregnancy and administer insulin at a dosage to

maintain euglycemia until prepregnant levels return in 3 to 4 weeks

(2) Breast-feeding is permitted as long as glucose control is maintained—hypoglycemia inhibits lactation and the letdown reflex

(3) Space next pregnancy, approximately 2 years, to allow for full physiologic recovery

c. Informing the gestational diabetic woman of the need to maintain a balance of nutrition and activity in order to avoid obesity since they are at increased risk for the development of gestational diabetes in future pregnancies and diabetes mellitus later in life

IX. Cardiac disease during pregnancy

A. Pregnancy places stress on the cardiovascular system as a result of plasma volume expansion which increases cardiac output and workload

B. The degree of cardiac dysfunction prior to pregnancy serves as the basis for pregnancy management—determination of cardiac status is made

1. Prior to pregnancy
2. At 3 months' gestation
3. At 7 months' gestation when blood volume is at its maximum and stress on the heart is greatest

C. Functional classifications of organic heart disease (New York State Heart Association, 1955) along with general recommendations for management are as follows

1. Class I
    a. Asymptomatic at normal levels of activity
    b. Management recommendations include
        (1) No limitations on activity
        (2) Limit stress
        (3) Additional rest periods at night (8 to 10 hours of sleep) and after meals (30 minutes)
        (4) Close health supervision during pregnancy with prompt treatment of infection
2. Class II
    a. Symptomatic with increased activity
    b. Management recommendations same as for Class I along with some activity limitations
    c. Hospitalization is likely as pregnancy reaches term
3. Class III

a. Symptomatic with ordinary activity
b. Approximately 30% of pregnant women in this class will experience cardiac decompensation
c. Management recommendations
(1) Moderate to marked activity limitations
(2) Bedrest for most of the day
d. Hospitalization is likely as pregnancy reaches the 7th to 8th month

4. Class IV
a. Symptomatic at rest
b. Pregnancy is not recommended but if it occurs
(1) Cardiac status must be improved early
(2) Early therapeutic abortion with regional anesthesia and prophylactic antibiotics may be required for the safety of the mother

D. Effects of cardiac disease on pregnancy

1. Women experiencing Class I and II cardiac disease generally experience an uneventful pregnancy as long as health supervision is provided and recommendations are followed
2. Women experiencing Class III and IV are at risk for severe cardiac decompensation resulting in adverse effects on the maternal-fetal unit
3. Problems encountered can include
a. Cardiac decompensation
b. Spontaneous abortion and stillbirth
c. Preterm labor and birth
d. Intrauterine growth retardation (IUGR)

E. Ongoing assessment of health status is required throughout pregnancy, labor, birth, and the postpartum period

1. Observe for signs of cardiac decompensation, with special emphasis
a. At 28 to 32 weeks' gestation when vascular volume reaches its peak and cardiac output-workload is greatest
b. During labor and birth when a woman must cope with the added stressors of pain and the work of giving birth
c. During the first 48 hours postpartum when vascular fluid volume increases with the reabsorption of extravascular fluid
2. Findings indicative of cardiac decompensation may appear gradually or suddenly
a. Decreasing energy level—fatigue increases with difficulty performing usual activities

b. Irregular, weak, rapid pulse rate (≥100/min)—woman may complain of palpitations
c. Alteration in respiratory pattern
   (1) Increase in respiratory rate (≥25/min)
   (2) Dyspnea with usual activities
   (3) Orthopnea
   (4) Moist, frequent cough
   (5) Crackles (rales) upon auscultation
d. Cyanosis of lips and nailbeds—a later sign
e. Progressive, generalized edema noted as
   (1) Weight gain
   (2) Swelling of face, eyelids, fingers, hands
   (3) Pitting edema of legs and feet

3. Antepartal monitoring to assess fetal status (see Chapter 4)

F. Management of the pregnant woman with cardiac disease

1. Pharmacologic measures
   a. Cardiac medications such as propranolol (Inderal), Lidocaine, digoxin (Lanoxin) to strengthen activity of the heart and enhance cardiac output
   b. Thiazide diuretics such as furosimide (Lasix) to reduce fluid retention
   c. Anticoagulant therapy with heparin to reduce clot formation
      ▼ Heparin, as a large molecule drug, does not cross the placenta whereas warfarin or coumadin do cross the placenta and affect the fetus
   d. Antibiotics such as ampicillin, gentamicin, amoxicillin to prevent infections, such as endocarditis; infections place added strain on the heart and increase its rate
2. Nutrition
   a. Balanced diet with calorie-nutrient increases to gain weight that meets the lower end of the recommended weight range, approximately 24 pounds; excessive weight gain will further increase cardiac workload
   b. Roughage to prevent constipation and straining at stool
   c. Sodium restriction may be required to reduce fluid retention—observe for signs of hyponatremia since sodium requirements increase with pregnancy
   d. Iron supplementation to prevent anemia since anemia would increase stress on cardiac function
3. Stress reduction and relaxation, rest
   a. During pregnancy

(1) Relaxation, stress management techniques incorporated into daily routine
(2) Involvement of family, friends, and homecare agencies to reduce household workload
(3) Balance periods of rest in the lateral position with periods of activity

b. During labor
(1) Prepared for labor by attendance at childbirth classes
(2) Regional anesthesia and comfort measures implemented
(3) Lateral position to enhance circulation
(4) Limitation on bearing down effort by using lateral position, episiotomy, low forceps or vacuum extractor
(5) Vaginal birth is generally considered to be the safest approach for all classes
(6) Class III and IV may require hospitalization prior to onset of labor to assure stability of cardiac condition and to induce labor

c. During the postpartum period—the goal is a healthy recovery
(1) Gradually increase activity from bedrest to out of bed as desired; observe effect of activity on woman's vital signs, color, stability
(2) Employ measures to prevent hemorrhage, infection, constipation
(3) Provide time for interaction with newborn, including a gradual increase in opportunities to care for newborn
(4) Implement discharge plans that include arrangements for help with household and infant care responsibilities in order to enhance recovery
(5) Evaluate effect of breast-feeding especially for women in Class III and IV
(6) Encourage use of birth control to space or prevent future pregnancies; sterilization may be recommended for Class II, III, and IV

X. Infection during pregnancy

A. An increased risk for infection may be greater during pregnancy

1. Risk results from
   a. Suppression of immunological system to prevent rejection of the fetus as foreign tissue

    b. Genitourinary adaptations to pregnancy
2. Risk for infection and severity of resulting complications increase among women who already exhibit physical and psychosocial risk factors. Examples: diabetes, limited access to health care, inadequate hygienic practices, unsafe sexual practices, nutritional deficits, stressful lifestyle, use of tobacco and drugs, previous history of infections.
3. Impact of systemic infections
    a. Elevation of maternal core temperature—fever
        (1) Increases fetal temperature, heart rate, basal metabolic rate, and oxygen consumption
        (2) Fetal anomalies, spontaneous abortion, IUGR, prematurity, and stillbirth are possible
    b. Pneumonia may be a complication with a resultant effect on oxygenation, hypoxemia
    c. Organisms causing the infection can cross the placenta and directly infect the fetus—viruses are especially harmful (Table 7-2)
        (1) First half of pregnancy—spontaneous abortion, anomalies
        (2) Second half of pregnancy—IUGR, stillbirth, preterm birth, neonatal infection
4. Impact of genital tract infections
    a. Origin of genital tract infections
        (1) Sexually transmitted diseases
        (2) Organisms normally present in the female genital tract, such as group B streptococcus (GBS)
            (a) Major infection responsible for neonatal morbidity and mortality
            (b) Present in the reproductive tract of as many as 35% of women and is most likely to cause problems among those women already exhibiting risk factors
            (c) IV antibiotics administered during labor to women with positive cultures, especially if at risk, has been found to be helpful in the prevention of neonatal problems
    b. Risk for direct infection of fetus as a result of
        (1) Transmission during passage through the birth canal as the fetus comes in contact with infected body substances: blood, vaginal secretions, feces
        (2) Intrauterine infection

Table 7-2. TORCH (Teratogenic) Infections

CHARACTERISTICS: Group of infections caused by organisms that can cross the placenta or ascend through birth canal and adversely effect fetal growth and development. These infections are often characterized by vague, influenza like findings, rashes and lesions, enlarged lymph nodes, and jaundice (hepatic involvement). In some cases the infection may go unnoticed in the pregnant woman yet have devastating effects on the fetus. **TORCH: T**oxoplasmosis, **O**ther, **R**ubella, **C**ytomegalo virus, **H**erpes simplex virus

Infection and Mode of Transmission	Nursing Implications for Client Care
T—Toxoplasmosis A protozoan infection transmitted by ▼ Handling raw meat, cat litter, or soil contaminated with cat feces ▼ Eating raw or inadequately prepared meat, animal products ▼ Eating inadequately washed vegetables that have come in contact with contaminated soil	Sulfa or clindamycin are the antiinfectives of choice. Teach client to ▼ Practice good handwashing technique ▼ Cook meat thoroughly ▼ Wash vegetables carefully ▼ Wear gloves or have someone else handle cat litter, soil, or raw meat
O—Other	
Hepatitis A (infectious hepatitis) A viral infection transmitted by ▼ Droplets ▼ Hands contaminated with oral or fecal material while eating ▼ Eating food handled by persons with contaminated hands	Administration of gamma globulin is recommended as a prophylactic measure after exposure Strict adherence to asepsis and good hygiene
Hepatitis B (serum hepatitis–HBV) A viral infection transmitted by contact with body substances containing blood ▼ Use of or injury by contaminated needles or syringes ▼ Sexual intercourse ▼ Handling of materials containing blood including transfusions, dressings, drainage ▼ Exposure during a splash or spray of blood as may occur during birth, surgery	Knowledge of and stict adherence to universal precautions are the major preventive measures Hepatitis B vaccine may be given to protect all persons including those at high risk for HBV such as healthcare workers; may be given to newborns and to high risk pregnant women Administration of hepatitis B immunoglobulin is recommended as a prophylactic measure after women have been exposed

Continued.

Table 7-2. TORCH (Teratogenic) Infections—cont'd

Human Immunodeficiency Virus (HIV)	
A retrovirus transmitted by contact with contaminated body fluids including blood and semen; infected pregnant women can infect fetus-newborn ▼ Transplacentally ▼ Contact with maternal blood, body fluids during labor and birth ▼ Ingestion of breast milk Infected pregnant women have increased susceptibility to other dangerous infections including other TORCH infections and reproductive tract infections	No known cure exists for HIV though many treatment measures are available to prolong life and well being Antiviral therapy with AZT has been found to decrease the fetal transmission rate from approximately 25% without AZT to approximately 8% with AZT Prophylactic treatment with trimethoprim (Proloprim) and sulfamethoxazole (Gantanol) is also recommended Prevention using universal precaution principles is critical
Syphilis A sexually transmitted disease (STD) caused by the spirochete, treponema pallidum. Transplacental transmission is possible after the 16th to 18th week of pregnancy resulting in stillbirth or congenital syphilis.	
R—Rubella (German or three-day measles)	
Viral infection transmitted by droplets	Rubella titres to determine immunity should be done prior to each pregnancy and rubella vaccine given if not immune. Pregnant women who are not immune ▼ Caution to avoid persons at risk for rubella, especially nonimmune young children ▼ Administer rubella vaccine *after* birth ▼ Caution to avoid pregnancy for at least 3 months after vaccination

Table 7-2. TORCH (Teratogenic) Infections—cont'd

C—Cytomegalovirus (CMV)	
Viral infection transmitted by contact with contaminated saliva, respiratory secretions, urine, semen, breast milk, blood, cervical-vaginal secretions Most often asymptomatic in the mother but produces severe fetal and neonatal effects including hemolytic anemia, jaundice, hydrocephaly-microcephaly, pneumonitis, mental retardation	Strict adherence to aseptic principles including universal precautions is of vital importance–healthcare workers are at increased risk
H—Herpes-Simplex Virus (genital herpes–HSV-2)	
A sexually transmitted viral infection that occurs when contact is made with contaminated genital secretions. Infected women can infect fetus ▼ Transplacentally especially during a primary infection when systemic findings occur and are most severe ▼ Contact with active lesions and contaminated secretions during passage through the birth canal	

(a) Infectious organisms weaken amniotic membranes, leading to premature rupture of the protective amniotic membranes

(b) Infectious organisms can then ascend into the uterus

(3) Transplacental transmission

c. Labor and birth are often complicated by infection

(1) Preterm birth may be precipitated by premature rupture of the membranes

(2) Cervix may be blocked by or fail to dilate adequately as a result of genital lesions, warts and scarring

(3) Cesarean section is often the delivery method of choice especially if cultures are positive and lesions are present

▼ Cesarean delivery must take place as soon as possible once membranes rupture to prevent ascent of organisms into the uterus

(4) Invasive procedures must be kept to a minimum
  (a) Limit number of vaginal examinations
  (b) Avoid use of internal monitoring
  (c) Cleanse newborn immediately after birth, before any invasive procedure is performed

d. Neonatal infection, with an early or late onset, can result in CNS (meningitis), respiratory (pneumonia), and sensory (blindness, deafness) involvement, mental retardation, chronic infection, and even death

5. Treatment options are limited by the potential for adverse effects on fetal well being

B. Diagnosis of infections during pregnancy

1. Specific findings may be limited and attributed to another cause or go unnoticed
2. Testing, including cultures of vaginal, cervical, and rectal secretions as well as serum antibody titres, can determine if exposure or infection has taken place and/or is present
3. Assessment for the presence of infection must continue throughout pregnancy to determine if
   a. High risk behaviors continue with reexposure to an infectious organism
   b. Treatment measures were effective

C. Prevention of infection is the best and safest approach!

1. Preconception counseling and care can provide
   a. Testing to determine exposure-immunity
   b. Immunizations
   c. Treatment without concern for fetal damage
   d. Reduction of high risk behaviors, such as unprotected sexual intercourse with multiple partners
2. Protective measures during pregnancy
   a. Hygiene-asepsis—handwashing, genital care, precautions when handling body substances
   b. Safe food preparation washing, cooking, and storage
   c. Avoidance of high risk situations or use of appropriate precautions (hygiene, universal precautions, safer sex practices) such as avoiding exposure to
      (1) Contaminated cat litter, soil, meat
      (2) Persons known to be infected or at risk for infection

(a) Sexual partner(s)
(b) Clients in ambulatory or in-hospital settings
(c) Young children especially if not immunized

D. Treatment approaches utilized are determined by the type of infection present with consideration given to the effect such treatment can have on fetal well being. Counseling and emotional support is of great importance if infection occurs and results in a strong possibility of congenital anomalies and fetal-newborn infection.

REVIEW QUESTIONS

1. Which of the following measures would be LEAST effective in reducing the stress associated with a high risk pregnancy?
   a. Educate the woman and her family regarding the health problem complicating pregnancy and the components of the treatment plan
   b. Encourage participation of both the woman and her family in the plan of care
   c. Arrange for home care if possible
   d. Reduce visiting hours, if hospitalization is required, to facilitate rest and relaxation

2. A pregnant African American woman, G 3 P 2002, is 38 years old. She is enrolling in Medicaid. She is married. Which of the following is NOT a risk factor for this woman?
   a. Age
   b. Need to use Medicaid to cover healthcare costs
   c. Race-minority status
   d. Status as a multiparous woman

3. A pregnant woman at 10 weeks' gestation calls the prenatal clinic to report that she is experiencing vaginal bleeding. What should the nurse's initial response be?
   a. "Describe your bleeding in terms of amount, duration, and characteristics"
   b. "Go to bed and rest for the remainder of the day and call if the bleeding continues"
   c. "Come into the clinic as soon as you can, so I can check you"
   d. "You are probably miscarrying. Bring in all your pads and come to the clinic now."

4. Signs of a threatened abortion are noted in a woman at 8 weeks' gestation. Which of the following is an appropriate management approach for this type of abortion?
   a. Prepare the woman for a D&C
   b. Place the woman on bedrest for at least one week and reevaluate
   c. Prepare the woman for a sonogram to determine the integrity of the gestational sac
   d. Comfort the woman by telling her that if she loses this baby she can try to get pregnant again in about one month

5. Which of the following is an expected assessment finding of a ruptured ectopic pregnancy in the fallopian tube?
   a. Sharp, bilateral abdominal pain
   b. Heavy bright red bleeding with the passage of large clots
   c. Tender abdominal mass
   d. Elevated BP and slow bounding pulse

6. Which of the following is UNCHARACTERISTIC of placenta previa?
   a. Implantation of the placenta in the lower uterine segment
   b. Severe pelvic pain
   c. Separation of the placenta as the cervix ripens
   d. Bright red bleeding, with amount dependent on degree of placental separation

7. A pregnant woman at 36 weeks' gestation is diagnosed with abruptio placenta. Assessment findings would include
   a. Placental location in the lower uterine segment
   b. Massive loss of bright red blood through the vagina
   c. Abdominal pain of increasing severity
   d. Rupture of the membranes

8. When assessing a pregnant woman, the nurse must be alert for risk factors associated with pregnancy induced hypertension (PIH). Which of the following would be a risk factor for PIH?
   a. Status as a multigravida
   b. Age between 25 and 32 years
   c. Diabetes mellitus
   d. Dietary deficiency of iron and magnesium

9. A woman with severe preeclampsia is being treated with an IV infusion of magnesium sulfate. This treatment will be evaluated as successful if
   a. BP is reduced to prepregnant baseline
   b. Deep tendon reflexes become hypotonic
   c. Seizures do not occur
   d. Diuresis reduces fluid retention

ANSWERS, RATIONALES, AND TEST-TAKING TIPS

Rationales | **Test-Taking Tips**

1. Correct answer: d

Women experiencing a high risk pregnancy often need the diversion and support that visitors can offer. Therefore, visiting hours should be individualized to meet the needs of the high risk pregnant woman.

Questions with the word "least" are better answered when the reading process includes rereading the question after initially reading through the responses. Only then should a selection be made; otherwise, the choice selected might focus on what is the best. Note that questions with "best" and "least" typically have four correct responses. You must then prioritize the responses.

2. Correct answer: d

An age of <15 years or >35 years would be considered a risk factor along with *b* and *c*. Primigravidas are at increased risk for complications during pregnancy.

If you had no idea, the best approach might be to cluster responses *a*, *b*, and *c* under demographic data. Response *d* falls outside of this category and would be the correct response.

3. Correct answer: a

Since the woman has provided very little information, the nurse must obtain specific data regarding the bleeding in order to determine the appropriate action. Responses *b* and *c* may be recommended depending on the data collected. While spontaneous abortion is certainly a possibility there is not yet enough information to make this judgement.

The key word in the question is "initial" which suggests use of the nursing process—do further assessment over the phone.

4. Correct answer: c

A D&C is not considered until signs progress to inevitable abortion, or expulsion of uterine contents is incomplete. Bed rest is recommended for 48 hours initially. Telling a woman she can get pregnant again soon is not a therapeutic response, since it discounts the importance of this pregnancy. If the pregnancy is lost she must be helped through the grieving process.

Again the approach to do further assessment will lead to the correct selection of response *c*.

5. Correct answer: c

Unilateral pelvic-abdominal pain, often referred to the shoulder, is expected. Bleeding is massive but internal, and accumulates in the abdominal cavity. Signs of hemorrhagic shock may appear with an increasing, thready pulse and a decrease in BP.

Key words in the question gives clues to the best response: "ruptured" may result in hemorrhage and shock and "ectopic" and "fallopian tube" suggest the location will be unilateral and internal, not external. Thus, responses *a*, *b*, and *d* can be eliminated.

6. Correct answer: b

Pain is not characteristic of this type of placental abnormality. Note that placenta previa typically involves painless bleeding. The bleeding in abruptio placenta is usually painful.

If you have no idea of the correct answer, cluster the responses. Responses *c* and *d* deal with separation, and response *a* with implantation; the only response left, option *b*, describes a client complaint of pain.

7. Correct answer: c

The placenta is located in the fundal portion of the uterus. Blood loss depends on degree of separation and

Recall that abruptio is a sudden separation so therfore logically the client will most likely have abdominal pain. Important words

may be overt or concealed depending on location of separation. Blood will appear dark red. Pain increases with continuing separation. Rupture of membranes is not associated with abruptio placenta.

to note are increasing severity which indicates that the clients situation will get worse which is what happens in this situation. The pain doesn't lesson or go away.

8. Correct answer: c

PIH is more common with first exposure to chorionic villi (primigravida) or increased amount of chorionic villi as with multiple gestations. Age of risk is <20 or >35 years. Protein and calcium deficiency have been associated with PIH.

If you have no idea of a correct answer, "Go with what you know" to make an educated guess. Of the given options, diabetes mellitus is the most associated with hypertension. Recall that diabetic clients may have multi system dysfunctions, especially with effects on the cardiac, vascular, and renal systems.

9. Correct answer: c

Magnesium sulfate is a CNS depressant given primarily to prevent seizures. A temporary decrease in BP can occur but is not the purpose for giving the medication. Hypotonia is a sign of an excessive serum level of magnesium. Diuresis is not an expected outcome from magnesium administration.

Because of the hemodilution effect from the excess water retention in severe preeclampsia the magnesium levels are low which may result in irritability of the muscles with tingling, twitching or tetany. Note that these findings are also characteristic of a low serum calcium. Associate findings of low magnesium with low calcium. Also, another approach is to take note of the key word *severe* and then match it up with the worst findings in the options which is seizures; make a logical guess that this is what is the expected effect.

CHAPTER 8

Parturition—The Process of Labor and Birth

STUDY OUTCOMES

After completing this chapter, the reader will be able to do the following:

- Define the key terms listed.
- Identify factors that initiate the process of labor.
- Identify the stages of labor.
- Contrast the characteristics of true labor contractions and those of false labor contractions.
- Describe the effects of uterine contractions on the process of labor.
- Describe the effects of abdominal muscle contractions as the secondary power of labor.
- Identify the landmarks and diameters of the fetal skull and the maternal pelvis.
- Describe the factors that influence the passage of the fetus through the maternal pelvis.
- Identify measures that can facilitate fetal passage through the pelvis.

KEY TERMS

Cardinal movements of labor Mechanism of labor whereby the powers of labor, combined with resistence from the passage, force the fetus to change the position of its head as it moves downward toward birth.

Cervical ripening Softening and thinning of the cervix in preparation for labor.

Dilatation Widening of the cervical os to 10 cm.

Effacement Thinning and shortening of the cervical canal.

Episiotomy Perineal incision performed to enlarge the vaginal outlet.

Fetal position Location of a set point on the fetal presenting part in a section-quadrant of the maternal pelvis; changes as fetus uses the cardinal movements of labor to pass through the pelvis.

Fetal presenting part Part of the fetus that enters the pelvic inlet first: head (cephalic), buttocks (breech), or shoulder.

Passage Maternal bony pelvis and soft tissues (lower uterine segment, cervix, vagina, introitus, pelvic floor muscles).

Passenger The fetus.

Powers of labor Forces which facilitate fetal descent and birth; namely, uterine contractions (primary power) and abdominal muscle contractions (secondary power).

Premonitory signs of labor Signs that signal the approach of the onset of labor.

CONTENT REVIEW

I. The process of labor: an overview

A. The process of labor usually begins between 38 and 42 weeks' gestation as a result of a combination of multiple factors from the maternal-fetal unit

1. Uterine stretch—the uterus has limited ability to enlarge and stretch; uterine irritability increases and contents are expelled once capacity is reached
2. Maternal estrogen-progesterone ratio changes
   a. Estrogen becomes more dominant
   b. Estrogen enhances uterine contractility by increasing the formation of oxytocin receptors and gap junctions

(pathways between myometrial cells that allow them to coordinate contractions) as pregnancy reaches term and during early labor

c. Uterus becomes more sensitive to oxytocin and prostaglandin—myometrial contractility increases

3. Prostaglandin activity increases and enhances
   a. Cervical ripening
   b. Uterine sensitivity to oxytocin—oxytocin in turn may enhance uterine sensitivity to prostaglandins
4. Fetal maturation, especially of the adrenal glands, may play a role in increasing prostaglandin activity

B. Premonitory signs of labor—period of prodromal labor

1. Signs which signal the approach of parturition
2. Present in varying degrees from woman to woman during the several days or even weeks before labor begins
3. Premonitory signs can include
   a. Lightening
   b. Weight loss (1 to 3 pounds) as a result of the change in the estrogen-progesterone ratio leading to a reduction in fluid retention
   c. Energy burst, nesting instinct—maternal desire to put all in readiness for the newborn
   d. False labor contractions (exaggeration of Braxton-Hick's)
      (1) Strong, uncomfortable
      (2) Irregular, nonprogressive in terms of intensity, frequency, or duration
      (3) Relieved with activity such as ambulation or changing of position
      (4) May enhance cervical ripening
   e. Bloody or pink show—passage of the cervical mucous plug (operculum); accompanies cervical ripening

C. Stages of labor and birth process—(Table 8-1)

1. First stage (cervical stage)—cervix effaces and dilates in preparation for the passage of the fetus
2. Second stage (delivery stage)—fetus descends through the birth canal and is delivered
3. Third stage (placental stage)—placenta (secundines) separates and is expelled
4. Fourth stage (recovery stage)—maternal stabilization during the first 1 to 2 hours after birth

Table 8-1. The Process of Labor and Birth

Stage of Labor	Expected Events	Duration	Assessment*
First Stage			
Focus: cervical effacement and dilatation (see Figure 8-1) *Powers:* uterine contractions			
1. Latent phase (L)	Progressive effacement Cervical dilatation: 0 cm to 2 to 3 cm	Average of 6 to 8 hours Nullipara: maximum of 20 hours Multipara: maximum of 14 hours	Fetal heart rate: every 30 to 60 minutes Maternal vital signs ▼ BP, pulse, respirations every 30 to 60 minutes ▼ Temperature every 4 hours until membranes rupture then every 2 hours Uterine contractions: every 30 to 60 minutes Vaginal show: every 30 to 60 minutes
2. Active phase—3 levels: Acceleration (A) Maximum slope (M) Transition-deceleration (D)	Progressive effacement Increasing intensity, frequency and duration of uterine contractions Rupture of membranes	Average of 3 to 6 hours	

2. Active phase levels			
Acceleration (A)	Cervical dilatation: 2 cm to 3 cm to 4 cm	Average of 2 to 3 hours	Fetal heart rate: assess every 15 to 30 minutes Maternal vital signs ▼ BP, pulse, respirations every 30 to 60 minutes ▼ Temperature as above Uterine contractions: assess every 15 to 30 minutes Vaginal show: assess every 30 minutes
Maximum slope (M)	Cervical dilatation: 4 cm to 8 cm to 9 cm	Average of ½ to 2 hours	Assessment frequency as for acceleration (A)
Transition-deceleration (D)	Cervical dilatation: 8 cm to 9 cm to 10 cm Fetal descent begins to accelerate at ▼ Nullipara: 1 cm/hour ▼ Multipara: 2 cm/hour	Average of 20 to 40 minutes Nullipara: maximum of 3 hours Multipara: maximum of 1 hour	Fetal heart rate: assess every 15 to 30 minutes Maternal vital signs ▼ BP, pulse, respirations every 15 to 30 minutes ▼ Temperature as above Uterine contractions: assess every 10 to 15 minutes Vaginal show: assess every 15 minutes

*Frequency of assessment is determined by the risk status of the maternal-fetal unit. More frequent assessment is required in high risk situations (i.e., if the range is every 30 to 60 minutes, then frequency for the high risk maternal-fetal unit would be every 30 minutes). Frequency of assessment and method of documentation are also determined by agency policy which are usually based upon the recommended standards of medical and nursing organizations. Always check the protocols of your agency.

Continued.

Table 8-1. The Process of Labor and Birth—cont'd

Stage of Labor	Expected Events	Duration	Assessment*
Second Stage			
Focus: fetal descent and birth *Powers:* uterine contractions coupled with abdominal muscle contractions	Progressive descent of fetus along with cardinal movements of labor	Average of 15 to 60 minutes Nullipara: maximum of 2 hours	Fetal heart rate: assess every 5 to 15 minutes
	Rate of descent ▼ Nullipara: 1 cm/hour ▼ Multipara: 2 cm/hour	Multipara: maximum of 1½ hours	Maternal vital signs: BP, pulse, respirations every 5 to 30 minutes Uterine contractions: assess every contraction Vaginal show: assess every 15 minutes
1. Early-latent: first phase	Transient decrease in intensity and frequency of contractions Time to rest and conserve energy until urge to push is felt	Average of 10 to 30 minutes	
2. Active-descent: second phase	Ferguson reflex is noted: rhythmic urge to bear down stimulated by fetal pressure against pelvic floor Active bearing down efforts begin	Average duration varies according to ▼ Parity ▼ Efficiency of bearing down effort ▼ Use of spinal or epidural anesthesia	

3. Transitional-perineal third phase	Perineal bulging Crowning Birth Use of interventions to facilitate birth ▼ Episiotomy ▼ Forceps ▼ Vacuum extractor	Average of 5 to 15 minutes	
Third Stage			
Focus: placental separation and expulsion *Powers:* uterine contractions and abdominal muscle contractions	Placental separation-signs of separation ▼ Bleeding: gush or trickle ▼ Fundal elevation to umbilicus ▼ Fundal shape becomes globular ▼ Cord advances and ceases to pulsate Placental expulsion ▼ Separated placenta falls into lower uterine segment ▼ Gentle pushing facilities expulsion ▼ Placenta is lifted out Episiotomy repair	Average of 15 to 30 minutes	Maternal vital signs: BP, pulse, respirations every 15 minutes Uterine contractions: palpate fundus ▼ Determine changes that indicate separation ▼ Ensure fundus remains firm to prevent hemorrhage; massage if bogginess is noted Placental assessment ▼ Completeness—fragments left in uterus could lead to hemorrhage and infection ▼ Condition: size, weight, presence of ischemic areas and signs of infection

Continued.

Table 8-1. The Process of Labor and Birth—cont'd

Stage of Labor	Expected Events	Duration	Assessment*
Fourth Stage			
Focus: physiologic stabilization of the woman following birth, and bonding of family with newborn ▼ Major concern of this stage is the prevention of hemorrhage and hypovolemic shock	Vital signs stabilize Fundus remains firm Bleeding moderate	Average of 1 to 2 hours Continues if vital signs do not stabilize and if bleeding is profuse	Maternal vital signs: ▼ BP, pulse, respiration every 15 minutes first hour and every 30 minutes second hour ▼ Temperature once or twice Postpartal check: as for vital signs ▼ Fundus ▼ Lochia ▼ Perineum—episiotomy ▼ Bladder Lower extremities: return of movement and sensation following epidural anesthesia

*Frequency of assessment is determined by the risk status of the maternal-fetal unit. More frequent assessment is required in high risk situations (i.e., if the range is every 30 to 60 minutes, then frequency for the high risk maternal-fetal unit would be every 30 minutes). Frequency of assessment and method of documentation are also determined by agency policy which are usually based upon the recommended standards of medical and nursing organizations. Always check the protocols of your agency.

II. Uterine contractions—primary power of labor

A. Regular, progressive uterine contractions signal the onset of true labor

B. Characteristics

1. Involuntary but enhanced with relaxation and activity
2. Four phases of a contraction
   a. Increment-crescendo
      (1) Pacemaker cells are activated; contraction begins in the fundus and radiates over the body of the uterus
      (2) As labor progresses a shorter period of time is required for a contraction to reach its acme
   b. Acme-apex
      (1) Maximum intensity of the contraction
      (2) As labor progresses the length of the acme increases
      (3) Decrement-decrescendo—gradual decrease in uterine activity
   c. Rest-relaxation
      (1) Reduction in uterine tone between contractions
      (2) Essential for restoration of blood flow through uterus and placenta
      (3) Rest periods become shorter as labor progresses
3. Fundal dominance—contractions begin, are most intense, and end in the fundus
4. Progressive—frequency, intensity, and duration increase as a result of a positive feedback cycle: during a contraction, fundal force pushes fetus downward against cervix, cervical impulses are sent to pituitary gland, oxytocin is secreted, increase in intensity and duration of next contraction occurs
5. Discomfort—characteristically begins in lower abdomen and back, then radiates over the entire abdomen; discomfort increases as contractions progress

C. Eight effects of uterine contractions

1. Division of uterus into two segments
   a. Fundus, also called the active segment—upper, contracting portion of the uterus that becomes thicker and more forceful as labor progresses; provides the force to push fetus downward
   b. Lower segment, also called isthmus or passive segment—thinner, more relaxed portion; expands to allow fetus to descend downward

   c. Physiologic retraction ring—separates upper contracting portion of the uterus from lower, more relaxed, stretchable portion
2. Effacement—lower uterine segment is pulled upward by uterine contractions and the descending fetus (Figure 8-1)
   a. Progress is expressed in percentages. Examples: 25% effaced, 50% effaced, 75% effaced, 100% effaced.
   b. Primigravida—effacement typically occurs prior to dilatation
   c. Multipara—effacement typically occurs simultaneously with dilatation
3. Dilatation—widening of the cervical os and canal from <1 cm to a full 10 cm as a result of the upward pull of the upper uterine segment and the downward pressure of the descending fetus during uterine contractions (see Figure 8-1)
   a. Amniotic membranes and fluid act as a dilating wedge prior to rupture of the membranes
   b. Fetal presenting part acts as a dilator after membranes rupture; fetal head tends to be a more effective dilator than the fetal buttocks
   c. Pattern of dilatation (see Table 8-1; Figure 8-1)
      (1) Parity of the laboring woman influences the rate of dilatation—nullipara dilates more slowly than the multipara

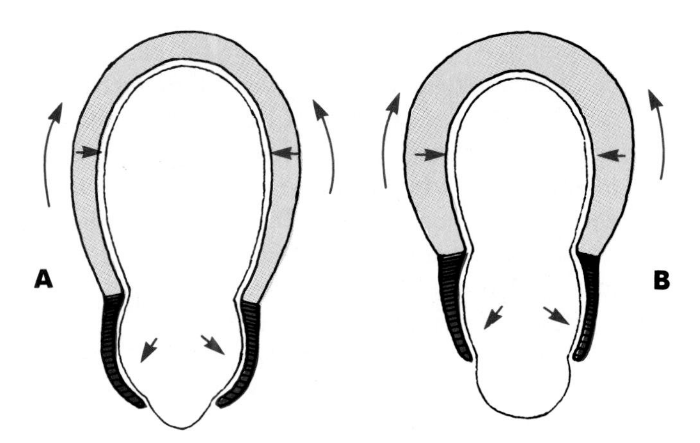

Figure 8–1. Lower uterine segment and cervix are pulled up (retracted) as the fetus and amniotic sac are pushed downward. **A**, Cervix is effaced and partially dilated. **B**, Cervical dilatation is complete. Cervix is being pulled upward as presenting part descends. Intrauterine space is decreasing. (From Willson JR, Carrington ER: *Obstetrics and gynecology*, ed 8, St Louis, 1987, Mosby. Bobak IM et al: *Maternity and gynecologic care: the nurse and the family*, ed 5, St Louis, 1993, Mosby.)

        (2) Rate of dilatation accelerates as uterine contractions progress in terms of frequency, duration, and intensity
4. Fetal progress
    a. Station or degree of descent is measured in cm above or below the ischial spines of the pelvis
    b. Rate of descent
        (1) Begins to accelerate during the transition-deceleration phase of the first stage of labor
        (2) Influenced by the laboring woman's parity—fetal descent is slower in the nullipara than in the multipara (see Table 8-1)
5. Rupture of membranes
    a. Opening of the amniotic membranes—membranous sac that encloses the amniotic fluid
    b. Timing
        (1) Most often occurs at the peak of a strong intense contraction during the active phase of the first stage of labor
        (2) May occur prior to the onset of labor
            (a) Premature rupture of the membranes (PROM) when they rupture at term (after the completion of the 37th week of pregnancy)—labor usually begins within 12 to 24 hours of rupture
            (b) Preterm premature rupture of the membranes (PPROM) when they rupture prior to the 38th week of pregnancy
    c. Types of rupture
        (1) Spontaneous rupture of membranes (SRM)
        (2) Artificial rupture of membranes (ARM)—amniotomy
            (a) An amnihook is guided toward the cervix and the membranes are ruptured
            (b) Goal—enhance uterine contractions thereby stimulating the progress of labor
                (i) Presenting part is considered more efficient as a dilator than the "bag of waters"
                (ii) Prostaglandin secretion is stimulated when membranes rupture
    d. Risks associated with membrane rupture
        (1) Intrauterine infection—the longer the membranes are ruptured prior to birth the greater the danger of infection

(2) Compression of the cord as a result of
(a) Prolapse of the cord—gush of fluid carries cord past presenting part where it can be compressed between the presenting part and the birth canal
(b) Loss of amniotic fluid reduces the cushioning effect of the fluid for the fetus
(3) See Chapter 11 for management
6. Uteroplacental blood flow alteration (see Chapter 10)
7. Placental separation and expulsion (third stage)
a. Contractions after birth decrease uterine size, allowing the site of implantation to become smaller, whereby the placenta is squeezed off the uterine wall and into the lower uterine segment where it is pushed or lifted out
b. Duration, signs of separation, and management are described in Table 8-1, p. 177
8. Prevention of postpartum hemorrhage—contracted uterus constricts and seals off blood vessels at the placental attachment site

III. Abdominal muscle contractions—secondary power of labor

A. Abdominal muscle contractions (pushing and bearing down efforts)—increase intraabdominal pressure; facilitate fetal descent and birth when combined with the primary force of uterine contractions

B. Abdominal muscle contractions are typically used during the second stage of labor
1. Cervix is fully dilated and effaced—pushing before the cervix is ready can damage the cervix and interfere with completion of dilatation
2. Urge to bear down is experienced—pushing before this urge is felt is less effective and can increase maternal fatigue

C. Correct technique is required to facilitate descent, conserve maternal energy, and prevent fetal hypoxia (see Chapter 9)

D. Abdominal muscle contractions can also be used during the third stage to facilitate the expulsion of the separated placenta

IV. The passage

A. Components of the passage
1. Bony pelvis
2. Soft tissues—lower uterine segment, cervix, vagina and introitus, and muscles of the pelvic floor

B. Bony pelvis—shape or type and size play a critical role in the ability of fetal skull and shoulders to pass

1. Shape or type
   a. Favorable for vaginal birth
      (1) Gynecoid-female pelvis—most common type of pelvis; rounded shape with adequate diameters accommodates the fetal skull and shoulders
      (2) Anthropoid pelvis—oval shape with longer anteroposterior diameter and more narrow transverse diameter; favorable especially if fetal skull is in the occiput posterior position
   b. Unfavorable for vaginal birth
      (1) Android-male pelvis—heart-shaped inlet with narrowed midpelvis and outlet diameters
      (2) Platypelloid pelvis—oval or flat shape with longer transverse diameter and narrower anteroposterior diameter
2. Size, diameters—measurement may be done in the first or third trimester using manual or ultrasound techniques
   a. Subpubic angle—should be at least 90 degrees since a rounded arch favors fetal passage into pelvis
   b. Inlet—upper border of true pelvis
      (1) Obstetric conjugate
         (a) Anteroposterior diameter extending from sacral promontory to posterior surface of symphysis pubis
         (b) Estimate during a vaginal examination by determining diagonal conjugate—measure from inferior border of symphysis pubis to sacral promontory and subtracting 1.5 cm from measurement
         (c) Adequate measurement—11 cm
      (2) Transverse diameter—at least 13 cm
   c. Midplane—curved pelvic cavity
      (1) Anteroposterior diameter—at least 11.5 cm
      (2) Interspinous diameter (transverse diameter between the ischial spines)—at least 10.5 cm
   d. Outlet—lower border of true pelvis
      (1) Anteroposterior diameter—at least 11.9 cm from lower border of symphysis pubis to tip of sacrum; coccyx can be pushed backward

(2) Intertuberous-transverse diameter (length from inner border of one ischial tuberosity to the other)—at least 8 cm

3. Enhancement factors—facilitate pelvic accommodation to the fetus
   a. Relaxin—corpus luteal hormone that facilitates slight expansion and mobility of pelvic joints
   b. Maternal position—squatting or sitting slightly can increase pelvic diameters

C. Soft tissues

1. Tissues of lower uterine segment, cervix, and vagina soften and become more stretchable during pregnancy to accommodate the fetus
2. Cervix effaces and dilates during the first stage of labor
3. Pelvic floor muscles guide fetus during its descent through the passage

V. The passenger—fetus must descend through the passage if vaginal birth is to occur; birth is accomplished by the interaction of the following factors

A. Size of the fetal skull

1. Diameters—average size at term is indicated
   a. *Biparietal diameter* (largest [widest] transverse diameter of the skull)—average of 9.25 cm
   b. Anteroposterior diameter passing through the pelvis is determined by the degree of extension or flexion of the fetal head
      (1) Suboccipitobregmatic (smallest diameter presented when the head is fully flexed)—average of 9.5 cm
      (2) Occipitofrontal (presented when the head is in moderate extension)—average of 12 cm
      (3) Occipitomental (presented when the head is in full extension)—average of 13.5 cm
2. Molding—bones of the skull, since they are not fused together, can overlap and allow the fetal skull to adjust to the diameters of the maternal pelvis; within a few days of birth the skull resumes its original shape

B. Fetal lie—relationship of the fetal spine to the maternal spine

1. Longitudinal-vertical lie—fetal spine and maternal spine are parallel to one another; seen with both cephalic and breech presentations (Figure 8-2A, B, C, E)

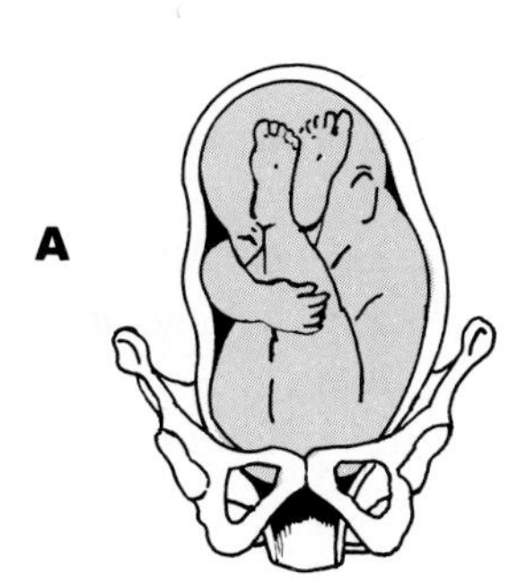

Frank breech

Lie: Longitudinal or vertical
Presentation: breech (incomplete)
Presenting part: sacrum
Attitude: flexion, except for legs at knees

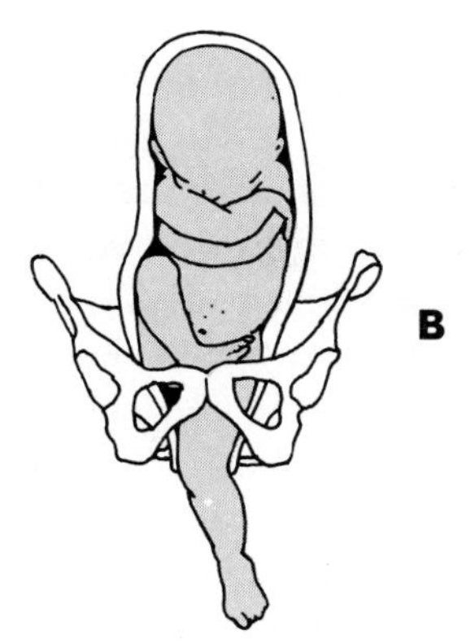

Single footling breech

Lie: Longitudinal or vertical
Presentation: breech (incomplete)
Presenting part: sacrum
Attitude: flexion, except for one leg extended at hip and knee

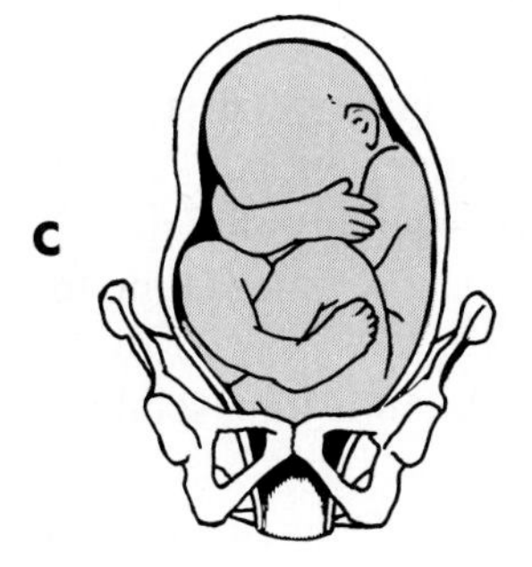

Complete breech

Lie: Longitudinal or vertical
Presentation: breech (sacrum and feet presenting)
Presenting part: sacrum (with feet)
Attitude: general flexion

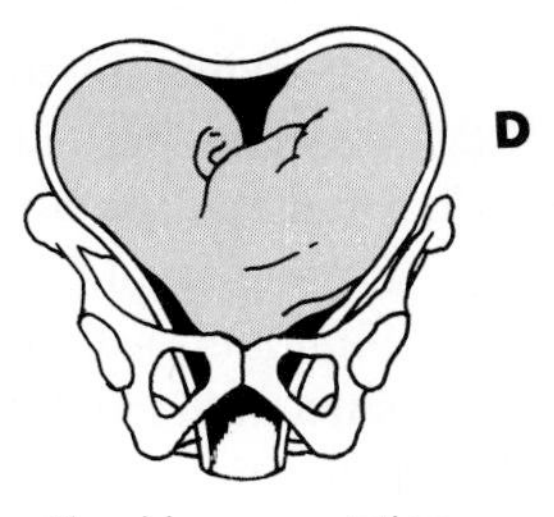

Shoulder presentation

Lie: Transverse or horizontal
Presentation: shoulder
Presenting part: scapula (Sc)
Attitude: flexion

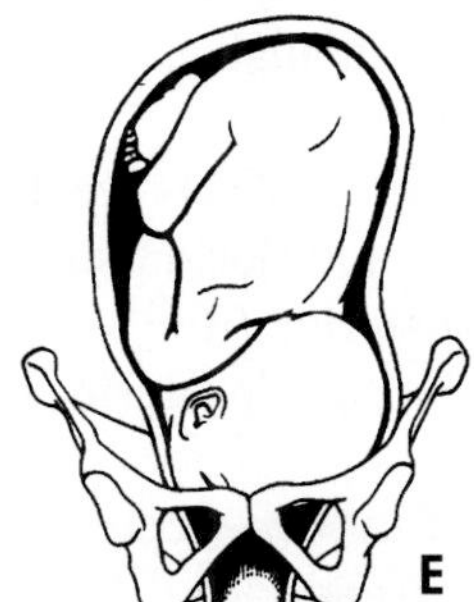

Figure 8–2. Fetal presentations. **A** to **C**, Breech (sacral) presentation. **D**, Shoulder presentation. **E**, Face presentation. (**A–D** from Bobak IM et al: *Maternity and gynecologic care: the nurse and the family*, ed 5, St Louis, 1993, Mosby. **E**, from *Instructor's manual to accompany maternity and gynecologic care: the nurse and the family*, ed 5, St Louis, 1993, Mosby.)

2. Transverse-horizontal lie—fetal spine and maternal spine are perpendicular (right angles) to one another; seen with shoulder presentation (Figure 8-2D)

C. Fetal attitude—relationship of the fetal parts to one another (see Figure 8-2)

1. General flexion—fetus accommodates to the size and shape of the uterus by assuming an oval shape (flexing its head and folding its limbs over its body)
   - ▼ Flexion of the head is a critical factor in the facilitation of a vaginal birth
2. Extension—fetal extension of the head increases the difficulty of birth and may result in a cesarean birth (see Figure 8-2E)

D. Fetal presentation—refers to the fetal part that enters the pelvic inlet first (see Figure 8-2); fetal presenting parts may be

1. Cephalic—head enters first; most common
   a. Vertex—head is fully flexed; area over the parietal bones presents first; vaginal birth is facilitated
   b. Face—head is fully extended and face presents first; vaginal birth is difficult and may be impossible
2. Breech—buttocks or foot, feet enter first—a more difficult vaginal birth since the head is delivered last with less time to accommodate to the pelvis
3. Shoulder—shoulder enters first; vaginal birth is impossible since fetus is in a transverse lie

E. Fetal position—location of a set point on the fetal presenting part in a section or quadrant of the maternal pelvis; fetal position changes as the fetus passes through the pelvis (see Figure 8-2)

1. Set points—vertex (occiput), face (mentum, chin), breech (sacrum), shoulder (scapula)
2. Examples
   a. Left occiput anterior (LOA)—vertex presentation with occiput in the left anterior quadrant of the maternal pelvis
   b. Right sacrum posterior (RSP)—breech presentation with the sacrum in the right posterior quadrant of the maternal pelvis

F. Cardinal movements of labor—occur concurrently with gradual downward progress

1. Engagement—fetal biparietal diameter passes through the pelvic inlet and reaches station zero at the level of the ischial spines

2. Descent—fetus forced downward as a result of pressure from the powers of labor and stretching of the lower uterine segment, cervix, and vagina; described in terms of station
3. Flexion—fetal head flexes during descent as resistance is encountered from the passage; smallest anteroposterior diameter can then pass through the pelvis
4. Internal rotation—fetal head turns to accommodate the diameters of the pelvic outlet and allow the biparietal diameter to pass between the ischial spines
   - ▼ Failure to rotate will likely halt the progress of descent and result in a cesarean birth
5. Extension—fetal head extends and is forced upward when it reaches the perineum; occiput is anterior and pivots beneath the symphysis pubis
6. External rotation, restitution and shoulder rotation—fetal head turns and realigns itself with its shoulders and spine, upon emerging from the pelvis; further rotation occurs as the shoulders move through the pelvis and are delivered from under the symphysis pubis (anterior) and then from over the perineum (posterior)
7. Expulsion—delivery of the fetal trunk follows the delivery of its head and shoulders

G. Medical interventions to facilitate birth

1. Episiotomy—controversy exists regarding its routine use
   a. Facilitates birth of the fetus
   b. Shortens the second stage of labor
   c. Prevents tearing of the perineum
2. Use of instruments
   a. Types of instruments
      (1) Forceps—metal instruments applied around the fetal skull
      (2) Vacuum extractor—cup is attached to the fetal skull at the occiput then suction is applied
   b. Instruments facilitate birth by
      (1) Assisting in internal rotation and/or descent especially when immediate birth is required in the presence of maternal or fetal distress
      (2) Augmenting maternal pushing efforts when these efforts are ineffective as a result of regional anesthesia, fatigue, heart disease

REVIEW QUESTIONS

1. Which of the following factors has been associated with the onset of labor?
   a. Progesterone dominates, increasing uterine contractility
   b. Estrogen stimulates the cervix to ripen
   c. Uterus becomes more sensitive to prostaglandins and oxytocin
   d. Fetal maturation increases oxytocin and estrogen secretion from the placenta

2. Cervical ripening refers to
   a. Softening and thinning
   b. Progressive dilatation
   c. Increasing vascularity
   d. Development of oxytocin receptors and gap junctions

3. A primigravida asks the nurse about signs she can look for that would indicate that the onset of labor is getting closer. The nurse should describe which of the following
   a. Weight gain of 1 to 3 pounds
   b. Quickening
   c. Period of fatigue and lethargy
   d. Bloody show

4. The nurse should tell a primigravida that the definitive sign indicating labor has begun would be
   a. Regular, progressive uterine contractions that increase in intensity with activity
   b. Lightening
   c. Rupture of membranes
   d. Passage of the mucous plug (operculum)

5. Which of the following characteristics is associated with false labor contractions?
   a. Painless
   b. Decrease in intensity with activity such as ambulation
   c. Regular pattern of frequency is established
   d. Progressive in terms of intensity and duration

6. The discomfort expected with true labor contractions is most accurately described by which of the following?
   a. Discomfort begins in the fundus and then radiates downward to the cervix
   b. Discomfort centers in the fundus of the uterus during the entire contraction
   c. Discomfort begins in the lower back and abdomen and then radiates over the entire abdomen
   d. Discomfort radiates outward from the umbilicus

7. Upon completion of a vaginal examination on a laboring woman, the nurse records: 25%, 5 cm, –1. Which of the following is a correct interpretation of the data?
   a. Fetal presenting part is 1 cm above the ischial spines
   b. Effacement is 5 cm from completion
   c. Dilatation is 25% completed
   d. Acceleration phase of the first stage of labor is about to begin

8. When monitoring the progress of a nulliparous woman who is in the first stage of labor, the nurse would expect which of the following?
   a. Latent phase is completed in less than 20 hours
   b. Acceleration phase averages 6 to 8 hours
   c. Phase of maximum slope averages 3 to 4 hours
   d. Deceleration or transition phase lasts no longer than 1 hour

9. A multiparous woman in labor has progressed to 8 cm and is entering the deceleration-transition phase of the first stage of labor. This phase should last no longer than
   a. 20 minutes
   b. 40 minutes
   c. 1 hour
   d. 3 hours

10. A primigravida asks the nurse when her membranes are most likely to rupture. The nurse should tell her
   a. Just before your labor begins
   b. During the latent phase of the first stage of labor between contractions
   c. During the active phase of the first stage of labor, usually at the peak of a contraction
   d. During the perineal phase of the second stage of labor as the head of the baby crowns

ANSWERS, RATIONALES, AND TEST-TAKING TIPS

Rationales	Test-Taking Tips
1. Correct answer: c Estrogen becomes more dominant, enhancing uterine contractility by forming oxytocin receptors and gap junctions in the myometrium. Prostaglandins are responsible for cervical ripening. Maturation of the fetus, especially of its adrenal glands, increases the production of prostaglandins.	Memory aid: match alphabetically by top or bottom of the alphabet the hormone and the action—*e*strogen—*c*ontractility enhances *p*rogesterone—*r*ipening of cervix.
2. Correct answer: a Progressive dilatation occurs once the cervix is ripe. Increasing vascularity occurs earlier in pregnancy and prepares the cervix for ripening as labor approaches. Oxytocin receptors and gap junctions are formed in the myometrium of the uterus.	Recall the sequence of events in a reverse alphabet: *v*ascularity increases; *r*ipening of cervix; *d*ilation progresses of cervix. Compare ripening of fruit when it becomes soft with the ripening of the cervix, which also becomes soft.
3. Correct answer: d Premonitory signs of labor include: weight loss of 1 to 3 pounds, a burst of energy or the nesting instinct, and passage of the mucous plug (operculum) or bloody show as the cervix ripens. Quickening is perception of fetal movement and occurs at 16 to 20 weeks' gestation.	Of the given responses, response *d* is the only one that suggests a change in normal progression of the pregnancy.

4. Correct answer: a

Progressive uterine contractions are the definitive sign of true labor. Responses *b* and *d* are premonitory signs indicating the onset of labor is getting closer. Rupture of membranes usually occurs during labor itself.

Response *a* gives the most information and has clues in the words "regular," " progressive," and "increased intensity."

5. Correct answer: b

While false labor contractions decrease with activity, true labor contractions are enhanced or stimulated. False labor contractions are painful. Responses *c* and *d* are characteristics of true labor contractions.

The important phrase to note in the stem is "false labor" and in the response is "decrease in intensity."

6. Correct answer: c

Radiation of discomfort from the lower abdomen and back to the entire abdomen is characteristic for most labors. For occiput posterior positions of the fetus, "back labor" with pain centered in the lower back is the expected finding.

If you narrowed it to responses *a* and *c*, reread the question which is asking for a "most accurate" description. Note that response *a* is a more narrow anatomical description of the event as compared to response *c* which is more broad. Between the two, response *c* is the most accurate.

7. Correct answer: a

Station of –1 indicates that the fetal presenting part is above the ischial spines, while engagement is station 0. Progress of effacement is referred to by percentages and dilatation by cm, with 10 cm indicating full dilatation.

If you have no idea of the correct response try this approach. Eliminate response *d* since it has nothing to do with the given data and the other responses include a part of the data. Eliminate responses *b* and *c* with the similar terms "completed" and "completion." Select response *a*.

8. Correct answer: a

Latent phase: 6 to 8 hours but never longer than 20 hours for the nullipara. Acceleration: 2 to 3 hours. Maximum slope: ½ to 2 hours. Deceleration-Transition: 20 to 40 minutes but never longer than 3 hours for the nullipara.

No specific test strategy. The important approach is to refrain from responding with increased tenseness or tiredness from the few questions like this that you have no inkling of the given data. Take a deep breath—relax—make a choice and go on to the next question.

9. Correct answer: c

The average duration is 20 to 40 minutes for both the nulliparous and multiparous woman. The maximum duration is 1 hour for the multipara and 3 hours for the nullipara.

If you have no idea of the correct answer, eliminate the extremes, options *a* and *d.* Of the remaining choices make a reasonable selection of option *c,* one hour since 40 minutes would be more difficult to track.

10. Correct answer: c

While membranes may rupture at any time before and during the labor process, they are most likely to rupture during the active phase of the first stage of labor. Membranes are often artificially ruptured, if they are still intact at the onset of the second stage of labor, to reduce the risk of fetal aspiration.

Note the words "peak of contraction" in response *c* and common sense suggests that is when rupture would occur; compare response *b* that states "between contractions" which is less likely since increased pressure is less at this time.

CHAPTER 9

Application of the Nursing Process during Parturition

STUDY OUTCOMES

After completing this chapter, the reader will be able to do the following:

- Discuss the key terms listed.
- Identify the components to be included in an assessment of a woman in labor.
- Describe assessment findings that indicate expected progress during parturition.
- State warning signs indicative of ineffective progress during parturition.
- Utilize the nursing process to address the common problems experienced by a woman in labor.
- Describe pain relief measures used during labor and birth.
- Discuss the goals and techniques of prepared childbirth.
- Describe nursing measures that are designed to facilitate the progress of labor and birth.
- State the nursing responsibilities for the third and fourth stages of labor.

KEY TERMS

Apgar score — Method used to determine newborn's immediate adaptation to extrauterine life by assessing heart rate, respiratory effort, muscle tone, reflex irritability, and color.

Bearing down effort — Effective use of abdominal muscle contractions with uterine contractions to facilitate descent and birth of the fetus during the second stage of labor.

Epidural block — Injection of an anesthetic agent and/or narcotic analgesic into the epidural space at the lumbar level to produce relief of pain related to the process of labor and birth.

Frequency of contractions — Timing from the beginning of one contraction to the beginning of the next contraction to determine how often they occur.

Low spinal (saddle) block — Injection of an anesthetic agent into the subarachnoid space at the lumbar level to produce loss of sensation from the uterus downward to the lower extremities.

Oxytocics — Medications which stimulate the uterus to contract thereby limiting blood loss.

Partogram — Labor graph used to compare the progress of an individual woman's labor in terms of dilatation and fetal descent with expected norms.

Prepared childbirth techniques — Use of relaxation exercises, breathing techniques, and effleurage to reduce pain, stress, and tension, and to enhance rest and conserve energy during labor and birth.

CONTENT REVIEW

I. Application of the nursing process—general guidelines

A. The nursing process should be used when managing the care of the woman in labor

1. Assessment guidelines
   a. Use a holistic approach—assess physical and psychosocial responses to childbirth
   b. Use a variety of sources to facilitate data collection
      (1) Prenatal records

(2) Coach or family is often an important source of data especially when the woman is in active labor

2. Prioritize data collection in terms of
   a. Condition of the woman in labor
   b. Phase of labor being experienced
3. Use an organized approach when admitting the woman in labor (Box 9-1)

Box 9-1. Admission of the Woman in Labor—Critical Data

Ask

When did your labor begin?
How have your contractions been progressing—how often, how long, how strong?
Has your water broken? When did it happen? What did the fluid look like?
Have you had any discharge from your vagina? When? What is it like? How much is there?
Have you noticed any change in your baby's movements recently?
When was the last time you ate or drank? What did you eat or drink?
How many times have you been pregnant? What was the result of each pregnancy?
What is your birth plan? Do you have a coach or someone with you?
What kind of health care did you have during your pregnancy?
Did you have any health problems during pregnancy? Do you have any now?
Is there anything else you think I should know?

Assessment Techniques

Inspect external genitalia and perform vaginal examination to determine
- Presence of lesions and signs of reproductive tract infections
- Presence of vaginal show or bleeding—if no active bleeding, continue with vaginal examination
- Cervical changes—consistency, effacement, dilatation, position
- Fetal presentation, position, station
- Condition of membranes—if ruptured test fluid (nitrazine test, ferning) and assess characteristics

Perform maternal vital signs—BP, pulse, respiratory rate and effort, breath and heart sounds, temperature
Attach external electronic fetal monitor to determine
- Pattern of uterine contractions
- Fetal heart rate pattern

Obtain specimens of blood and urine for laboratory testing
Determine overall emotional status of woman in labor and her coach-family

4. Assess maternal-fetal unit with increased frequency as labor progresses since vulnerability to complications becomes greater; early detection and prompt intervention are critical
   - ▼ Hospital policy often determines the frequency and type of assessments to be made as labor progresses

B. Nursing diagnoses reflect the common problems encountered during the process of labor and birth

1. Pain and discomfort
2. Fatigue
3. Risk for fluid deficit
4. Altered elimination patterns
5. Risk for infection
6. Fear and anxiety

C. Nursing diagnoses commonly encountered during parturition, along with selected client outcomes, nursing interventions, and evaluation criteria are described in Table 9-1

D. A nursing approach that projects calmness, confidence, and concern will enhance the laboring woman's own confidence in the nursing care she receives and facilitate the ability of her coach to provide support and guidance in childbirth techniques

E. Documentation is a critical nursing responsibility when caring for the woman in labor—all data collected AND nursing actions taken as a result of data analysis must be fully and accurately documented

II. Assessment of the woman in labor

A. Obtain a nursing history—components include

1. Current labor events
   - a. Onset
   - b. Show or passage of mucous plug
   - c. Rupture of membranes—when, characteristics of fluid
   - d. Uterine contractions—intensity, frequency, duration
   - e. Changes in character of fetal movements
   - f. Time and nature of most recent meal or oral intake
2. Birth plan—consider cultural implications and whether plan is realistic
   - a. Childbirth techniques to be used, such as Lamaze
   - b. Anticipated support group participation in the process of labor. Examples: who will be the coach, who will be present for the birth, who will not be present.

Table 9-1. Common Nursing Diagnoses Encountered during Parturition

Client Outcomes	Nursing Interventions	Evaluation Criteria
A. Acute pain related to the process of labor and birth		
Client will Cooperate with measures offered to enhance her level of comfort Use techniques learned in childbirth classes to cope with pain experienced during labor and birth Experience pain reduction with the use of relief measures	Provide comfort measures to enhance relaxation, reduce anxiety, and increase effectiveness of pharmacologic relief measures ▼ Back massage, counterpressure at sacrum using tennis balls, fist, heel of hand ▼ Cold packs at sacrum, warm packs at lower abdomen-sacrum ▼ Cold, moist cloth on forehead ▼ Frequent change of position, ambulation ▼ Hygienic care: perineal cleansing, shower, sponge bath ▼ Oral care Encourage use of techniques learned in childbirth classes—provide praise and positive reinforcement for efforts (Box 9-2) ▼ Relaxation techniques, guided imagery, focal points ▼ Effleurage—gentle stroking of abdomen to soothe and distract ▼ Breathing techniques	*Client* Worked with coach when performing breathing techniques during contractions Stated breathing techniques and Nubain were effective in taking the edge off the pain Used guided imagery to relax between contractions Accepted need for Nubain to reduce pain and regain control

Continued.

Table 9-1. Common Nursing Diagnoses Encountered during Parturition—cont'd

Client Outcomes	Nursing Interventions	Evaluation Criteria
	Demonstrate simple breathing and relaxation techniques if no prior instruction Institute alternative measures for pain relief, relaxation, and stress reduction as appropriate to client and facilities available including ▼ Biofeedback ▼ Acupressure ▼ Transcutaneous electrical nerve stimulation (TENS) ▼ Hydrotherapy—warm showers, jacuzzi Administer analgesics safely (Table 9-3) Employ appropriate assessment and supportive measures during regional block anesthetics (see Table 9-3)	

B. Fatigue related to ineffective progress of labor

Client's labor will progress according to expected standards Client will participate in measures designed to enhance the process of labor and birth Client's energy level will be sufficient for effective bearing down efforts during the second stage of labor	Employ measures to enhance rest and conserve energy ▼ Create a calm, restful environment ▼ Encourage relaxation techniques, visual imagery, music ▼ Provide opportunities for enjoyable diversional activities ▼ Utilize hydrotherapy—warm showers, jacuzzi ▼ Use measures to reduce anxiety Employ measures to facilitate the process of labor ▼ Frequent periods of ambulation — Gravity pushes fetus against cervix facilitating fetal rotation, cervical dilatation, progress of contractions — Pelvic diameters increase slightly when upright — Diversion and relief of discomfort are enhanced ▼ Alternate positions, emphasizing upright positions every ½ to 1 hour—take into consideration woman's comfort level and wishes (Box 9-3)	Vaginal examinations indicated ▼ Cervical dilatation—1.5 cm/hr ▼ Fetal descent—2 cm/hr Latent phase lasted 16 hours, active phase 3.5 hours and transition 1.5 hours Uterine contractions progressed to ▼ Strong intensity—75 mm Hg with resting pressure of 15 mm Hg ▼ Duration of 65 to 75 seconds ▼ Frequency every 2 to 3 minutes Laboring woman ▼ Ambulated for 15 minutes every 30 to 45 minutes until 7 cm dilated ▼ Alternated positions between lateral and semirecumbent every 45 minutes ▼ Demonstrated effective bearing down efforts during each contraction of the descent phase of the second stage of labor Duration of second stage of labor was appropriate for parity

Continued.

Table 9-1. Common Nursing Diagnoses Encountered during Parturition—cont'd

Client Outcomes	Nursing Interventions	Evaluation Criteria
	▼ Nipple stimulation to increase secretion of endogenous oxytocin; consult unit protocol — Stimulate only one nipple to avoid hyperstimulation — Stimulate for short periods between contractions—stop when contraction begins and when pattern is established ▼ Maintain caloric and fluid intake with oral and/or IV fluids Assure that active labor is established before analgesics or spinal block anesthetics are administered (see Table 9-3) Employ measures to prevent premature pushing before cervix is fully dilated and effaced and urge to push is experienced ▼ Explain why pushing must be avoided ▼ Reduce pressure against perineum by the use of a lateral position ▼ Encourage use of a pant and blow breathing pattern to prevent pushing when urge to bear down is felt Assist woman with bearing down effort at appropriate times	Spontaneous vaginal birth was accomplished without the use of forceps or vacuum extraction

C. Risk for fluid deficit related to limitation on oral intake during parturition

Client will		*Client*
Maintain fluid and electrolyte balance Experience limited nausea and vomiting Exhibit no signs of fluid deficit or overload	Explain purpose of restricted oral intake during labor Monitor hydration status ▼ Intake and output ▼ Assess for signs of fluid deficit or overload Prevent or treat nausea and vomiting ▼ Limit oral intake (see below) ▼ Use relaxation and comfort measures to decrease stress and anxiety ▼ Prepare to administer as ordered — Antiemetics such as prochlorperazine maleate (Compazine) — Tranquilizers such as promethazme Hcl (Phenergan) Institute oral intake restrictions as recommended—for example ▼ Latent phase—small amounts of — Low residue, high energy solids such as dry toast or crackers with honey or jelly — Glucose source—lollipops — Full liquids	Exhibited signs of good hydration ▼ Oral mucous membranes moist—no thirst ▼ Chest sounds clear ▼ Urine light yellow—specific gravity at 1.020 ▼ Skin turgor resilient ▼ BP, pulse, respirations within normal limits ▼ Oral temperature stable at 98.9° F Tolerated moderate amounts of clear liquids then ice chips during latent and active phase of labor Experienced mild nausea with small amount clear emesis × 1 during transition phase Progressed through labor in accordance with expected norms

Continued.

Table 9-1. Common Nursing Diagnoses Encountered during Parturition—cont'd

Client Outcomes	Nursing Interventions	Evaluation Criteria
	▼ Active-transition phase — Small amounts of clear liquids — Ice chips Initiate intravenous fluids as ordered ▼ When progress of labor slows ▼ When signs of dehydration begin to appear ▼ When oral fluids are not tolerated Intravenous fluids with or without 5% glucose in an electrolyte solution at 100 to 150 cc/hr are used to replace fluid-electrolyte losses and provide calories for energy Glucose is never used when rapid infusions are required; 0.9% normal saline or lactated ringers would be used	

D. Alteration in elimination—bowel and bladder related to changes in gastrointestinal and urinary function during pregnancy and parturition

Client will Empty lower bowel-rectum Void at least 100 cc every 2 to 3 hours Experience no bladder distension	Administer fleets enema if client reports no recent bowel movement, for example within the last 12 to 24 hours ▼ Assess client for contraindications to administration: bleeding, progress of labor, fetal status—presence of problems or impending birth ▼ Stay with client after administration since an enema often stimulates uterine contractions Enemas are used less frequently than in the past Assist client to void every 2 hours—measure urine and observe its characteristics: color, clarity, odor, amount, level of protein, glucose, ketones Utilize measures to facilitate voiding including upright position, privacy, running water, warm water poured over vulva-perineum, blowing bubbles with a straw in a glass of water Palpate-percuss bladder for distension Catheterize as needed ▼ Insert between contractions ▼ Place fingers in vagina and press fetal part upward if passage of catheter is impeded	*Client* Reported bowel movement of moderate amount soft brown stool 8 hours before onset of labor Voided approximately every 2 hours 150 to 200 cc of clear, yellow urine Exhibited no bladder distension upon palpation of lower abdomen

Continued.

Table 9-1. Common Nursing Diagnoses Encountered during Parturition—cont'd

Client Outcomes	Nursing Interventions	Evaluation Criteria
E. Risk for infection related to process of labor and rupture of amniotic membranes		
Client will progress through labor and birthing without developing an infection	Utilize universal precautions and regular handwashing. Risk of exposure to blood and body fluids is high Limit frequency of vaginal examinations Perform perineal care with greater frequency as show increases Utilize principles of asepsis when performing vaginal examinations: ▼ Cleanse vulva and perineum before and after examination ▼ Utilize surgical asepsis for examination—sterile glove and lubricant Utilize surgical asepsis for insertion of internal monitors Wear clean scrub clothing when working in labor Utilize measures to decrease number of invasive procedures ▼ Facilitate spontaneous voiding ▼ Assist with bearing down efforts ▼ Prevent prolonged labor Prepare perineal area with a mini shave (shave hair at lower vulva and over perineum)—used less often today	Client exhibited no signs of infection upon assessment ▼ Temperature stable at 99° F ▼ Maternal pulse and FHR remained within normal range ▼ Show exhibited only expected musty odor ▼ Urine clear, no dysuria

F. Moderate level of anxiety related childbirth experience

Client's level of anxiety will be maintained at a mild to moderate level Client and coach will work together effectively as a team Client will participate in measures designed to reduce anxiety and enhance relaxation	Encourage and guide couple in their use of childbirth techniques ▼ Provide positive reinforcement ▼ Review techniques they have learned as needed ▼ Help them get started and to advance techniques as labor progresses ▼ Do not interrupt during a contraction Review birth plan with woman and coach—ensure staff awareness of and respect for birth plan Facilitate relaxation using comfort measures and relaxation techniques Administer medications as needed ▼ Sedatives such as seconal may be given during the latent phase to help the client to rest or sleep until labor is more active Never give barbiturates once labor is active and progressing since profound depression of newborn can occur if drug is still in its system at birth ▼ Tranquilizers such as Phenergan can reduce anxiety and help client to relax	*Client* Demonstrated a reduction in her level of anxiety with successful use of guided imagery, breathing techniques, and focal point under the direction of her coach Dozed between contractions following the administration of Phenergan during the latent phase of her labor *Client and coach* Responded in a positive manner to comfort and labor facilitation measures provided by the healthcare team Openly expressed concerns and fears regarding labor and their ability to continue to cope as labor progressed

Continued.

Table 9-1. Common Nursing Diagnoses Encountered During Parturition—cont'd

Client Outcomes	Nursing Interventions	Evaluation Criteria
	Use a calm, confident, nonjudgmental caring approach—implement measures that reflect a sensitivity to the culture of the woman ▼ Touch—physical contact reassures, comforts, implies acceptance ▼ Encourage expression of feelings ▼ Maintain privacy and modesty ▼ Allow client to be herself—express self, deal with pain, make sounds during pushing ▼ Support and encourage coach Keep woman and coach informed of progress and events ▼ Explain procedures, equipment, routine; orient to room ▼ Simple teaching as needed in early labor especially if unprepared for childbirth ▼ Give progress reports in positive terms, for example — 2 cm dilated but already 50% effaced NOT only 2 cm dilated and still a long way to go — Contractions more intense and are doing more effective work NOT contractions more painful	

Box 9-2. Prepared Childbirth

Purpose

Provide information to reduce fear of the unknown

Teach childbirth techniques which

- ▼ Reduce stress and tension
- ▼ Conserve energy and enhance rest
- ▼ Reduce perception of pain
- ▼ Decrease need for pharmacologic pain relief measures in terms of amount, frequency, type

Create a satisfying childbirth experience that enhances cooperation among the woman in labor, her coach and family, and the healthcare team

PREPARED CHILDBIRTH TECHNIQUES: initiated at the beginning of the third trimester when motivation is highest; repeated practice will facilitate the mindset that effectiveness is possible

Relaxation Exercises

Consciously relax tense body parts as directed by the touch of the coach

Rhythmic breathing

Guided imagery—use of mental pictures to perceive

- ▼ Events of labor such as cervix opening, contractions pushing fetus downward
- ▼ Pleasant places or experiences that are special and relaxing to the woman in labor

Pain management techniques—reduce perception of pain through the use of increasingly complex distracting activities

Breathing techniques—deliberate, conscious breathing methods requiring concentration; techniques become more rapid, shallow, and complex as labor progresses

Focal point—focusing on a favorite picture or object to enhance concentration while performing breathing techniques

Effleurage—rhythmic stroking of the abdomen by the woman while she is performing a breathing technique and focusing on a focal point

c. Expectations regarding parturition events include
   (1) Analgesia, anesthesia
   (2) Role of the nurse
   (3) Monitoring—external, internal, none at all
   (4) Invasive techniques—IVs, episiotomy, enemas
   (5) Position for birth; where it will take place

3. Prenatal history
   a. Current pregnancy
      (1) Prenatal care received

Table 9-2. Assessment of Newborn Using the APGAR Score

I. APGAR Score—Performed at 1 and 5 Minutes after Birth

Sign Assessed	*Score Assigned* 0	1	2
Heart rate	Not present/absent	Less than 100 beats per minute	Greater than 100 beats per minute
Respiratory *effort*	Not present/absent	Weak, slow, irregular respirations	Cries vigorously
Muscle tone	Flaccid/limp	Some flexion of arms and legs, limited movement	Actively moving, good range of motion
Reflex irritability	Unresponsive when stimulated	Minimal response or grimace when stimulated	Cries, coughs, sneezes in response to stimulation
Color	Cyanotic, pale	Body pink with blue hands and feet (acrocyanosis)	Fully pink, including hands and feet

II. Interpretation of Scores and Recommended Actions

Score	*Interpretation*	*Recommended Action*
8 to 10	Reassuring—good initial response to birth	Basic newborn care Suction to maintain patent airway Prevent heat loss Facilitate bonding with parents
3 to 7	Mild to moderate depression or asphyxia	Support respiratory effort as indicated ▼ Gentle stimulation; ventilation with bag, oxygen administration ▼ Oro-nasopharyngeal suction ▼ Administer narcotic antagonist
0 to 2	Severe depression or asphyxia	Insert endotracheal tube, oxygenate Initiate cardiopulmonary resuscitation Administer narcotic antagonist (Narcan), epinephrine, glucose, sodium bicarbonate with arterial blood gas results

Table 9-3. Pharmacologic Measures to Manage Discomforts of Labor and Birth

Pharmacologic Measures	Effects on Maternal-Fetal Unit	Nursing Considerations
I. Systemic Analgesics		
Types Meperidine (Demerol) ▼ Dose: 50-100 mg (IM)* 25-50 mg (IV)* ▼ Peak: 40-60 min (IM) 2-10 min (IV) ▼ Duration: 2-4 hr (IM/IV) Fentanyl (Sublimaze) ▼ Dose: 50-100 mcg (IM) 25-50 mcg (IV) ▼ Peak: 20-30 min (IM) 3-5 min (IV) ▼ Duration: 1-2 hr (IM) 30-60 min (IV) Nalbuphine (Nubain) ▼ Dose: 0.2 mg/kg (IM) 0.1-0.2 mg/kg (IV) ▼ Peak: 1 hr (IM), 30 min (IV) ▼ Duration: 3-6 hrs (IM/IV) IV administration preferred to IM since a smaller dose is required, with a faster onset and more reliable effect	Maternal effects ▼ CNS depression—BP and respirations decrease ▼ Slowing of uterine contractions if given before labor is well established in the active phase and cervix is dilated at least 4 cm ▼ Takes edge off of pain and sedates allowing woman to — Regain control — Rest between contractions — Reduce anxiety and tension — Experience a more positive, comfortable labor ▼ Maternal relaxation can enhance labor and facilitate fetal descent Fetal-newborn effects ▼ Direct effect of analgesic—drug crosses placenta and is metabolized slowly — CNS depression of fetus and of newborn if given within 2 hours of expected birth	Assess need for analgesic and effectiveness of nonpharmacologic pain relief measures Assess before and after administration ▼ Maternal-fetal vital signs ▼ Phase of labor ▼ Need and effectiveness Do not give if ▼ Labor is not established or birth is anticipated in 1 to 2 hours ▼ Signs of fetal hypoxia are noted ▼ Maternal BP or respirations are decreased Enhance effectiveness by ▼ Reducing environmental stimuli ▼ Providing comfort measures and opportunity to rest ▼ Explaining beneficial effects related to mother, fetus, and labor Institute safety measures—bedrest, siderails, call light

*IM—intramuscular, IV—intravenously

Continued.

Table 9-3. Pharmacologic Measures to Manage Discomforts of Labor and Birth—cont'd

Pharmacologic Measures	Effects on Maternal-Fetal Unit	Nursing Considerations
Tranquilizers, when administered in combination with analgesics potentiate the analgesic's action and require a smaller analgesic dose	— Transitory decrease in variability related to mild hypoxia (see Chapter 10) — Respiratory depression after birth — Decreased alertness and responsiveness of newborn—may persist for ≥24 hours ▼ Indirect effect of analgesic is related to fetal response to a decrease of maternal BP and/or respiratory rate	▼ Keep a narcotic antagonist such as Narcan in readiness for administration to a depressed neonate: 0.1 mg/kg via umbilical vein; may be repeated every 2 to 3 minutes for 3 doses
II. Nerve Block Anesthesia		
Local infiltration anesthesia—anesthetic agent is injected into perineal tissue during the second stage of labor just prior to birth and/or during the third stage of labor	Maternal effects ▼ Interrupts conduction of pain impulses from the perineum prior to performance of an episiotomy and during repair of episiotomy and lacerations ▼ No relief of pain associated with contractions ▼ Allergic (systemic/local) reaction can occur Fetal/newborn effects: none	Determine presence of maternal allergies to local anesthetic agents Provide client support and explanations Assess for signs of allergic reactions Assess perineal area for ecchymosis, edema, erythema

Pudendal block—between contractions, anesthetic agent is injected near the ischial spines in order to anesthetize the pudendal nerve during the second stage of labor just prior to birth	Maternal effects ▼ Pain relief in clitoris, labia majora and minora, perineum ▼ No effect on pain associated with uterine contractions ▼ Bearing down reflex may be reduced ▼ Effective pain relief for the use of low forceps or vacuum extractor, for performance of an episiotomy, and repair of an episiotomy and lacerations ▼ Allergic reaction (systemic-local) can occur Fetal-newborn effects: none	Assist with bearing down efforts—pushing Assess for hematoma formation Assess perineal area for ecchymosis, edema, erythema Assess for signs of allergic reactions Provide client support and explanations
Epidural block—between contractions, anesthetic agent is injected into the epidural space at level L2 to L4 Anesthetic agent such as bupivacaine can be administered alone or in combination with a narcotic analgesic such as fentanyl Onset occurs within 10 to 20 minutes Single injection can be used during second stage for vaginal or cesarean birth	Maternal effects ▼ Hypotension: most common complication; a drop of >25% from baseline or <90 mm Hg systolic pressure would result in a BP that would be inadequate to maintain placental perfusion ▼ Respiratory depression may occur — When given with narcotic — If dura mater is punctured profound depression, even respiratory arrest can occur	Assess maternal-fetal status prior to procedure Prepare woman for and support her during the procedure ▼ Explain what to expect ▼ Have her void prior to procedure ▼ Assist into position — Sitting on side of bed or delivery table with feet on a stool and back curved by leaning forward supported by nurse — Modified Sims position, with head supported on small pillow, back curved, and legs flexed

Continued.

Table 9-3. Pharmacologic Measures to Manage Discomforts of Labor and Birth—cont'd

Pharmacologic Measures	Effects on Maternal-Fetal Unit	Nursing Considerations
Continuous infusion can be accomplished by inserting a catheter into the epidural space and connecting it to an infusion pump during active phase when ▼ Contractions are well established ▼ Cervix is dilated at least — 5 to 6 cm: nullipara — 3 to 4 cm: multipara Level of analgesia-anesthesia achieved is dosage dependent Duration of action ranges from 30 minutes to 4 hours depending on agent used, i.e., bupivacaine has the longest duration of 2 to 4 hours Contraindications include: coagulation disorders, infection at injection site, maternal hypotension or shock	▼ Decreased to loss of sensations to the uterus, bladder, and perineum ▼ Depression of contractions especially if given too early can prolong labor ▼ Decreased sensation and motor function to lower extremities ▼ Relaxation of muscles including perineum ▼ Limitation on urge to bear down and ability to push effectively may occur; this increases the need for the use of forceps, vacuum extractor, and episiotomy — Dosage may be decreased or stopped in second stage to facilitate bearing down effort — Local anesthesia would be used if episiotomy is performed ▼ Allergic (systemic/local) reactions Fetal/newborn effects: primarily an indirect effect related to fetal response to maternal respiratory depression and hypotension, and to a prolonged labor requiring invasive medical procedures	▼ Assist to maintain position without movement during procedure; use touch; keep her informed of what is occurring, what she will feel ▼ Assist to supine position for 5 to 10 minutes after injection for equal diffusion of agent then assist to a lateral position Monitor maternal-fetal effects ▼ Electronic monitoring of maternal heart beat and BP is often used for continuous epidural infusions ▼ Respiratory rate-effort—every 15 minutes ▼ Continuous electronic monitoring of FHR pattern and contractions ▼ Effectiveness of pain relief—watch for break through pain ▼ Bladder function for distention—every 30 minutes ▼ Sensation-motor function in lower extremities—every hour ▼ Site of infusion, line, pump Maintain IV infusion to ensure adequate hydration—woman who is adequately hydrated and receives a loading IV infusion is less likely to experience hypotension

- Prehydrate with 500 to 1000 cc of a balanced salt solution (0.9% NS) with no glucose over 15 to 30 minutes prior to induction
- Continue infusion at 125 to 150 ml per hour

Intervene if hypotension occurs: increase rate of IV, raise legs (10 to 20 degrees), give oxygen via mask (8 to 10 L/min), prepare to administer a vasopressor such as ephedrine IV

Intervene if respiratory depression occurs—respirations slow to ≤12: give oxygen via mask (8 to 10 L/min), prepare to administer narcan (0.4 mg to 2 mg IV, repeat every 2 to 3 minutes as needed up to a total of 10 mg) if depression is related to use of a narcotic analgesic, and raise head of bed approximately 30 degrees to facilitate breathing; resuscitation is initated if woman is unresponsive to above measures

Prepare to augment labor if progress slows—pitocin, nipple stimulation, and assist with pushing

Continued.

Table 9-3. Pharmacologic Measures to Manage Discomforts of Labor and Birth—cont'd

Pharmacologic Measures	Effects on Maternal-Fetal Unit	Nursing Considerations
		Change position from side to side every hour to equalize effect and avoid reduction in BP Protect legs from injury Encourage voiding every 2 hours—catheterize as ordered if unable to void
Low spinal (saddle) block—between contractions anesthetic agent is injected into the subarachnoid space at level L3, L4, or L5 where it mixes in the spinal fluid and settles into the lower spine. Inducted during the second stage when birth is imminent—fetal head at perineum Onset in 1 to 2 min with a duration of 1 to 3 hours Effective for vaginal or cesarian birth	Maternal effects ▼ Hypotension ▼ Respiratory depression if anesthetic agent rises in spinal fluid ▼ Loss of sensation to uterus, bladder, and perineum ▼ Loss of sensation and motor function to lower extremities ▼ Loss of bearing down reflex increases use of forceps, vacuum extractor, episiotomy ▼ Spinal headaches as a result of leakage of spinal fluid during induction ▼ Allergic reactions (systemic-local) Fetal-neonatal effects: primarily indirect effect related to the fetal response to maternal hypotension, respiratory depression, and invasive procedures required for birth	Assess maternal-fetal status prior to procedure Prepare woman for and support her during the procedure ▼ Explain what to expect ▼ Assist into sitting position as for epidural block; sometimes lateral position is used with HOB in low fowlers ▼ Assist to maintain position without movement ▼ Maintain upright position for time prescribed—the longer upright the lower the level of the anesthesia, for example — Change to supine with lateral tilt immediately for cesarean — Maintain for 2 to 5 minutes for vaginal birth to allow the heavy anesthetic to settle in and become adherent in lower back

		Return to supine position with small pillow under shoulders and under hip Raise legs together and carefully place in stirrups—protect from injury Monitor maternal-fetal effects ▼ Maternal BP, pulse, respirations, FHR pattern every 2 minutes (1st 10 minutes) then every 5 to 10 minutes ▼ Urinary function, comfort level, and legs Maintain IV infusion as for epidural
III. General Anesthesia		
Intravenous and/or inhalation induction of anesthesia resulting in loss of body sensation and consciousness Used primarily for emergency cesarean birth or vaginal birth requiring emergency intervention Administered just prior to birth to limit fetal exposure since anesthetic agent crosses placenta rapidly	Maternal effects ▼ Vomiting with aspiration related to decreased gastric emptying time and loss of gag reflex ▼ Loss of consciousness—unable to participate in the birth ▼ Uterine relaxation increases risk of postpartum hemorrhage Fetal-newborn effects and their duration depend on depth of anesthesia, dosage used, and length of time under anesthesia ▼ CNS depression ▼ Hypoxia—altered FHR pattern ▼ Postnatal respiratory depression ▼ Decreased newborn responsiveness, limiting interaction, sucking	Record time and nature of recent oral intake Complete ongoing assessment of maternal-fetal status Administer an alkalinizing agent such as Bicitra to decrease acidity of gastric contents thereby preventing aspiration pneumonitis (15 to 30 ml, every 2 hours during labor or 1 hour before induction) Place wedge under hip, tilt to side to prevent vena caval pressure Apply cricoid pressure during induction until endotracheal tube is in place—depress cricoid cartilage 2 to 3 cm downward with fingers to occlude esophagus

Box 9-3. Maternal Positions During Labor and Birth

Semirecumbent Position

Sitting with upper body elevated to at least a 30 degree angle, place wedge or small pillow under hip to prevent vena caval compression and reduce incidence of supine hypotension

The greater the angle of elevation the more gravity or pressure is applied to enhance fetal descent, progress of contractions, and widening of pelvic dimensions

Convenient for care measures and external fetal monitoring

Lateral Position

Alternate between left and right side-lying position, providing abdominal and back support as needed for comfort—current research indicates there is no significant difference in cardiac output between the right or left side-lying position

Removes pressure from the vena cava and back—enhances uteroplacental perfusion and relieves backache

Easier to perform back massage or counter pressure

Associated with less frequent more intense contractions

External fetal monitoring may be more difficult

May be used as a birthing position

Upright Position

Gravity effect enhances contraction cycle and fetal descent: fetus increases pressure on cervix, cervix is pulled upward facilitating effacement and dilatation, impulses from cervix to pituitary gland increase, oxytocin secreted in greater amount, contraction intensified with more forceful downward pressure on fetus

Fetus is aligned with pelvis and pelvic diameters are widened

Effective upright positions include

- ▼ Ambulation
- ▼ Standing and leaning forward with support from coach, end of bed, back of chair; relieves backache and facilitates counterpressure-back massage
- ▼ Sitting up in bed, chair, birthing chair
- ▼ Squatting

**Hands and Knees Position—ideal position for posterior positions of the presenting part*

Assume an "all fours" position in bed or on a covered floor

Relieves backache characteristic of "back labor"

Facilitates internal rotation of the fetus: increases mobility of coccyx, increases pelvic diameters, and applies the force of gravity to turn the fetal back and rotate the head

Assess the effect of each position on the laboring woman's comfort and anxiety level, progress of labor, and fetal heart rate pattern. Alternate positions every 30 minutes to one hour.

(2) Effectiveness of physical and psychosocial adaptations to pregnancy including baseline health status data, such as vital signs
(3) Difficulties encountered during pregnancy
(4) Expected date of birth (EDB)—weeks' gestation
(5) Results of laboratory and diagnostic testing
  (a) CBC especially hematocrit, hemoglobin, white blood cell count, platelets
  (b) Blood type, Rh factor, antibody screens
  (c) Urinalysis and urine cultures
  (d) Cultures and tests for reproductive tract infections
  (e) Special tests including sonogram, chorionic villi sampling, amniocentesis, nonstress test, biophysical profile, contraction stress test
(6) Impressions of the pregnancy experience
(7) Childbirth classes attended

b. Previous experiences with pregnancy and parturition including outcomes
  (1) Gravida, para—TPAL
  (2) Maternal health problems during pregnancy
  (3) Occurrence of complications during labor—hemorrhage, prolonged-protracted phases of labor, fetal presentation-position problems (breech, face, posterior position), fetal distress, failure to progress, cephalopelvic disproportion
  (4) Required augmentation-induction of labor
  (5) Birth by cesarean section
  (6) Client impressions of previous experiences
  (7) Newborn health problems

c. Presence of current risk factors
  (1) Diabetes
  (2) Anemia, cardiovascular disorders, hypertension
  (3) Reproductive tract infections
  (4) Pregnancy induced hypertension (PIH)
  (5) Limited or nonexistent support group

B. Assess the reproductive changes that occur during parturition—uterine contractions, cervical changes with fetal progress, condition of amniotic membranes, characteristic of vaginal discharge

1. Uterine contractions
  a. Characteristics to be assessed
    (1) Frequency—timing from the beginning of one contraction to the beginning of the next contraction,

indicates how often the contractions are occurring, such as q 2 min, q 5 min

(2) Duration—timing from the onset of the contraction until it ends indicates how long the contraction lasts

(3) Intensity—determines the strength of the contraction

(4) Resting tone—determines degree of fundal relaxation during the rest phase between contractions and the duration of the rest period

b. Assessment techniques

(1) Assess a series of several contractions and rest periods in order to determine overall pattern

(2) Frequency of assessment is determined by stage of labor, condition of maternal-fetal unit, and labor events. Example: induction-augmentation.

(3) Palpation method

(a) Place hand over fundus and use fingers to assess

(i) Changes in tone and intensity—degree fingers can be indented into fundus. Example: boardlike fundus with no indentation = strong intensity.

(ii) Frequency and duration

(b) Occasionally palpate entire uterus to note differences in tone from fundus to lower uterine segment

(4) External monitor method

(a) Place tocotransducer over the fundus

(b) Determines frequency and duration of contractions but not intensity

(c) Palpate uterus occasionally to determine overall uterine tone and to confirm monitor data

(5) Internal monitor method

(a) Insert intrauterine pressure transducer into the uterus through the cervix

(b) Determines frequency, duration, intensity, and resting tone

(c) Palpate uterus occasionally to determine overall uterine tone and to confirm monitor data

c. Expected findings

(1) Gradual progression in frequency, duration, and intensity

(2) Regular pattern is established but may become irregular during the transition phase of the first stage of labor

(3) Frequency—average of q 2 to 5 minutes; should not occur more frequently than every 2 minutes since adequate rest periods will not occur

(4) Duration—no longer than 90 seconds

(5) Rest periods—at least 30 seconds; relaxation of fundus palpated

(6) Intensity if using internal monitoring

(a) During a contraction—<100 mm Hg with an average of 50 to 75 mm Hg

(b) Rest period—resting pressure average of 15 mm Hg

d. Warning signs

(1) Failure to progress or establish a regular pattern

(2) Frequency—more frequent than every 2 minutes

(3) Duration—>90 seconds

(4) Limited to no relaxation of the fundus palpated during the rest period

(5) Rest periods—<30 seconds

(6) Intensity if using internal monitoring

(a) During a contraction—>100 mm Hg

(b) Resting pressure—>15 mm Hg

2. Cervical changes and fetal progress through the birth canal

a. Vaginal examination

(1) Characteristics to assess

(a) Signs of reproductive tract infections such as erythema, edema, discharge, lesions; determine during first examination upon admission

(b) Cervical characteristics

(i) Cervical consistency—soft or firm

(ii) Degree of effacement (%) and dilatation (cm)

(iii) Cervical position—posterior, midline, anterior

(c) Condition of amniotic membranes—intact, bulging, ruptured

(d) Fetal characteristics

(i) Presentation and position

(ii) Degree of descent—station, bulging of perineum, crowning with advanced fetal descent
(iii) Presence of molding

(2) Vaginal examination technique
 (a) Explain procedure, purpose, and describe results to client and coach
 (b) Strict asepsis to prevent infection
 (c) Cleanse vulva-perineum before and after the examination as needed; wear clean gloves for cleansing
 (d) Use sterile gloves and water-based lubricant to perform the examination
 (e) Note maternal and fetal responses during and following the examination

(3) Frequency—perform examination only as needed to reduce danger of infection and limit maternal discomfort

(4) Recommended timing of examinations
 (a) Admission
 (b) Following rupture of membranes once fetal condition is assessed
 (c) Prior to administration of analgesic, anesthetic to determine degree of dilatation and progress of labor
 (d) Presence of FHR pattern indicative of distress. Example: variable deceleration—check for cord prolapse.
 (e) When contraction pattern and maternal behavior indicate progress in labor has been made. Examples: increased frequency and intensity of contractions, perineal pressure and urge to bear down.

▼ VAGINAL EXAMINATIONS ARE NOT PERFORMED WHEN FRANK BLEEDING IS PRESENT—bleeding may be the result of a placental previa, implantation of placenta in lower uterine segment that is separating. ACTION MUST BE TAKEN IMMEDIATELY.

▼ Notify physician

▼ Prepare for possibility of immediate delivery

b. Leopold's maneuvers—systematic palpation of the abdomen to determine fetal presentation, position, fetal movement

c. Partogram—labor graph used to compare an individual woman's progress in labor with an expected labor pattern
   (1) Graphs of expected labor patterns related to cervical dilatation and fetal descent are available for nulliparousand multiparous women
   (2) Data gathered during vaginal examinations related to cervical dilatation and fetal descent are superimposed on the appropriate graph
   (3) Expected finding—progress of labor reflects norms for a nulliparous or multiparous woman
   (4) Warning sign—progress of cervical dilatation and fetal descent deviate from the expected norm
      (a) Prolonged latent phase
      (b) Protracted or arrested active phase
      (c) Failure of descent
      (d) Precipitous labor

3. Condition of amniotic membranes
   a. Determine status—intact, bulging, ruptured
      (1) Vaginal examination
      (2) **Nitrazine test**—distinguish between urine and amniotic fluid by using test paper to determine the pH of the fluid expelled
         (a) Dark blue (positive)—alkaline result indicating amniotic fluid
         (b) Remains yellow (negative)—acidic result indicating urine
      (3) **Ferning**
         (a) Smear fluid onto a glass slide
         (b) Use microscope to detect presence of amniotic fluid crytalization which results in a characteristic fernlike pattern
   b. Determine characteristics of amniotic fluid expelled—amount, color, clarity, consistency (thick or thin), odor
   c. Determine time of occurrence—birth should take place within 24 hours of rupture to reduce risk of exposure of fetus and uterine cavity to infection
   d. Expected findings
      (1) Clear, slightly yellow—resembles very dilute urine
      (2) Faint, fleshy or musty odor

e. Warning signs
   (1) Thick, cloudy, foul odor—infection
   (2) Thick, green—recent passage of meconium by the fetus related to recent hypoxia or a breech presentation
   (3) Yellow—bilirubin or hypoxia over 36 hours ago
   (4) Wine—bleeding
f. Nursing actions upon rupture of membranes
   (1) Assess FHR pattern—immediately and 5 minutes later; FHR pattern should continue to exhibit reassuring characteristics (see Chapter 10)
   (2) Perform vaginal examination, following assessment of fetal status, to determine
      (a) Presence of cord prolapse
      (b) Progress in cervical effacement, dilatation, fetal descent
   (3) Assess characteristics of fluid
   (4) Assess maternal BP, pulse, and respirations
   (5) Monitor maternal temperature orally q 2 hr between contractions—increased danger of infection with rupture of membranes
   (6) Provide comfort measures
      (a) Keep woman clean and dry
      (b) Reassure regarding her condition and that of her fetus
   (7) May need to have activity restricted to prevent prolapse of the cord

4. Characteristics of vaginal discharge, show
   a. Assess frequently throughout labor
   b. Expected findings
      (1) Pink to bloodtinged, sticky, mucoidtype discharge
      (2) Faint fleshy or musty odor
      (3) Gradual increase as cervical changes and fetal descent progresses
      (4) Total estimated blood loss (EBL) at the time of vaginal birth is approximately 300 cc
   c. Warning signs
      (1) Frank bleeding
         (a) Bright red blood may be indicative of placenta previa

(b) Dark red blood may be indicative of abruptio placenta, premature separation of a placenta that is implanted in the upper uterine segment

(2) Foul odor—infection

C. Assess the degree of pain and discomfort experienced during the process of labor and birth—considered to be a major stressor of childbirth; assessment includes

1. Source and location of pain experienced

▼ Never assume that pain experienced by the woman in labor is originating from the labor process; for example, chest pain might occur from cardiac problems or pulmonary embolism

2. Expected characteristics of pain experienced during childbirth are

a. Pain related to contractions

(1) Intermittent

(2) During a contraction, pain begins in the back and radiates over the entire abdomen as blood vessels are compressed and uterine muscle cells become hypoxic

(3) During the rest period, pain of contraction diminishes

b. Pain related to lower uterine and pelvic pressure

(1) Nerves and organs are compressed and tissues of cervix, vagina, and perineum are stretched by the descending fetus as labor advances

(2) Pain extends into rest period between contractions

c. Pain related to occiput posterior position of the fetal head results in back pain as occiput presses against sacrum

d. Pain severity increases as labor advances

(1) Contractions intensify, become more frequent, last longer

(2) Rest periods are shorter

(3) Fetal descent accelerates, increasing pressure and soft tissue stretching

e. Effects of pain on the maternal-fetal unit

(1) Alteration in maternal vital signs—elevated BP, pulse, and oxygen use; hyperventilation

(2) Anxiety, fear, and muscular tension occur—may impede labor, uteroplacental perfusion, descent, and magnify the pain sensation

(3) Negative impressions of labor may be formed

3. Effectiveness of relief measures
4. Factors influencing pain experience—degree to which each factor influences labor depends on each circumstance of a woman in labor
    a. Availability of support system-coach—many women in labor report that the presence of a supportive person is a critical factor influencing their ability to cope with the process of labor
        (1) Willingness and ability of the coach to assist the woman during the labor and birth process
        (2) Cultural influence on roles played by coach and family
    b. Unique pain tolerance, threshold and cultural patterns of response to pain
    c. Physical condition at onset of labor—higher energy levels and better health status strengthen ability to respond to pain in a more effective manner
    d. Personal expectations regarding the pain of labor
        (1) Primigravida—fear of unknown, stories heard, expects the worst
        (2) Previous experiences with parturition influences what to expect now
        (3) Realistic or unrealistic preparation for pain and effectiveness of relief measures learned in childbirth education classes
        (4) Views of labor as a natural process or as a medically directed process
    e. Length of labor and ease of birth as influenced by
        (1) Status as a nullipara or multipara
        (2) Fetal presentation and position
        (3) Need for augmentation-induction with oxytocin (Pitocin)
    f. Acceptance of the pregnancy itself
    g. Openness to a variety of measures to relieve pain

D. Assess status of oxygenation and circulation during parturition

1. Maternal BP, pulse, respirations
    a. How to assess
        (1) Use consistent technique. Examples: same arm, same position to allow for comparison.
        (2) Assess between rather than during contractions

b. When to assess
   (1) Recommended frequency according to stage of labor and risk status
   (2) Increased frequency is indicated by
      (a) Baseline range changes, such as pattern of rising or decreasing BP
      (b) FHR patterns indicative of fetal distress or stress (see Chapter 10)
      (c) Administration of medications such as sedatives, tranquilizers, analgesics, anesthetics (epidural, spinal), CNS depressants, antihypertensives
      (d) Procedures instituted for suppression, initiation, or augmentation of labor
c. Expected findings
   (1) Remain close to the client's own baseline range established during pregnancy
   (2) Slight elevations may be noted as a result of pain, fatigue, stress, or dehydration
   (3) Slight decreases may occur when client relaxes, such as following pharmacologic pain relief measures
   (4) Heart beat should remain strong and regular to maintain adequate cardiac output
   (5) Respirations should be of normal depth, regular, effortless, and quiet with no adventitious sounds noted upon auscultation to ensure adequate oxygenation
   (6) BP should remain within normal range to ensure adequate uteroplacental perfusion
d. Warning signs
   (1) Increasing rate and decreasing volume of the pulse (rapid, thready) and decreasing BP are associated with hemorrhage
      (a) Placenta previa
      (b) Abruptio placenta
   (2) Increasing BP could be indicative of pregnancy induced hypertension (PIH)—>140/90 or an increase of 30/15 mm Hg over client's prepregnant baseline
   (3) Decreasing BP (<100 mm Hg systolic) may occur as a result of spinal blocks anesthesia (epidural, low spinal)

(4) Decreasing rate and depth of respirations (hypoventilation) may occur as a side effect of analgesic or anesthetic administration limiting oxygenation
(5) Dyspnea, rales, cough could be indicative of pulmonary edema accompanying cardiac decompensation

2. Effectiveness of breathing techniques used during contractions
   a. Ability to use techniques with contractions
   b. Effectiveness of techniques in pain relief
   c. Ability to avoid hyperventilation associated with
      (1) Rapid, shallow breathing techniques used in advanced labor
      (2) Pain, fear, anxiety
   d. Hyperventilation—rapid, deep respiratory pattern causes carbon dioxide level to fall resulting in respiratory alkalosis; woman experiences lightheadedness, dizziness, tingling in extremities
   e. Remedy for hyperventilation—raise carbon dioxide level by rebreathing exhaled air using a paper bag, cupped hand, a rebreather mask if on oxygen
3. Circulatory status to extremities
   a. Temperature—bilaterally warm
   b. Capillary refill—rapid, <3 seconds
   c. Presence of edema, varicosities—may interfere with adequate tissue perfusion and venous return
      (1) Signs of thrombophlebitis—if present, risk for pulmonary embolism exists
      (2) Pulmonary embolism findings of sudden onset of chest pain and sudden increased respiratory effort
4. Laboratory tests
   a. Review tests done during the antepartal period and results
   b. Complete blood count
   c. Type and cross match as indicated. Examples: presence of signs indicating placental previa, history of hemorrhage with a previous pregnancy.

E. Assess nutritional-fluid and electrolyte status during parturition

1. Gastric motility and emptying time are decreased during labor and require a limitation of oral food and fluid intake to
   a. Reduce incidence of nausea and vomiting

b. Prevent aspiration of vomitus and airway obstruction should general anesthesia be required

2. Assess
   a. Presence of nausea, vomiting, epigastric distress
   b. Extent of diaphoresis—expect increase during transition phase and second stage
   c. Body temperature
      (1) Every 4 hours then every 2 hours after membrane rupture
      (2) Elevated temperatures, >99.6° F (orally) may indicate dehydration or infection
   d. Signs of energy depletion
      (1) Fatigue
      (2) Slowing in the progress of labor
   e. Signs of dehydration
      (1) Dry, sticky oral mucous membranes, thirst
      (2) Decreased urinary output; urine concentrated—specific gravity >1.030
      (3) Elevated body temperature
      (4) Decreased turgor

F. Assess elimination patterns during parturition

1. Bowel—character and time of last bowel movement; an empty rectum
   a. Facilitates descent of fetus and bearing down efforts
   b. Minimizes passage of fecal material that can contaminate birth canal
2. Urinary—distended bladder can inhibit fetal descent and suppress uterine contractions
   a. Obtain clean voided midstream specimen for analysis and culture if indicated; use dipstick to test urine for protein, acetone, and glucose, repeating as indicated every 2 to 4 hours
   b. Observe for signs and symptoms of urinary tract infection
   c. Assess throughout labor to ensure that bladder is being emptied
      (1) Frequency—at least every 2 hours
      (2) Amount and characteristics of urine—expect at least 100 cc of clear, yellow urine at each voiding
      (3) Assess bladder for distension by palpating and percussing over lower abdomen above symphysis pubis; with distention woman complains of tenderness or pain

- ▼ Greater emphasis on urinary assessment should occur when sensitivity to bladder fullness is diminished during
  - ▼ Regional anesthetics—low spinal, epidural block
  - ▼ Advanced labor—intensifying contractions and pelvic pressure as fetus descends

G. Assess physical activity and rest during parturition

1. Energy level—assess for signs of fatigue and growing exhaustion which can interfere with effective pushing in the second stage of labor
2. Degree of muscular tension or relaxation
3. Ability to attain and maintain positions that facilitate cardiac output, uteroplacental perfusion, and progress of labor
4. Desire to participate in activities that reduce tension and conserve energy
   a. Diversional activities and ambulation in early labor
   b. Relaxation measures to rest between contractions

H. Assess integument—note alterations in integrity

1. Rashes, lesions
2. Lacerations, bruises
3. Track marks indicative of drug abuse

I. Assess psychosocial reactions related to the process of labor and birth—emotional state affects progress

1. Ongoing assessment is required since maternal emotional status and mood changes as labor progresses
   a. Latent phase—excited, anxious, talkative, ambivalent regarding ability to cope with labor; "in control"
   b. Active phase—introverted, less responsive, decreased attention span, intense concentration on work of labor, some loss of control may occur along with growing irritability
   c. Transition phase—decreased confidence, loss of control, desire to give up and go home, fear of death for self and fetus; does not want to be touched and rejects help from the coach
   d. Second stage—renewed energy and purpose, "second wind," rewarded with perception of progress in fetal descent with each bearing down effort
2. Assessment of the mother
   a. Mood, effect
   b. Level of fear and anxiety
   c. Attention span; level of alertness and orientation
   d. Body posture and movements indicative of tension

e. Ability and desire to work with the labor process rather than against it
f. Degree of effectiveness in use of childbirth techniques
g. Willingness to participate in techniques designed to enhance the process of labor and ensure a positive outcome. Examples: willing to change positions, receptive to medications and fetal monitor.

4. Assessment of the coach
   a. Effectiveness in providing support and encouragement in the use of childbirth techniques
   b. Ability to work together with the laboring woman and the healthcare team
   c. Response to labor events and behaviors of laboring woman
   d. Status in terms of fatigue, hunger or thirst, anxiety, need for support

III. Common nursing diagnoses encountered during parturition, along with selected client outcomes, nursing interventions, and evaluation criteria are described in Table 9-1

IV. Nursing responsibilities during the third stage of labor focus on mother and newborn

A. Mother

1. Assess
   a. Vital signs—BP, pulse, respirations
   b. Consistency of fundus, blood loss
   c. Signs of placental separation
2. Assist with bearing down effort to expel separated placenta (Box 9-4)
3. Administer oxytocic medications
   a. Pitocin IV 10 to 20 units mixed in intravenous solution or 10 units slowly IV push as directed by the physician or midwife
   b. Methylergonovine maleate (Methergine) 0.2 mg IM—assess BP before and 5 to 15 minutes after administration since hypertension can occur; it is not given to women already hypertensive, such as when BP ≥140/90
4. Inform client and coach regarding progress of recovery
5. Facilitate bonding between newborn and parents

Box 9-4. Bearing Down Effort (BDE)—Pushing

What: during the second stage of labor effective use of abdominal muscle contractions, the secondary force or power of labor, combined with uterine contractions to facilitate descent and birth of the fetus. Emphasis is placed on women responding to their own, natural urge to push

When: Phase one of the second stage of labor—early-latent (10 to 30 minutes)

- ▼ Transient decrease in intensity-frequency of uterine contractions
- ▼ Assist laboring woman to rest in a position of comfort and conserve energy until the natural urge to push is felt
- ▼ Provide emotional support and encourage use of relaxation techniques

Phase two of the second stage of labor—active-descent (average duration varies according to parity, efficiency of bearing down effectively, and use of spinal or epidural (anesthesia)

- ▼ Ferguson reflex occurs: fetal presenting part descends—pelvic floor is distended—stretch receptors are stimulated—rhythmic urge to push or bear down is felt
- ▼ Assist laboring woman into position and coach the BDE with contractions

Phase three of the second stage of labor—transition-perineal (5 to 12 minutes)

- ▼ Birth is imminent as perineal bulging, then crowning occurs, vulva surrounds largest diameter of the fetal head
- ▼ Assist laboring woman to reduce or equalize forces during delivery of the fetal head
  - —Pant to avoid abdominal muscle contraction during a uterine contraction
  - —Gentle, steady BDE between contractions

How: assume position that will facilitate BDE and birth during second stage of labor phases two and three—change positions to enhance effectiveness

- ▼ Upright: squatting on bed or side of bed; sitting on toilet, birthing chair, birthing bed
- ▼ Semirecumbent with knees and legs lower than heart and assuming a C posture with shoulders curved forward and knees pulled up when BDE begins
- ▼ Lateral—descent slower but perineum more relaxed; raise and support upper leg during BDE
- ▼ Lithotomy—least effective since effect of gravity is not realized and cardiac workload is increased; legs must be raised and placed into stirrups together

Breathing during the bearing down effort

- ▼ Take two deep cleansing breaths at the onset of the contraction to allow it to reach its acme-peak
- ▼ Take a breath, hold it for a couple of seconds to start the push, then push vigorously while exhaling (open-glottis pushing)—push in short periods of approximately 7 seconds
- ▼ Take breaths between BDEs
- ▼ Take two deep cleansing breaths at the end of the contraction and assume a position of rest and comfort

Prolonged breath holding while pushing (valsalva maneuver), for periods of more than 6 seconds, can decrease maternal BP or heart rate and reduce uteroplacental perfusion leading to fetal hypoxia

B. Newborn

▼ WEAR GLOVES WHEN HANDLING NEWBORN UNTIL FULLY CLEANSED OF BODY FLUIDS AND SUBSTANCES

1. Immediate assessment of newborn adaptation to extrauterine life—Apgar score (see Table 9-2)
   a. Determine score at 1 and 5 minutes; 5 minute score is usually considered to be more reflective of the newborn's ability to adapt to extrauterine life
   b. Continue to 10 minutes if condition is unstable and first two scores are low
   c. Apgar score, cardiopulmonary and thermoregulatory status, and circumstances of labor and birth (signs of fetal distress or stress and passage of meconium) guide the care of the newborn immediately after birth and the need for resuscitation measures
2. Maintain airway patency
   a. Suction mouth then nose as required using bulb syringe
      (1) Used for initial suction at delivery of head and after birth if newborn is stable, with a good Apgar score, no meconium present in amniotic fluid, and airway patency is achieved
      (2) Compress bulb, insert along side of mouth, and release compression slowly
      (3) Suction each nostril
      (4) Continue until airway patent—breathing, crying sounds clear
   b. Suction oro-nasopharynx (mouth first then nose) using mechanical suction
      (1) Used when
         (a) Apgar scores are low and respirations are depressed
         (b) Amniotic fluid was meconium stained; danger if meconium is aspirated since meconium destroys lung tissue
         (c) Airway secretions are copious and cannot be cleared adequately with the bulb syringe
      (2) Set at low suction—<100 mm Hg
         (a) Lubricate sterile suction catheter (8 to 12 french) with sterile water
         (b) Insert with suction off
         (c) Apply suction as tube is removed

(d) Limit each suction attempt to <5 seconds and oxygenate well between attempts

(3) Limit frequency and perform gently to prevent trauma to delicate mucous membranes

▼ Use of the DeLee mucous trap with suction applied by the mouth of the caregiver is no longer recommended

c. Use Trendelenburg position of 15 to 30 degrees to facilitate drainage of lung fluid by gravity

3. Administer oxygen as required by newborn's condition
   a. Mildly depressed—whiffs of oxygen over nose
   b. Moderately depressed—tight mask
   c. Severely depressed—endotracheal tube is inserted to facilitate administration of oxygen
4. Cardiopulmonary resuscitation (CPR) measures may be required for the severely depressed neonate
5. Maintain body temperature
   a. Institute heat conservation measures
      (1) Dry skin
      (2) Use warming measures when assessing newborn and providing care including resuscitation measures
         (a) Place under radiant heat warmer
         (b) Skin to skin contact with mother
         (c) Wrap in warmed blankets
   b. Assess body temperature using thermistor probe of radiate heat warmer
6. Assess general health status
   a. Ongoing assessment of vital signs
      (1) Apical heart beat
      (2) Respiratory effort, rate, pattern, breath sounds
      (3) Temperature
   b. Assess cord
      (1) Obtain cord blood samples for
         (a) Blood type and Rh
         (b) Direct coombs test
         (c) Serological testing (syphilis)
         (d) Acid-base status
      (2) Vessels—2 arteries, 1 vein (Figure 9-1)
      (3) Placement and security of the clamp
   c. Measurements—head and chest circumference, length, weight

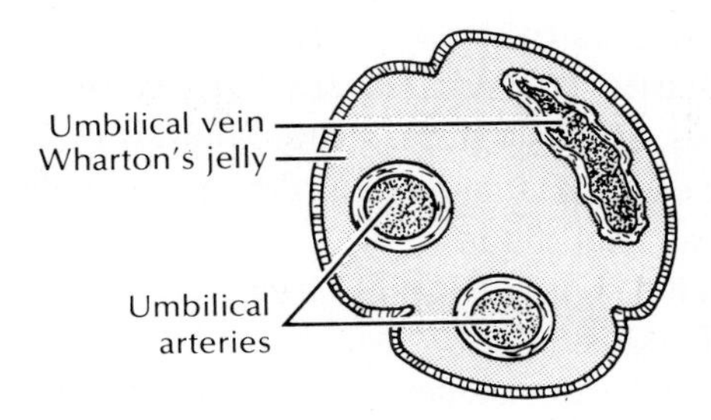

Figure 9-1. Cross section of umbilical cord. Note collapsed appearance of thin-walled umbilical vein and contour of thicker, muscular-walled arteries. (From Bobak IM et al: *Maternity and gynecologic care: the nurse and the family,* ed 5, St Louis, 1993, Mosby.)

   d. Posture, movement
   e. Condition of integument—color, injuries, peeling
   f. Presence of visible anomalies such as cleft lip and palate, absent or deformed limbs, spinal defects
   g. Elimination—bowel or bladder
   h. Gestational age
7. Institute identification measures
   a. Attach matching ID bands
      (1) Newborn—wrist and ankle
      (2) Mother—wrist
   b. Footprint newborn and fingerprint mother
8. Administer medications
   a. Eye prophylaxis—prevention of ophthalmia neonatorum, infection of eyes as a result of exposure to gonorrhea and/or chlamydia during passage through the birth canal
      (1) Cleanse eyes from inner to outer canthus with sterile water
      (2) Instill erythromycin or tetracycline ointment into conjunctival sac of each eye; do not flush eyes after instillation of ointment
      (3) Instillation may be delayed for approximately 1 hour in order to facilitate eye contact with parents—encourages attachment and bonding
   b. Inject vitamin K (Aquamephyton) 0.5 to 1 mg IM into lateral aspect, middle third of vastus lateralis muscle of thigh to prevent clotting problems associated with absence of intestinal bacteria needed to synthesize vitamin K

V. Nursing responsibilities during the fourth stage of labor—first one to two hours following birth

1. Assess recovery status—first hour every 15 minutes; second hour every 30 minutes; third hour and thereafter as indicated by maternal status
   a. Vital signs—BP, pulse, respirations
   b. Fundus
      (1) Consistency—firm or boggy
      (2) Height—above, below, at umbilicus
      (3) Location—midline or deviated to the right or left
   c. Lochia
      (1) Amount
         (a) Degree of pad saturation and time elapsed. Example: pad half saturated in 1 hour.
         (b) Scant, light, moderate, profuse (Figure 9-2)
      (2) Characteristics—type-stage, presence of clots, odor
         ▼ ALWAYS CHECK UNDER BUTTOCKS FOR POOLING OF LOCHIA
   d. Perineum—episiotomy and/or lacerations
      (1) R—redness
      (2) E—ecchymosis
      (3) E—edema
      (4) D—drainage
      (5) A—approximation
      (6) Indications of hematoma formation—presence of swelling, intensifying perineal pain or pressure, sensation of need to defecate, and alteration in vital signs which reflect a significant blood loss

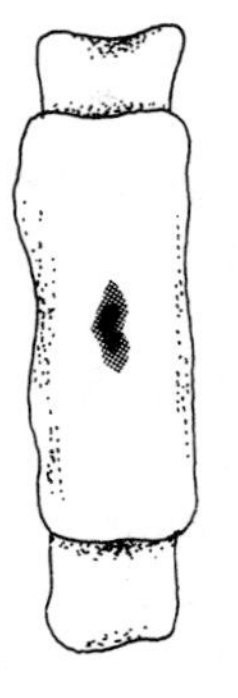
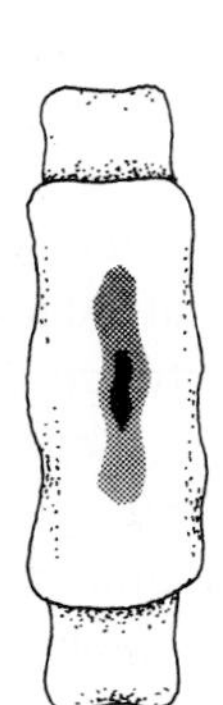
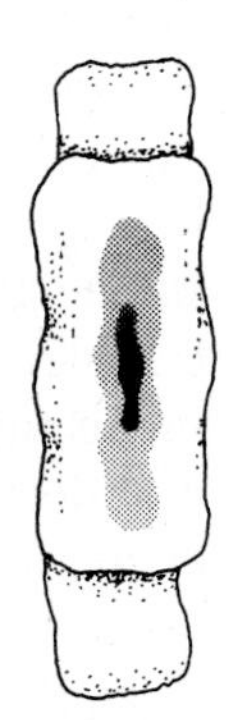
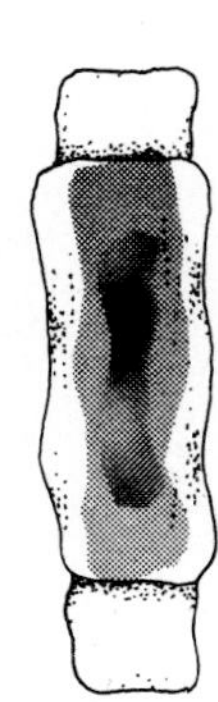

Figure 9-2. Peripad saturation volumes. (From Bobak IM et al: *Maternity nursing,* ed 4, St Louis, 1995, Mosby.)

e. Signs of hypovolemic-hemorrhagic shock
    (1) Alteration in vital signs
        (a) Increasing pulse rate, decreasing strength and volume—pulse becomes rapid, weak, and thready
        (b) Narrowing of pulse pressure followed by hypotension
        (c) Increasing respiratory rate, decreasing depth
    (2) Altered sensorium—anxious and restless, irritable, lightheaded, "feels funny, nauseous," "sees stars"
    (3) Profuse blood loss
        (a) Lochia—saturation of peri pad within 15 minutes
        (b) Sensation of intense pain or pressure in perineum with or without swelling
    (4) Cool, pale integument

2. Additional assessments
    a. Urinary elimination
        (1) Amount of urine—at least 100 cc per voiding
        (2) Bladder distention—must be avoided; a distended bladder
            (a) Elevates fundus above umbilicus and pushes it off midline; deviated to right or left
            (b) Inhibits uterine contraction with an increased risk of blood loss
    b. Progress in recovery from anesthesia
        (1) Spinal block—return of movement and sensation to lower extremities, sensation of bladder fullness
        (2) General anesthesia—return of consciousness and gag reflex
    c. Presence of pain—severity, location
    d. Temperature—elevation usually indicative of dehydration, especially after long labors
    e. Level of fatigue
    f. Hunger and thirst
    g. Baseline assessment of the breasts
    h. Responses to experience of birth and to the newborn

3. Implement measures to prevent hemorrhage
    a. Massage fundus when boggy—massage only until firm, then stop (Figure 9-3)
    b. Administer oxytocics (Pitocin, Methergine) as ordered
    c. Keep bladder empty

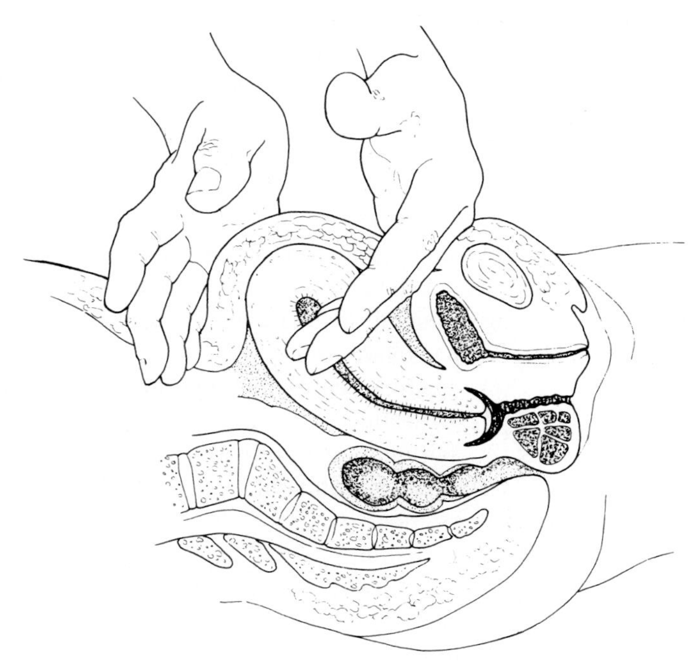

Figure 9-3. Palpating fundus of uterus during first hour after birth. Note that upper hand is cupped over fundus; lower hand dips in above symphysis pubis and supports uterus while it is massaged gently. (From Bobak IM et al: *Maternity nursing,* ed 4, St Louis, 1995, Mosby.)

4. Take action if signs of hemorrhagic shock are noted
    a. Stay with client—call for help
    b. Massage fundus if boggy, expel clots with downward pressure on firm fundus, and administer oxytocics
    c. Raise legs from hip
    d. Start or increase rate of IV infusion that contains no medications
    e. Administer oxygen via mask at 8 to 10 liters/minute
5. Provide for client comfort and safety
    a. Assist with hygienic measures
        (1) Oral care
        (2) Sponge bath
        (3) Peri care including cleansing, ice packs, and topical anesthetics; sitz baths are usually initiated after the first 24 hours
        (4) Clean, dry clothing and bedding
    b. Administer analgesics as needed

c. Facilitate rest
d. Provide food or fluids at end of this stage when physiologic stability is firmly established
e. Institute safety measures
    (1) Raise siderails, bed in low position
    (2) Assist with ambulation until woman can move safely on her own
        (a) Determine that sensation and motor function have been restored
        (b) Move to upright position slowly
        (c) Dangle feet at side of bed for several minutes; assess for dizziness
        (d) Assist to standing position if dizziness is not present
        (e) Support during ambulation

6. Provide opportunities for newborn-parent interaction

REVIEW QUESTIONS

1. A nullipara experienced a normal pregnancy and has exhibited no risk factors. It is recommended that during the latent phase of the first stage of labor, the nurse should assess
   a. Fetal heart rate every 30 to 60 minutes
   b. Maternal BP, temperature, pulse, and respirations every 2 to 4 hours
   c. Uterine contractions every 2 hours
   d. Vaginal show every 2 hours

2. A pregnant couple has formulated a birth plan and are reviewing it with the nurse at an expectant parents' class. Which of the following aspects of their birth plan would be considered unrealistic and require further discussion with the nurse?
   a. "My husband and I have agreed that my sister will be my coach since he becomes anxious with regard to medical procedures and blood. He will be nearby and check on me every so often to make sure everything is okay."
   b. "We plan to use the techniques taught in the Lamaze classes to reduce the pain experienced during labor"
   c. "We want the labor and birth to take place in a birthing room. My husband will come in the minute the baby is born."
   d. "We do not want the fetal monitor used during labor since it will interfere with movement and doing effleurage"

3. To determine the frequency of uterine contractions, the nurse should
   a. Time from the onset of the contraction until it ends
   b. Time from the beginning of one contraction until the end of the next
   c. Time from the onset of one contraction until the onset of the next
   d. Time from the end of one contraction until the end of the next

4. Which of the following statements is INACCURATE concerning the assessment of uterine contractions during labor?
   a. Place hand over fundus in order to palpate uterine frequency, intensity, and duration
   b. Determine intensity by placing tocotransducer over the fundus
   c. Use palpation to confirm monitor data
   d. Palpate entire uterus on a regular basis to determine overall uterine tone and symmetry

5. The nurse assessed the internal monitor tracing for a series of three uterine contractions while caring for a woman in the active phase of the first stage of labor. Which of the following findings is a warning sign requiring further assessment and intervention?
   a. Average duration of 50 to 60 seconds
   b. Frequency of every 2 to 2 ½ minutes
   c. Average resting tone of 18 to 20 mm Hg
   d. Average intensity during the acme of the contraction of 75 to 80 mm Hg

6. When performing vaginal examinations on women in labor the nurse should be guided by which of the following principles?
   a. Cleanse the vulva and perineum before and after the examination as needed
   b. Wear a clean glove lubricated with tap water to reduce discomfort
   c. Perform the examination every hour during the active phase of the first stage of labor
   d. Perform immediately if bleeding is present

7. The nurse would perform a nitrazine test to
   a. Determine if blood is present in the amniotic fluid
   b. Distinguish between amniotic fluid and urine by testing the pH
   c. Distinguish between maternal feces and meconium
   d. Determine the specific gravity of urine

8. Which of the following is an expected finding when assessing amniotic fluid?
   a. Deep yellow color
   b. Absence of odor
   c. Ferning
   d. Cloudiness with particles of cellular debris

9. A laboring woman's amniotic membranes have just ruptured. The immediate action of the nurse would be to
   a. Assess the FHR pattern
   b. Perform a vaginal examination
   c. Inspect the characteristics of the fluid
   d. Assess maternal temperature along with pulse, respirations, and BP

ANSWERS, RATIONALES, AND TEST-TAKING TIPS

Rationales	Test-Taking Tips
1. Correct answer: a	
For a low risk woman in labor, FHR, maternal BP, pulse, respirations, uterine contractions, and vaginal show are all assessed at least every 60 minutes until a change in status should occur. Temperature is assessed every 4 hours until the membranes rupture, then every 2 hours.	If you have no idea, cluster responses *b, c,* and *d* under the time indicated in hours and eliminate. Response *a* is in terms of minutes which is a better action.
2. Correct answer: d	
Responses *a, b,* and *c* are all realistic. Both partners have agreed on the father's role during labor that is best for them. Since monitoring is essential to assess fetal well being, it is not a factor that can be determined by the couple. The nurse should fully explain its importance.	The important word to keep in mind as the responses are read is "unrealistic." Also note that response *d* is the only response that describes what they "don't want"; the other responses can be clustered with what they want.
3. Correct answer: c	
Response *a* refers to duration; *b* and *d* do not reflect timing of uterine contraction characteristics.	Note the key word in the question is "frequency." This is onset to the onset of an event; associate this with other types of events like frequency of angina for the cardiac client.
4. Correct answer: b	
A tocotransducer can only assess duration and frequency. An intrauterine pressure transducer provides the most accurate	Important is to note the word "inaccurate" in the question or else you may have selected a correct technique. For this type of question the recommendation

measurement of intensity in terms of mm Hg. Palpation gives a gross assessment of intensity. Responses *a, c,* and *d* describe appropriate techniques for contraction assessment.

is to reread the question after the responses have been reviewed. A true-false approach can also be used—identify responses *a, c,* and *d* are true and then response *b* must be incorrect.

5. Correct answer: c

Rest periods should be at least 30 seconds with a resting tone of 15 mm Hg or less; responses *a, b,* and *d* all fall within the expected findings of frequency every 2 to 5 minutes, duration <90 seconds, contraction intensity <100 mm Hg or an average of 50 to 75 mm Hg.

Use the true-false approach with identification that responses *a, b,* and *d* seem to be true and reasonable findings. Therefore, response *c* is the correct answer.

6. Correct answer: a

Sterile gloves and lubricant must be used to prevent infection. Vaginal exams are only performed as needed to limit maternal discomfort and reduce the risk of infection. Examinations are never done by the nurse if vaginal bleeding is present since it could result in further separation of a placenta previa.

Key words in the responses give clues to make them incorrect: in response *b* the words "clean tap water"; this contradicts the goal to prevent infection; in response *c* the words "examination every hour"; this contradicts the guideline to intervene based on patient need; and response *d* "if bleeding perform immediately"; this defies common sense to refrain from further stimulation if bleeding occurs as in this situation.

7. Correct answer: b

Nitrazine test paper evaluates the pH of fluid thereby helping to distinguish between amniotic fluid (turns paper dark blue—alkaline) and urine (no color change—acid).

Think anatomy and that the urethra and the vaginal canal are in close proximity. Then associate that the need will be to distinguish between the fluids from each.

8. Correct answer: c

Amniotic fluid creates a crystallized ferning pattern when spread on a glass slide and viewed under a microscope. Amniotic fluid should be clear, and pale yellow with a faint musty odor. Dark yellow could indicate bilirubin or a hypoxic episode more than 36 hours ago. Cloudiness could indicate infection.

The key words in the question are "expected finding." Look for normal findings.

9. Correct answer: a

While *b, c,* and *d* are all important they should be done after the FHR pattern is assessed. Compression of the cord could occur after rupture leading to fetal hypoxia as reflected in alterations in the FHR pattern, characteristically variable decelerations.

Recall that in the event of a change in the laboring process the fetus is a priority.

CHAPTER 10

Assessment of Fetal Responses to Labor and Birth

STUDY OUTCOMES

After completing this chapter, the reader will be able to do the following:

- Define the key terms listed.
- Describe the stressors affecting the fetus during labor and birth.
- Compare fetal heart rate auscultation and electronic fetal monitoring (external and internal).
- State the recommended frequency for assessing the fetal heart rate pattern during labor and birth.
- State the guidelines that should be followed for the documentation of fetal assessment data.
- Describe the expected assessment findings related to reassuring fetal heart rate patterns.
- Identify signs of fetal distress.
- Describe baseline alterations in fetal heart rate.
- Describe periodic alterations in fetal heart rate.
- Discuss measures effective in preventing and treating fetal distress.

KEY TERMS

External fetal monitoring Noninvasive method of continuously or intermittently monitoring uterine contractions and FHR patterns using a tocotransducer and an ultrasound transducer.

Internal fetal monitoring Invasive method of continuously monitoring uterine contractions and FHR patterns using an intrauterine pressure transducer and a cardiotachometer.

Nonreassuring FHR pattern FHR changes that reflect the warning signs of mild hypoxia.

Ominous FHR pattern FHR changes reflective of severe hypoxia and worsening fetal distress or stress.

Reassuring FHR pattern FHR reflective of fetal well being, adequate oxygenation, and expected responses to the stress of labor.

CONTENT REVIEW

I. Major fetal-neonate stressors of the labor and birth process

A. Major stressors of the labor and birth process alter placental perfusion, inhibiting gas exchange, leading to fetal hypoxia, hypercapnia, and acidosis with an altering of fetal-neonatal heart rate patterns

B. Major stressors of the labor and birth process include

1. Uterine contractions
   a. Blood flow through the placenta decreases or stops especially during the peak-acme of the contraction
   b. Blood pooled in intervillous spaces provides a limited reserve for fetal gas exchange
   c. Rest phase of a contraction is critical to restore blood flow and efficient gas exchange
   d. Stress increases as duration, intensity, and frequency of contractions progress and rest periods become shorter with advancing labor
   e. Uterine hyperstimulation can occur spontaneously or during augmentation or induction of labor
2. Medications administered to the laboring woman
   a. Regional analgesics-anesthetics (epidural, spinal) can lower maternal BP and interfere with placental perfusion

   b. Narcotic analgesics can lower maternal BP and respiratory rate and interfere with placental perfusion and the level of oxygen available to the fetus
3. Maternal position
   a. Supine position—pressure on inferior vena cava leads to hypotension and limits placental perfusion
   b. Cord compression can occur depending on cord location and maternal position
4. Maternal stress response
   a. Fear and anxiety can impede the labor process and interfere with maternal respirations
   b. Mother hyperventilates and experiences difficulty relaxing
   c. Placental perfusion and level of oxygen available to the fetus are impaired with hyperventilation
5. Ineffective pushing technique
   a. Prolonged breath holding (valsalva maneuver) alters maternal oxygenation and inhibits circulation—decreased preload and cardiac output
   b. Placental perfusion and level of oxygen available to the fetus are decreased
6. Impaired placental development and function
   a. Maternal health problems and habits during pregnancy can effect placental development
      (1) Pregnancy induced hypertension (PIH), diabetes
      (2) Smoking, inadequate nutritional intake
   b. Natural aging of the placenta which begins at approximately 36 weeks' gestation creates a problem when the pregnancy is postterm—postmaturity syndrome can result

C. Management of labor and birth must emphasize

1. Frequent assessment of FHR patterns throughout the labor and birth process to facilitate early detection and prompt treatment of hypoxia
2. Frequent assessment of maternal vital signs and the progress of labor to identify the degree of stress experienced by the fetus
3. Implementation of measures to prevent the occurrence of fetal hypoxia include
   a. Maternal relaxation techniques and frequent position changes
   b. Safe and effective administration of drugs
   c. Bearing down efforts that utilize open-glottis pushing

II. Assessment of FHR pattern—primary method for determination of fetal health status and fetal response to the labor and birth process

A. Goals of assessment

1. Early detection of mild fetal hypoxia
2. Prompt intervention for prevention of fetal damage from advancing hypoxia and acidosis

B. Assessment methods

1. Auscultation—use of fetoscope or doppler
   a. Determine site of maximal intensity of fetal heart sounds
      (1) Use Leopold's maneuvers—determine presentation and position
      (2) Locate curved fetal back
   b. Place fetoscope or doppler over fetal back if possible—adjust placement until most distinct sounds are heard
   c. Assess maternal pulse to differentiate between uterine souffle and funic souffle
   d. Count FHR
      (1) During a uterine contraction and for 30 seconds afterwards to determine effect of uterine contraction on FHR pattern. Did it increase or decrease, how much, and for how long?
      (2) Count between contractions for 30 to 60 seconds to determine baseline rate and rhythm
      (3) Recount during several contractions and rest periods to confirm presence of fetal distress or stress when significant changes have been noted in the FHR pattern
   e. Recommended frequency—adjust frequency according to
      (1) Stage and phase of labor
      (2) Condition of fetus. Example: increase assessment frequency if signs of hypoxia begin to occur.
      (3) Maternal condition and status of pregnancy. Example: more frequent monitoring is required for the high risk woman and pregnancy.
      (4) Labor events—FHR pattern should be assessed before and after
         (a) Procedures—enema, catheterization, vaginal examinations
         (b) Administration of medications such as sedatives, tranquilizers, analgesics, and anesthetics

(c) Initiation of labor suppression, induction, or augmentation measures
(d) Maternal activity—position change, ambulation, emesis, voiding
(e) Rupture of membranes—spontaneous or artificial—immediately afterwards and then 5 minutes later

2. External fetal monitoring—commonly used in low risk pregnancies to monitor uterine contractions and FHR patterns may be continous or intermittent
   a. Tocotransducer—device placed on abdomen over uterine fundus to assess duration and frequency of uterine contractions. NOTE: intensity or resting tone is not measurable using this method.
   b. Ultrasound transducer—device placed on abdomen over site of maximal intensity of fetal heart sounds (use location method stated above) to assess FHR pattern. NOTE: apply conduction gel to surface of transducer.
   c. Transducers attached to abdomen using belts
      (1) Readjust placement as needed since maternal and fetal position changes can interfere with accurate monitoring
      (2) Assess for signs of skin irritation and maternal discomfort as labor progresses
      (3) Massage reddened areas and reapply approximately once per hour
   d. Support measures are required since monitoring can be frightening
      (1) Discuss rationale for external monitoring and equipment used
      (2) Describe data collected by using monitor strip to show fetal heart pattern and uterine activity
      (3) Encourage coach to use monitor strip to facilitate guidance of prepared childbirth breathing techniques by noting the beginning, peak, and end of a contraction
   e. Portable monitors and intermittent monitoring can be used to reduce time spent in bed—maternal activity including ambulation and frequent position changes enhance the process of labor
3. Internal fetal monitoring—commonly used in high risk pregnancies since greater accuracy is obtained; it is an

invasive, continous monitoring of uterine contractions and FHR pattern

a. Intrauterine pressure transducer—inserted into amniotic fluid in the uterus; senses changes in uterine pressure during and between contractions; assesses intensity, duration, and frequency of uterine contractions as well as resting tone
b. Cardiotachometer—attached to fetal presenting part using a spiral electrode; continuous assessment of FHR pattern including short- and long-term variability; more complete and more accurate than external monitoring
c. Insertion of transducer and cardiotachometer requires
    (1) Ruptured membranes
    (2) Sufficient fetal descent
    (3) Cervical dilatation
d. Risk for infection is present—assessment for signs of infection and measures to prevent infection are critical
e. Support measures related to monitoring, as described above, should be instituted

4. External and internal fetal monitoring can be used in combination
    a. Tocotransducer for external monitoring of uterine contractions
    b. Cardiotachometer for internal monitoring of FHR patterns
        ▼ Monitor strips must be evaluated and findings documented following the same frequency guidelines used for auscultation of the fetal heart rate

III. Baseline FHR

A. Average baseline FHR at term—rate per minute 120 to 160; determination is made when there is no stress or stimulation affecting the fetus

1. During prenatal evaluation of FHR pattern
2. During labor between uterine contractions

B. Variability—normal irregularity of cardiac rhythm as a result of mature functioning of autonomic nervous system (ANS) which can balance cardiodeceleration (parasympathetic) and cardioacceleration (sympathetic); results in a characteristic fluctuation of the baseline

1. Short-term variability (STV)—change in FHR from one beat to the next as a result of differences in the interval between consecutive heart beats; usual fluctuation of 6 to 10 beats per minute

2. Long-term variability (LTV)—rhythmic and cyclical fluctuations of the FHR occurring in waves; usually 3 to 5 waves or cycles per minute
3. Variability requires electronic monitoring for assessment
   a. External monitoring can determine long-term variability
   b. Internal monitoring is the most accurate method of determining both short- and long-term variability

B. Alterations in the baseline FHR

1. Alteration in variability
   a. Often the first sign of fetal distress or stress is a reduction in variability
      (1) Minimal variability—3 to 5 beats per minute
      (2) Smooth-fixed baseline—absence of variability; 0 to 2 beats per minute
      (3) Common causes include
         (a) Hypoxia and acidosis
         (b) Use of CNS depressants and regional anesthesia
         (c) Congenital anomalies
         (d) Extreme prematurity
            ▼ A temporary decrease in long-term variability lasting approximately 20 to 30 minutes can occur during a fetal sleep state
2. Tachycardia
   a. FHR >160 beats per minute or 30 beats per minute above baseline FHR
   b. Duration of 10 minutes or longer
   c. Common causes can include
      (1) Early hypoxia
      (2) Medications such as Ritodrine, Terbutaline
      (3) Maternal infection, fever including chorioamnionitis
      (4) Maternal hyperthyroidism
3. Bradycardia
   a. FHR <120 beats per minute or 30 beats per minute below baseline FHR
   b. Duration of 10 minutes or longer
   c. Common causes can include
      (1) Late hypoxia
      (2) CNS depressants and regional anesthetics (spinal, epidural)
      (3) Alteration in perfusion through cord or placenta related to such factors as maternal hypotension, cord compression

IV. Periodic alterations in FHR—FHR changes defined in terms of their relationship to uterine contractions, namely timing, shape, and repetitiveness (Figure 10-1)

A. Acceleration (15 beats per minute)—occurs with contractions, fetal movement, vaginal examinations; indicate fetal well being

B. Early deceleration (Figure 10-1A)—not indicative of fetal distress or stress

1. FHR decreases (rarely below a FHR of 100) as a result of fetal head compression which stimulates vagus nerve to slow heart
2. Onset—early in contraction before acme-peak
3. Duration—short, with recovery to baseline by end of contraction
4. Shape—uniform
5. Occurrence—repetitious; occurs with each contraction
   a. Between 4 to 7 cm dilatation
   b. Second stage of labor

C. Late deceleration (Figure 10-1B)—indicative of fetal distress or stress when persistent

1. FHR decreases (rarely below a FHR of 100) as a result of interference with uteroplacental blood flow related to such factors as maternal hypotension, analgesic-anesthetic use, placental abnormalities, uterine hyperactivity
2. Onset—late in the contraction, after the acme-peak
3. Duration—long with recovery to baseline extending into rest period
4. Shape—uniform
5. Occurrence—repetitious; occurs with each contraction; influenced by intensity, duration, frequency of contractions

D. Variable deceleration (Figure 10-1C)—indicative of fetal distress or stress when moderate to severe and persistent

1. FHR decreases as a result of cord compression related to such factors as cord prolapse, maternal position, cord around fetal neck, short or knotted cord, oligohydramnios
2. Onset, duration (length of time from onset to recovery), depth of deceleration: variable—depends on degree and duration of the compression (partial, complete, brief, prolonged); classified as mild, moderate, or severe
3. Shape—variable usually with sudden drop in FHR (U or V shape)
4. Occurrence—late in labor with ROM, fetal descent, pushing

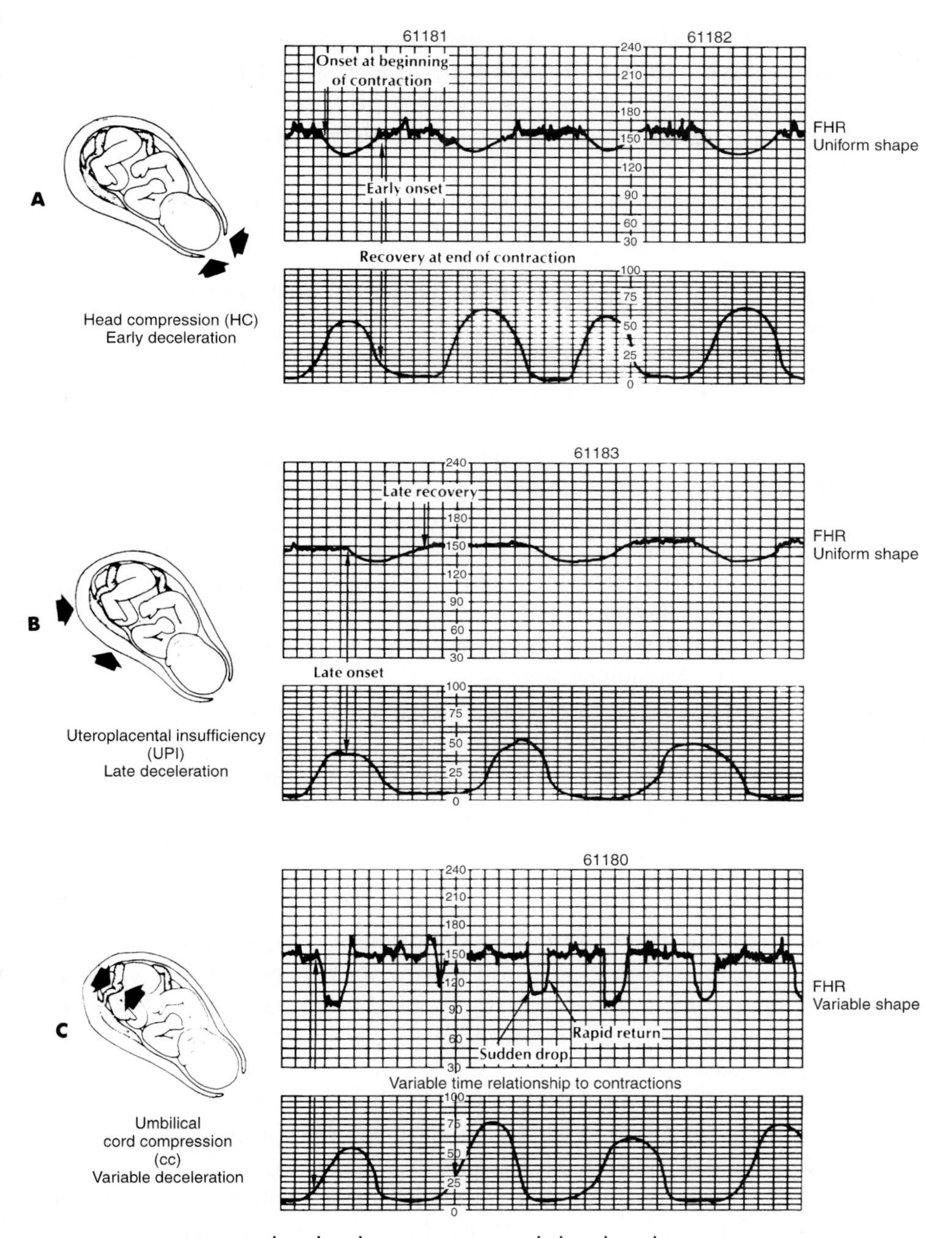

Figure 10-1. **A,** Early decelerations caused by head compression. **B,** Late deceleration caused by uteroplacental insufficiency. **C,** Variable deceleration caused by cord compression. (From Bobak IM et al: *Maternity and gynecologic care: the nurse and the family*, ed 5, St Louis, 1993, Mosby.)

V. Expected assessment findings related to fetal responses to the process of labor and birth—characteristics of a reassuring FHR pattern

A. **Baseline FHR of 120 to 160 beats per minute**

B. **Average baseline variability**

C. **Accelerations of FHR with fetal movement or contractions**

D. **Early decelerations and mild variable decelerations**

VI. Assessment findings indicative of fetal distress or stress

A. **Nonreassuring FHR patterns—warning of mild hypoxia**
   1. Progressive increase or decrease in baseline
   2. Baseline tachycardia; FHR >160
   3. Progressive decrease in baseline variability

B. **Ominous FHR patterns—reflect severe hypoxia and worsening fetal distress or stress**
   1. Moderate to severe variable decelerations
      a. FHR decreases below a rate of 70, for longer than 30 seconds
      b. Slow return to baseline
      c. Variability decreases
   2. Late decelerations especially if
      a. Persistent and prolonged
      b. Accompanied by a rising baseline or decreasing variability
   3. Smooth-fixed baseline especially if associated with late decelerations
   4. Severe bradycardia—a FHR of <100

C. **Acidosis—determined by obtaining a sample of fetal blood from presenting part and testing its pH, performed to assess degree of fetal hypoxia and its impact on acid-base balance when FHR patterns indicate the presence of distress or stress**
   1. 7.25 to 7.35 indicates acid-base is in balance
   2. 7.20 to 7.24 indicates a preacidotic state—repeat in approximately 15 to 30 minutes
   3. Less than 7.20 indicates acidosis and the need for intervention
      ▼ Cord blood analysis can be performed after birth to determine pH, PCO_2, PO_2, bicarbonate, and base deficit; confirms presence of fetal distress or stress during parturition; evaluates newborn status at time of birth, including need for intervention to support respiration

D. Additional signs of fetal distress or stress which accompany abnormal FHR patterns

1. Meconium stained amniotic fluid in a cephalic presentation. NOTE: may normally occur in breech presentations.
   a. Hypoxia increases intestinal peristalsis and relaxes anal sphincter
   b. Fetus passes meconium—thick, dark green fecal substance found in fetal intestines
2. Change in pattern of fetal movement—excessive fetal movement followed by cessation of movement
   a. Movement increases with passage of meconium
   b. Hypoxia depresses fetus and decreases movement

VII. Measures effective in the prevention and treatment of fetal distress or stress

A. Prevention

1. Alter maternal position on a regular basis, at least every 30 minutes to 1 hour
   a. Sitting, ambulation
   b. Lateral position supports BP and cardiac output
   c. Semifowlers position—use wedge to tilt to side
   d. Avoid supine position
2. Use stress reduction methods to reduce anxiety, enhance relaxation, and maintain an effective respiratory pattern
3. Teach and encourage effective pushing technique—use cleansing breaths, catch breaths, and open-glottis pushing

B. Treatment measures—depend on underlying cause of fetal distress or stress

1. Enhance cardiac output and uteroplacental circulation
   a. Turn to side-lying position—decreases pressure on inferior vena cava
   b. Maternal position change can remove pressure on cord
2. Increase circulating blood volume
   a. Raise legs
   b. Start or increase rate of IV fluids
3. Oxygenate blood—administer oxygen with a tight face mask at 10 to 12 liters/minute
4. Reduce uterine hyperactivity
   a. Stop Pitocin infusion
   b. Administer tocolytics (medications which suppress contractions) as needed. Example: terbutaline (Brethine) 0.25 mg subcutaneously.

5. Initiate prompt intervention for cord prolapse
   a. Measures to reduce pressure on cord
      (1) Elevate presenting part with gloved hand
      (2) Change maternal position to elevate hips—modified Sims, Trendelenburg, knee-chest
      (3) Distend bladder above symphysis pubis—insert Foley catheter and fill bladder with approximately 750 ml of warm sterile normal saline
         (a) Elevates fetal presenting part
         (b) Inhibits uterine contractions
   b. Measures to maintain integrity of the cord
      (1) Wrap protruding cord in sterile compresses wet with warm sterile normal saline
      (2) Never attempt to reinsert cord
      (3) Administer oxygen, start or increase IV fluids
6. Administer narcotic antagonist (Narcan) to mother if delivery is imminent or to neonate via cord after birth
7. Reduce cord compression related to oligohydramnios by instilling warm, sterile normal saline into uterus; this is termed amnioinfusion
8. Reduce maternal fever

VIII. Documentation related to fetal health status must reflect

A. Assessment of FHR pattern

1. According to recommended frequency for low and high risk pregnancies and policy-protocol of agency
2. Before and after significant labor events

B. For auscultation—description of FHR pattern should include

1. Rate and rhythm
2. Presence or absence of changes related to uterine contractions or significant labor events

C. For electronic monitoring

1. Documentation in nurses notes—description of monitor tracings must be recorded on a regular basis including average baseline FHR, degree of variability, presence of accelerations or decelerations
2. Documentation directly on tracing—maternal vital signs, status, and position changes, pushing, fetal movement, significant labor events, adjustments in monitor or transducers
3. Attach tracing to client chart or record according to agency policy since it is a legal component of the chart or record

D. All actions taken in terms of
1. Identified fetal distress patterns
2. Outcomes of the actions taken
3. Record in nurses notes and on monitor strip if applicable

E. Follow hospital-agency policy when documenting FHR patterns
1. What to document
2. When to document—frequency
3. Where to document—nurses notes, tracing
4. How to handle tracing after birth—stay with client chart, filed on labor unit

REVIEW QUESTIONS

1. The point of maximum intensity of the FHR should be identified to facilitate accurate placement of the ultrasound stethoscope, fetoscope, or ultrasound transducer. Which method should be used to identify the point of maximum intensity?
   a. Vaginal examination
   b. Leopold's maneuvers
   c. Ritgen's maneuver
   d. Effleurage

2. When the fetal position is LOA, the point of maximum intensity of the FHR would be located in the _______ quadrant of the maternal abdomen
   a. Left upper
   b. Right upper
   c. Left lower
   d. Right lower

3. When evaluating the FHR and uterine contraction tracing from an external fetal monitor, the nurse should understand that
   a. Contraction intensity, duration, and frequency are determined
   b. Long- and short-term variability are fully and accurately assessed
   c. Data recorded on tracings is influenced by changes in both the maternal and fetal positions
   d. Abdominal palpation of the uterus during and between contractions is not necessary

4. The nurse caring for women in labor should recognize that fetal tachycardia is most likely the result of
   a. Fetal movement
   b. Maternal hypotension
   c. Elevation in maternal core temperature, i.e., fever
   d. Administration of narcotic analgesics

5. When assessing an FHR tracing, the nurse notes a decrease in the baseline rate from 155 to 120. The rate of 120 persists for more than 10 minutes. The nurse could attribute this decrease in baseline to which of the following factors?
   a. Maternal hyperthyroidism
   b. Initiation of epidural anesthesia that resulted in maternal hypotension
   c. Maternal infection accompanied by fever
   d. Alteration in maternal position from semirecumbent to lateral

6. Upon review of a fetal monitor tracing, the nurse notes that for several contractions the FHR decelerates as a contraction begins but returns to baseline just before it ends. The nurse should
   a. Describe the finding in the nurse's notes
   b. Reposition the woman on to her side
   c. Call the physician for instructions
   d. Administer oxygen at 10 to 12 liters/minute with a tight face mask

7. Which of the following measures would be INEFFECTIVE in preventing fetal distress or stress?
   a. Alternate maternal position every 30 minutes to 1 hour
   b. Coach prepared childbirth breathing techniques
   c. Assist woman to relax by providing comfort measures
   d. Encourage use of the valsalva maneuver to increase the rate of fetal descent during the second stage of labor

8. Late deceleration patterns are noted when assessing the monitor tracing of a woman whose labor is being induced with an infusion of Pitocin. The woman is in a side-lying position and her vital signs are stable and fall within a normal range. Contractions are intense, last 80 seconds, and occur every 2 to 2½ minutes. The nurse's immediate action would be to
   a. Change the woman's position
   b. Stop the Pitocin
   c. Elevate the woman's legs
   d. Administer oxygen via a tight mask at 10 to 12 liters/minute

9. Following rupture of membranes, a prolapse of the cord was noted upon vaginal examination. Which of the following would be a recommended action to prevent cord compression?
   a. Place woman in a supine position and elevate legs from the hips
   b. Insert a Foley catheter to keep the bladder empty
   c. Keep the protruding cord moist with warm sterile normal saline compresses
   d. Attempt to reinsert the cord

ANSWERS, RATIONALES, AND TEST-TAKING TIPS

Rationales	Test-Taking Tips
1. Correct answer: b Leopold's maneuvers is a system of abdominal palpation to identify fetal presentation, position, and location of fetal parts. Point of maximum intensity (PMI) is usually found over the curved back of the fetus. Ritgen's maneuver is used to control birth of the head. Effleurage is rhythmic stroking of the abdomen for relaxation and distraction during a contraction.	Remember Leo*p*old's the *p*arts, *p*resentation, and *p*osition are *p*alpated of the fetus. Let the letter *p* be a clue.
2. Correct answer: c When presentation is breech the PMI is in the upper quadrants while for cephalic presentations it is found in the lower quadrants. Right or left quadrant is determined by the location of the fetal back.	LOA is Left Occipital Anterior position of the fetus. This means the head tends to be the presenting part. Thus, narrow the responses to options *c* or *d* that have lower in them. then select the same side of the position of the back, left, in this case since the fetal heart rate is better auscultated over this area of the fetal back.
3. Correct answer: c Internal monitoring is required to accurately determine intensity of contractions and short-term variability. External monitors can assess duration and frequency of contractions and long-term variability. Maternal and fetal movement require relocation	The question is asking about both the fetus and the mother, FHR and contractions. Therefore, if you have no idea of the correct answer select a response where both are taken into consideration, option *c*.

of the transducers. Periodic assessment using palpation and ultrasound stethoscope is important since mechanical failure of the monitor can occur, interfering with accuracy of data.

4. Correct answer: c

Fetal movement should result in an acceleration of FHR which is limited in duration and remains within the normal range. Responses *b* and *d* result in bradycardia.

Recall that fetal heart rate response to maternal hypotension is opposite (it slows) of what the mothers heart rate does; in hypotension the mothers heart rate increases. Make an educated guess by application of a general concept—fever results in an increased heart rate.

5. Correct answer: b

Fetal bradycardia is the pattern described and results from the hypoxia that occurs when uteroplacental perfusion is reduced by maternal hypotension. Responses *a* and *c* could result in baseline tachycardia. Assumption of a lateral position enhances placental perfusion and should result in a reassuring FHR pattern.

Recall maternal hypotension results in fetal bradycardia. See rationale for additional strategies.

6. Correct answer: a

An early deceleration pattern from head compression is described. No further action is required. Options *b, c,* and *d* would be implemented when nonreassuring or ominous changes are noted.

Important words that guide to do no further action: "several contractions," "returns to baseline." The findings are not constant for frequency and deviations from baseline in which case action would be needed.

7. Correct answer: d

Valsalva maneuver or closed-glottis pushing has been associated with a decrease in maternal blood preasure which reduces uteroplacental perfusion and leads to fetal hypoxia. Responses *a, b,* and *c* all decrease maternal stress and discomfort thereby enhancing uteroplacental circulation.

Associate the key words "valsalva maneuver" with a decrease in cardiac output and then blood pressure drop. Think of the cardiac client who is taught not to strain. The same response would be found in the laboring mother. Thus, response ***d*** is the ineffective action.

8. Correct answer: b

Late deceleration patterns noted are most likely related to alteration in uteroplacental perfusion associated with the strong contractions described. The immediate action would be to stop the Pitocin infusion. The woman is already in an appropriate position for uteroplacental perfusion. Elevation of the legs would be appropriate if hypotension were present. Oxygen is appropriate but not the immediate action.

Use common sense in that if a medication is being given and a negative response occurs, the immediate action is to slow or stop the medication.

9. Correct answer: c

Recommended positions to elevate the hips are modified Sims, Trendelenburg, or knee-chest. A distended bladder has a beneficial effect by elevating the presenting part and inhibiting uterine contractions. Never attempt to reinsert the cord since it may be injured.

Recognize that responses *a* is the position for shock. Make an educated guess that response *c* is the best since it provides an action for the problem of the prolapsed cord.

CHAPTER 11

Complications Associated with Labor and Birth

STUDY OUTCOMES

After completing this chapter, the reader will be able to do the following:

- Define the key terms listed.
- Describe the effects of childbirth complications on the maternal-fetal unit.
- Identify typical nursing diagnoses associated with childbirth complications.
- Discuss essential nursing care measures related to
  - dysfunctional labor
  - suppression of labor
  - induction and augmentation of labor
- Describe preoperative and postoperative nursing care measures related to cesarean birth.

KEY TERMS

Augmentation of labor Methods used to enhance existing uterine contractions to facilitate the progress of labor.

Cesarean birth Transabdominal delivery of the fetus through an incision into the abdomen and uterus.

Dystocia Labor that is abnormal, dysfunctional, difficult as a result of ineffective uterine contractions (powers), fetal problems (passenger), or pelvic inadequacy (passage).

Induction of labor Stimulation of the onset and progress of labor.

Postmaturity syndrome Newborn exhibits the detrimental effects of placental insufficiency from a prolonged pregnancy.

Preterm labor Begins after 20 to 24 weeks' gestation but before the end of 37 weeks' gestation.

Prolonged-postterm pregnancy Lasts 42 or more weeks.

Tocolytics Medications that suppress labor.

CONTENT REVIEW

I. Application of the nursing process to childbirth complications

A. A labor that does not conform to expected norms increases the level of stress experienced by the pregnant woman and her family

1. Feelings of powerlessness and a loss of control occur as labor becomes a more managed, medically oriented event rather than an anticipated natural experience
2. Self-confidence and self-esteem are diminished as the pregnant woman feels unable to secure safe passage for her baby
3. Fear and anxiety occur as concern for the safety of the maternal-fetal unit begins to rise—a realistic fear since the incidence of morbidity-mortality increases with complications of childbirth and their management
4. Stress and the body's response to it further interfere with the progress of childbirth

B. The nursing process is the framework for the organization of nursing management for complications of childbirth

1. Thorough, ongoing, frequent assessment of the health status of the maternal-fetal unit and the progress of labor (Box 11-1) is critical to determine

Box 11-1. Assessment Measures to Determine the Status of the Maternal-Fetal Unit and the Progress of Labor

Maternal Status

Circulatory status—BP, apical-radial pulse, signs of thrombophlebitis
Respiratory status—rate, regularity, depth, and effort of respirations, breath sounds
Hydration status—I&O, weight, edema, signs of fluid excess or deficit
Signs of infection—fever, maternal and fetal tachycardia, malodorous vaginal discharge, malaise
Level of pain or discomfort and effectiveness of relief measures
Emotional status—expressions of fear, anxiety, stress

Fetal Status

Fetal heart rate pattern using ausculation or electronic monitoring as appropriate
Fetal presentation, changes in station and position
Signs of fetal distress: nonreassuring-ominous FHR pattern, passage of meconium

Progress of Labor

Uterine activity—characteristics and progress of uterine contractions
Cervical changes—ripening, effacement, dilatation
Pattern of labor progress—use of a partogram

▼ Vaginal examinations, to determine progress of cervical change and fetal descent, are performed only as warranted and not at a set frequency, in order to prevent infection. This is especially important once membranes are ruptured.

a. Baseline data prior to the initiation of treatment measures such as labor suppression, augmentation, or induction
b. Expected effects and identification of side effects continuously during treatment
c. Psychosocial effects of the treatment plan on the pregnant woman and her family

2. Nursing diagnoses (Table 11-1) reflect the physical and psychosocial effects of
   a. Dysfunctional or difficult labor
   b. Preterm onset of labor
   c. Prolonged pregnancy
   d. Required medical management, surgical intervention
3. Nursing interventions must emphasize
   a. Measures to enhance or facilitate the labor process including comfort, nutrition-hydration, activity-positioning

Table 11-1. Selected Nursing Diagnoses Related to Complications Associated with Labor and Birth

Maternal-Family Nursing Diagnoses	Fetal-Newborn Nursing Diagnoses
Ineffective Breathing Pattern Related to Depressant effects of magnesium sulfate Pulmonary edema associated with administration of ritodrine Experience of incisional discomfort when taking deep breaths	*Impaired Gas Exchange Related to* Aging of placenta associated with prolonged pregnancy Hyperstimulation of the uterus associated with Pitocin induction of labor Compression of umbilical cord associated with oligohydramnios Aspiration of meconium
Decreased Cardiac Output Related to Tachycardia associated with administration of terbutaline	*Risk for Fetal Injury Related to* Macrosomia requiring operative birthing measures Intrauterine infection
Fluid Volume Excess Related to Fluid retention associated with administration of ritodrine	*Alteration of Nutrition—< than Body Requirements Related to* Ineffective feeding behaviors associated with high magnesium levels Ineffective breast-feeding associated with maternal pain and fatigue following cesarean section
Risk for Infection Related to Premature rupture of amniotic membranes Alteration in skin integrity following cesarean birth	*Risk for Neonatal Injury Related to* Hypoglycemia associated with prolonged pregnancy
Pain Related to Hypertonic uterine contraction pattern Abdominal-uterine incision associated with cesarean birth	
Fatigue Related to Interruption of sleep patterns associated with prolonged labor process CNS irritability associated with ritodrine (Yutopar) administration	

Continued.

b. Safe, knowledgeable implementation of treatment protocols ordered by the healthcare provider, such as the obstetrician, nurse-midwife
c. Emotional support of the pregnant woman and family including explanations of interventions and descriptions of progress

Table 11-1. Selected Nursing Diagnoses Related to Complications Associated with Labor and Birth—cont'd

Maternal-Family Nursing Diagnoses	Fetal-Newborn Nursing Diagnoses
Anxiety Related to Preterm onset of labor Required medical management of labor Prolonged pregnancy Lack of knowledge concerning labor induction and its effects	
Situational Low Self-Esteem Related to Perceived inability to secure safe passage for self and fetus	
Altered Family Processes Related to Limitation placed on maternal role performance as part of treatment regime to prevent preterm birth	

d. Detailed, ongoing documentation of observations made, actions taken, and outcomes of actions

4. Evaluation criteria will determine effectiveness of intervention plan—evaluation criteria can include
   a. Preterm labor was suppressed
   b. Uterine activity and progress of cervical dilatation approximated expected labor induction patterns
   c. Active labor was initiated following a period of therapeutic rest for a prolonged latent phase with hypertonic uterine contractions
   d. Fetal heart rate patterns remained reassuring
   e. Anxiety level of laboring woman and family remained at a mild to moderate level

II. Dystocia

A. Uterine dystocia

1. Contributing factors, many of which relate to mismanagement of labor, include
   a. Pharmacologic interventions
      (1) Analgesics, anesthetics, sedatives administered too early in labor or in too large a dose
      (2) Pitocin improperly regulated

b. Activity level during labor
   (1) Limitation on position change and activity
   (2) Bedrest
c. Limitation on fluid and nutrient intake during labor leading to dehydration and energy depletion
d. Bladder and bowel distention
e. Uterine factors
   (1) Malformations
   (2) Over distention related to fetal macrosomia, multiple gestation, hydramnios
   (3) Repeated stretching as with grandmultiparity
   (4) Rigid cervix
f. Fetal factors
   (1) Malpresentation
   (2) Fetopelvic (cephalopelvic) disproportion
   (3) Fetal anomalies such as hydrocephalus

2. Two types of contractions characteristic of dystocia
   a. Hypotonic uterine contractions
      (1) Infrequent (<3 within 10 minutes), irregular contraction pattern
      (2) Mild or low intensity
         (a) Intrauterine pressure catheter— <25 mm Hg
         (b) Palpation—limited fundal tone
      (3) Typically occur
         (a) During active phase in the first stage of labor following a normal latent phase
         (b) Among multiparous women
      (4) Results in a protracted-arrested active phase
   b. Hypertonic uterine contractions
      (1) Painful, strong, but ineffective uterine contractions that lack fundal dominance—uncoordinated, asymmetrical in tone
      (2) Short rest period between contractions with an increase in uterine resting tone
      (3) Typically occur during latent phase of labor of a nulliparous woman; may be related to the higher level of anxiety in first time labors
      (4) Results in a prolonged latent phase
3. Four patterns of dysfunctional labor—classified according to the phases of the first stage of labor as identified by Friedman and determined by plotting labor progress on a partogram
   a. Prolonged latent phase

- (1) Duration of >20 hours (nullipara) or >14 hours (multipara)
- (2) Typically noted in combination with hypertonic contractions
- (3) Management
    - (a) Therapeutic rest—use of narcotic analgesics, tranquilizers, or sedatives and comfort or relaxation measures to facilitate a rest period of 4 to 6 hours; following rest, the active phase of labor usually begins
    - (6) Augmentation of labor when cervix is ripe by using nipple stimulation, amniotomy, or intravenous Pitocin

b. Protracted active phase—duration of the active phase of labor is prolonged as a result of the slowing of dilatation and/or fetal descent

- (1) Nullipara
    - (a) Cervical dilatation— <1.2 cm/hr
    - (b) Fetal descent— <1 cm/hr
- (2) Multipara
    - (a) Cervical dilatation— <1.5 cm/hr
    - (b) Fetal descent— <2 cm/hr
- (3) Typically noted in combination with hypotonic contractions
- (4) Management
    - (a) Rule out cephalopelvic (fetopelvic) disproportion—fetal head is unable to fit though pelvis if head is too large and/or pelvis is too small
    - (b) Institute labor augmentation methods if pelvis is adequate for fetal passage

c. Arrested active phase—progress stops in terms of dilatation and/or fetal descent

- (1) Absence of progress in dilatation for >2 hours during the active phase
- (2) Absence of progress in fetal descent for >1 hour during active phase
- (3) Failure of descent—lack of descent during deceleration phase and second stage of labor
- (4) Frequently associated with cephalopelvic (fetopelvic) disproportion
- (5) Management as for protraction—be prepared for birth by cesarean section

d. Precipitous labor—rapidly paced labor with delivery within 3 hours or less of onset
   (1) Often associated with
      (a) Intense, frequent contractions that may occur with Pitocin administration or cocaine use
      (b) Low resistance of maternal tissues resulting in a more rapid pace of dilatation and fetal descent
   (2) May result in a precipitous, unattended delivery accompanied by tearing of maternal tissue, early placental separation, and fetal cranial damage
   (3) Management
      (a) Slowing of labor using tocolytics
      (b) Planned induction of labor at term to control the onset and progress of labor

B. Passenger dystocia

1. Fetal injury is a major concern related to
   a. Trauma associated with medical interventions to accomplish birth such as external versions, forceps, vacuum extractor, cesarean section
   b. Hypoxia associated with cord prolapse or compression
2. Contributing factors
   a. Fetal size
      (1) Excessively large and/or hard bony skull associated with hydrocephalus, postmaturity syndrome, limits ability of head to mold during passage through the pelvis
      (2) Macrosomia—large (for gestational age) fetus resulting from increased intrauterine growth often associated with poorly controlled pregestational or gestational diabetes
   b. Multiple gestations
   c. Fetal presentation-position
      (1) Occiput posterior position—increased internal rotation arc required to bring occiput in line with symphysis pubis
      (2) Face presentation—extension of neck presents larger cephalic diameters for passage through the pelvis; neonatal facial bruising and edema result if vaginal delivery is accomplished
      (3) Shoulder presentation—transverse lie—fetus is horizontal with its spine perpendicular to maternal spine and shoulder presenting first

(4) Breech presentation—fetal buttocks or foot or feet present first—major dangers result from
  (a) Prolonged labor related to slower dilatation—buttocks less effective as a dilator since they are soft and fit less closely than the head to the cervix
  (b) Hypoxia related to cord compression—cord prolapse occurs more frequently
  (c) Passage of fetal head, which has less time to mold and accommodate to the pelvis
  (d) Passage of meconium into the amniotic fluid is more common as abdomen and buttocks are compressed during passage through birth canal
  (e) Aspiration of amniotic fluid and meconium since breathing can begin with emergence of body before head is delivered and respiratory passages suctioned

3. Management of fetal dystocia—major determining factors: size of maternal pelvis and condition of the maternal-fetal unit; management approaches
   a. Maternal pelvis adequate for passage of fetus
      (1) Forceps and vacuum extractor used to facilitate internal rotation and delivery of fetal head
      (2) Maternal positioning used to facilitate rotation and descent. Example: a hands and knees position can facilitate internal rotation when fetal head is in the occiput posterior position.
      (3) External version can be attempted after 37 weeks' gestation to change fetal presentation from breech or shoulder to cephalic by gentle pressure over the abdomen following administration of terbutaline subcutaneously and epidural anesthesia
   b. Maternal pelvis is inadequate, borderline, or doubtful (nullipara)—cesarean section is the delivery method of choice

III. Preterm labor

A. Incidence and significance

1. Occurs in 5 to 15% of all births
2. Accounts for 75 to 80% of all neonatal mortality primarily related to immature respiratory function

B. Contributing factors

1. Previous history of preterm labor or birth

2. Demographic factors
    a. Age (<17 or >34)
    b. Race—African American
    c. Low socioeconomic status
    d. Inadequate prenatal care
    e. Unmarried
    f. Low educational level
3. Lifestyle factors
    a. Inadequate nutrition, including anemia, hyperemesis
    b. Poor hygienic practices, unsafe sex practices
    c. Substance abuse with tobacco, alcohol, or cocaine
    d. Inability to cope with stressors in life
4. Health problems
    a. Infections of genitourinary tract or systemic infections especially accompanied by fever
    b. Chronic health problems such as diabetes, hypertension
5. Uterine factors
    a. Abnormalities such as incompetent cervix, malposition, fibroids
    b. Conditions which interfere with myometrial blood flow such as overdistention with multiple gestation or hydramnios (excessive amniotic fluid)
    c. Uterine trauma associated with surgery, childbirth injuries, accidents
    d. Premature rupture of the membranes

C. Detection of preterm labor

1. Early detection of the signs of preterm labor is important since labor suppression methods are more successful if major cervical changes have not occurred; initiation of treatment once dilatation is >4 cm results in limited success
2. Signs of preterm labor may be difficult to detect since they are often vague and nonspecific; diagnosis of preterm labor is based primarily on the uterine contraction pattern presented and changes in the cervix
3. Signs of preterm labor
    a. Uterine contractions
        (1) Frequency of 1 every 10 minutes or less
        (2) Duration of ≥30 seconds
        (3) Persist for at least one hour
        (4) Regular pattern of increasing intensity, duration, and frequency is developed
        (5) Often painless, with a sensation of tightening or tingling

b. Cervical changes
   (1) Ripening (softening and thinning)
   (2) Effacement up to 80%
   (3) Dilatation up to 2 cm
c. Discomfort—characteristics of discomfort vary
   (1) Constant or intermittent low back pain
   (2) Abdominal-menstrual like cramping with or without diarrhea
   (3) Gastrointestinal upset with nausea and vomiting
   (4) Pelvic pressure that is constant or intermittent; may seem like the fetus is pressing down
   (5) General feeling of uneasiness—that things are not quite right
d. Vaginal discharge—sudden change in the character or amount of vaginal discharge; increase in amount, more watery, clear to pale pink or bloody, passage of mucous plug

4. All patients especially those at high risk must be taught how to detect the early signs of preterm labor

D. Conservative measures to suppress preterm labor—primarily successful if cervical changes are not occurring or advaneed

1. At home—when signs of labor are detected, the client should
   a. Empty bladder
   b. Drink 3 to 4 glasses of water, 6 to 8 ounces each
   c. Lie down in a lateral recumbent position—enhances uteroplacental perfusion and reduces pressure on cervix
   d. Continue to count contractions, which should subside
   e. If contractions are not suppressed within 1 hour the client should be admitted for evaluation and treatment
2. In hospital
   a. Bedrest in the lateral recumbent position
   b. Intravenous hydration taking care to avoid hypervolemia
   c. Oral intake may be limited. Example: NPO except for ice chips sparingly.
   d. Regular voiding to prevent bladder distension
   e. Measures to enhance relaxation and reduce stress such as emotional support, relaxation techniques, and explanations of procedures and progress—stress interferes with labor suppression
   f. Gather baseline data in anticipation of tocolytic therapy
      (1) Maternal status
         (a) Cardiac and respiratory status including vital signs, heart and breath sounds, and respiratory effort

(b) Health status including signs of infection
(c) Hydration status including weight, I&O, edema
(d) CNS status—LOC, orientation, deep tendon reflexes (DTR), signs of irritability, restlessness
(e) Lab-diagnostic tests—ECG, CBC, clean catch urine specimen for analysis and bacteria screen (bacteria are associated with preterm labor), serum electrolytes and glucose level

(2) Fetal status—apply external monitor to assess FHR patterns noting reassuring and nonreassuring or ominous patterns
(3) Status of labor—signs of labor and status of cervix through vaginal exams; use sterile speculum and limit number, since vaginal exams increase risk of infection and stimulate cervix

E. Pharmacologic approaches to suppress labor—if conservative measures are not successful tocolytics are administered

1. Criteria must be met prior to initiation of tocolysis
   a. Fetus—healthy at 20 to 36 weeks' gestation; no signs of distress, severe intrauterine growth retardation (IUGR), or major anomalies incompatible with life
   b. Mother must be relatively healthy without active hemorrhage or significant bleeding, intrauterine infection, severe pregnancy induced hypertension, or health problems incompatible with the tocolytic drug being used. Example: heart disease incompatible with ritodrine (Yutopar) or terbutaline (Brethine).
   c. Definitive signs of preterm labor have been confirmed
2. Tocolytic medications currently in use
   a. Beta-sympathomimetics and magnesium sulfate are the most common tocolytics used today (Table 11-2)
   b. Routes of administration
      (1) Intravenous and subcutaneous administration—most effective method
      (2) Oral administration is often less effective related to
         (a) Poor compliance in terms of timing and missed doses
         (b) Limited absorption via the GI system
         (c) Gastrointestinal side effects such as nausea, vomiting, GI distress
         (d) Contraction breakthrough within 3 weeks of initiation of oral administration from

Table 11-2. Tocolytics—Administration and Nursing Implications

Principles of Administration	Nursing Implications
Beta Adrenergic Stimulant	
A. Ritodrine (Yutopar). Only drug approved by the FDA for labor suppression. Used less often due to side effects especially with intravenous use	
Administration of $Beta_2$ Adrenergic Stimulant	**Implications Related to Administration of Both $Beta_2$ Adrenergic Stimulant**
Administration of Ritodrine **Intravenous Route**	
Prepare ritodrine solution by mixing 150 mg of ritodrine in 500 cc of 5% dextrose in ½ normal saline, for a concentration of 0.3 mg/ml (some authorities advocate dextrose free solutions since hyperglycemia can occur); label the bag Attach ritodrine solution to a controller-pump Piggyback ritodrine solution to the primary line at the port closest to the IV insertion site (port most proximal to the client) Begin infusion and increase rate according to the following guidelines ▼ Starting rate—0.05 to 0.1 mg/min ▼ Increase rate in increments of 0.05 mg/min every 10 to 20 minutes until the desired response is obtained (uterine contractions cease or there are <4 in 1 hour), side effects become intolerable, or the maximum dosage of 0.35 mg/minute is reached	Assessment of maternal-fetal unit and progress of labor must be made throughout the period of treatment with the most frequent and thorough assessment during intravenous administration (see Box 11-1) Observe for specific side effects related to administration of beta-sympathomimetics ▼ Maternal—fetal tachycardia and palpitations with skipped beats ▼ Alteration in BP with widening pulse pressure progressing to hypotension ▼ Fluid volume excess progressing to pulmonary edema ▼ Transient hyperglycemia with increased insulin secretion and metabolic acidosis ▼ Transient hypokalemia ▼ Nausea and vomiting

Continued.

Table 11-2. Tocolytics—Administration and Nursing Implications—cont'd

Principles of Administration	Nursing Implications
Beta Adrenergic Stimulant—cont'd	
A. Ritodrine (Yutopar)—cont'd	
▼ Document maternal-fetal-labor status at each increment on chart or flow sheet and monitor strip Maintain at effective rate for approximately 60 minutes then begin to decrease if suppression is maintained, at 0.05 mg/min every 30 minutes until the lowest effective dose is achieved but not lower than 0.05 to 0.1 mg/min; maintain at this lower rate for 12 to 24 hours Begin oral tocolytics 30 minutes prior to discontinuing the infusion	▼ CNS irritability—tremors, nervousness, agitation, restlessness ▼ Neonatal glucose imbalance may occur during the first 24 hours following birth Observe for signs of *intolerable side effects* requiring that treatment be discontinued and physician notified ▼ Maternal heart rate >140 beats per minute, cardiac dysrhythmias ▼ Fetal heart rate >180 beats per minute ▼ BP <90/60
Oral Route 10 to 20 mg every 2 to 4 hours for the first 24 hours 10 to 20 mg every 4 to 6 hours maintenance with no more than 120 mg in 24 hours—must be taken on time with food to limit gastrointestinal distress Check pulse prior to each dose—acceptable range of 90 to 110 beats per minute; hold if pulse is >110 beats per minute	▼ Signs of pulmonary edema, chest pain Keep propranolol (Inderal) 0.5 to 1 mg at the bedside for emergency administration (IV push over 1 minute) when toxic effects appear especially related to cardiac function Limit fluid intake to 100 cc/hour
Report ▼ Drug side effects such as palpitations, pulse >120 BPM, chest pain, dyspnea, tremors, and nervousness ▼ Signs of labor ▼ Signs of infection	Maintain strict asepsis to prevent infection especially if membranes are ruptured Intervene to minimize effects of bedrest ▼ Assist with TED stockings, ROM exercises to lower extremities to prevent pooling of blood ▼ Alternate position ▼ Cough and deep breathe

Beta Adrenergic Stimulant—cont'd

A. Ritodrine (Yutopar)—cont'd

Provide comfort measures, emotional support, relaxing diversions

Provide homecare support and follow-up using telephone contact and home visitation on a weekly or biweekly basis

B. Terbutaline (Brethine) More commonly used than ritodrine especially subcutaneously via a continuous pump infusion

Administration of Terbutaline

Intravenous Route

Mix 5 mg of terbutaline in 500 ml of an IV solution and add to primary infusion as specified for ritodrine

Begin infusion at 2.5 to 20 mcg/min increasing at a rate of 5 mcg/min every 10 minutes until desired response is obtained, side effects are intolerable, or a maximum dose of 80 mcg/min is reached

Maintain at effective dosage for 12 to 24 hours then gradually reduce dosage and begin oral or subcutaneous administration

Oral Route

2.5 mg every 4 hours or 5 mg every 6 to 8 hours

Follow same principle as for oral ritodrine

Continued.

Table 11-2. Tocolytics—Administration and Nursing Implications—cont'd

Principles of Administration	Nursing Implications
Beta Adrenergic Stimulant—cont'd	
B. Terbutaline (Brethine)—cont'd	
Subcutaneous Route Injection of 0.25 mg every 4 hours Terbutaline pump increases contraction breakthrough time to 6 weeks thus prolonging pregnancy; provides ▼ Continuous maintenance (low) dose of 0.05 mg to 0.1 mg/hour ▼ Bolus dose of 0.25 mg every 4 to 6 hours according to client's unique contraction pattern (determined over a 24-hour period using an external monitor); hold for pulse >110 beats per minute ▼ Approximately 3 mg/24 hours are administered Teach woman/family principles of treatment including ▼ Use of pump—change of syringe, rotation of site (every 3 to 4 days), adjustment of dosage ▼ Site assessment for signs of infection ▼ Self-assessment for signs of labor and side effects of terbutaline	

Magnesium Sulfate

Along with terbutaline is a first-line drug for suppression of labor. Effective with fewer side effects than the beta-sympathomimetics

Administration of Magnesium Sulfate

Intravenous Route

Prepare a loading dose of 4 to 6 g of magnesium sulfate in 100 to 250 ml of IV solution and administer via infusion pump over 15 to 20 minutes. NOTE: one dose of terbutaline 0.25 mg subcutaneous may be given just prior to the loading dose since magnesium sulfate has a slower onset than other tocolytics.

Continue infusion at 1.5 to 2 g/hr, increasing by 0.5 to 1 g every 30 minutes until desired effect is obtained, side effects become intolerable or a maximum of 3 Gm/hour has been reached

Continue at effective dosage rate for approximately 12 to 24 hours

Begin oral tocolytics 30 to 60 minutes prior to discontinuing the infusion

Monitor urine output since an output <25 cc/hr increases likelihood of hypermagnesemia

Oral Route

Magnesium oxide—200 mg every 3 to 4 hours

Magnesium gluconate—1 g every 2 to 4 hours

Implications Related to Administration of Magnesium Sulfate

Assessment of maternal-fetal unit and progress of labor at frequent intervals especially during intravenous administration (see Box 11-1)

Observe for specific findings indicating hypermagnesemia

- ▼ Transient flushing, sweating at start of treatment
- ▼ Depression of CNS as noted in
  - — Diminished level of consciousness and deep tendon reflexes (DTR), drowsiness
  - — Check DTR every hour
- ▼ Depressed cardiac and respiratory function
  - — Check respirations every hour
  - — Check for hypotension
  - — Assess breath sounds taking note for signs of pulmonary edema
- ▼ Gastrointestinal distress—nausea and vomiting
- ▼ Hypermagnesemia—evaluate serum magnesium levels which should be maintained between 6 to 8 mg/dL (4 to 7 mEq/L)
- ▼ Hypocalcemia—paresthesia, dizziness, tetany

Continued.

Table 11-2. Tocolytics—Administration and Nursing Implications—cont'd

Tocolytic	Principles of Administration	Nursing Implications
Magnesium Sulfate—cont'd		
As effective as oral ritodrine or terbutaline with fewer side effects though nausea, vomiting, diarrhea can occur		▼ Neonatal hypermagnesemia—especially if maternal levels rose above 8 mEq/L; noted as transient lethargy and poor feeding behavior after birth Alert for *intolerable side effects* requiring that treatment be discontinued and physician notified ▼ Respiratory rate < 12 RPM ▼ Absence of DTR ▼ Severe hypotension ▼ Serum magnesium above therapeutic level Keep Ca gluconate (1 g of a 10% solution) at the bedside for emergency administration IV push over 5 to 10 minutes for CNS depression and diminished respirations Additional care measures include comfort, emotional support, diversional activities, and minimizing effects of bedrest

desensitization of receptor sites and increasing tolerance to the effects of the drug

3. Second-line tocolytic drugs currently under study and used when first-line drugs are ineffective include
    a. Indomethacin—a prostaglandin inhibitor
    b. Nifedipine—a calcium channel blocker

F. Health teaching and supportive measures for the client at risk for preterm birth

1. Medication instructions—include when and how to take prescribed medications, assessment measures to be done prior to the dose, signs of toxicity and what to do if they appear, terbutaline subcutaneous pump maintenance (see Table 11-2)
2. Signs of labor—assessment measures to include how to use a home monitoring system
    a. Assume lateral recumbent position and assess for uterine contractions for 1 full hour twice a day
    b. Palpate uterine fundus with fingertips taking note of muscle tightening OR apply external monitor over fundus—records uterine activity and stores data for later telephone transmission
    c. Record time, frequency, duration, and perceived intensity of uterine contractions experienced
    d. Take note of any associated signs of labor
    e. Report findings during daily telephone contact with a nurse—daily contact accompanied by earlier detection of preterm labor has been effective in reducing preterm births as a result of prompt, successful treatment
3. Actions to take if signs of labor are noted
4. Measures to prevent the onset of preterm labor and cope with required lifestyle changes
    a. Balance activity and rest by pacing activities and taking frequent rest periods in the lateral recumbent position—for some clients bedrest may be required
    b. Avoid lifting
    c. Take a leave of absence from job
    d. Prevent stimulation of uterine contractions by changing sexual activity to prevent orgasm and stimulation of the cervix
    e. Avoid stimulation of nipples
    f. Prevent genitourinary tract infection (associated with premature rupture of membranes and onset of labor)
        (1) Genital hygiene after voiding or elimination
        (2) Void every 2 hours to keep bladder empty

g. Maintain nutrient and fluid balance and appropriate weight gain
    (1) Avoid long periods without food
    (2) Maintain daily fluid intake of 2 to 3 liters
    (3) Avoid caffeine
h. Reduce stress by engaging in pleasant, distracting activities, relaxation techniques
i. Involve family in treatment regime
j. Cooperate with referrals to homecare agencies

IV. Spontaneous rupture of the membranes before the onset of labor

A. Types

1. Premature rupture of the membranes (PROM)—rupture of membranes after the completion of the 37th week of gestation with labor usually beginning within 12 to 24 hours
2. Preterm premature rupture of the membranes (PPROM)—rupture of membranes before the 38th week of gestation
    a. Labor is less likely to begin
    b. Tear may heal and membranes reseal if rupture was small

B. Contributing factors

1. Reproductive tract infections including STDs, chorioamnionites, group B streptococcus infection since microorganisms can weaken the amniotic membranes
2. Increased intrauterine pressure as a result of hydramnios, multiple gestation
3. Lifestyle habits including poor dietary practices, smoking
4. Fetal anomalies and malpresentations

C. Complications

1. Risk for infection—membranes no longer protect uterine cavity and fetus
2. Fetal hypoxia as a result of cord compression
    a. Prolapse of the cord
    b. Decreased amounts of amniotic fluid to cushion cord

D. Management

1. Determine
    a. Exact time of rupture
    b. Characteristics of fluid—amount, color, and odor; confirm that fluid is amniotic by performing
        (1) Nitrazine test—alkaline reaction
        (2) Fern test—ferning pattern appears when fluid dries on a glass slide

c. Gestational age of the pregnancy
d. Maturitiy of the fetus by collecting fluid and test for L/S ratio and presence of phosphatidylglycerol (Pg); rupture of membranes may facilitate lung maturation by enhancing surfactant production

2. Watchful waiting may be instituted if tear is small with minimal fluid loss if pregnancy is preterm, and if signs of infection are absent; management includes
   a. Ongoing assessment of the maternal-fetal unit for signs of infection and labor
   b. Infection control measures with scrupulous hygiene practices, limitation on frequency of vaginal examination, and prophylactic antibiotics
   c. Labor suppression with tocolytics
3. Prevent onset of preterm labor and cope with required lifestyle changes (see discussion of preterm labor)
4. Administer corticosteriods (Betamethsone) to stimulate maturation of the fetal lungs if preterm birth becomes inevitable
5. Labor may be induced if pregnancy is at term and labor does not begin spontaneously

V. Prolonged-postterm pregnancy

A. Incidence and significance

1. Occurs in 3 to 14% of all births
2. Accounts for over 15% of all perinatal deaths with ⅓ of these deaths occurring before labor and ⅔ occurring during the process of labor and birth

B. Complications

1. Dystocia related to
   a. Uterine factors—ineffective contraction patterns
   b. Fetal factors—macrosomia with large head and shoulders and limited molding ability of head
   c. Pelvic factors—pelvis unable to accommodate macrosomic fetus
2. Postmaturity/dysmaturity syndrome
   a. Placental function peaks at 36 weeks and the aging process begins; aging limits ability of placenta to supply fetus with oxygen and nutrients, resulting in
      (1) Alteration in gas exchange leading to fetal hypoxia as indicated by
         (a) Nonreassuring FHR patterns such as late decelerations and diminished baseline variability

(b) Passage of meconium with thickening of amniotic fluid—increases danger of meconium aspiration and infection, dries the umbilical cord, and stains the skin green (recent) to yellow (chronic)
(c) Increased RBC production that results in a high incidence of neonatal hyperbilirubinemia

(2) Alteration in nutrition leading to
(a) Fetal weight loss with a decrease in subcutaneous tissue
(b) Dry, cracked, peeling skin (desquamation) which is loose and wrinkled
(c) Muscle wasting
(d) Increased incidence of neonatal hypoglycemia as glucose stores are used up prior to birth

b. Amniotic fluid begins to decrease after 38 weeks' gestation (oligohydramnios) and leads to
(1) Cord compression—less fluid to cushion cord
(2) Nonreassuring FHR patterns such as variable decelerations and diminished variability

C. Management

1. Testing to confirm gestational age and determine status of maternal-fetal unit
   a. Determine week of occurrence for quickening, auscultation of fetal heart sounds with doppler or fetoscope
   b. Examine fetus and uterine structures using diagnostic ultrasound, taking note of
      (1) Fetal size—biparietal diameter, femur length
      (2) Calcification of fetal skeleton
      (3) Amount of amniotic fluid
      (4) Degree of placental aging—grading of placenta
   c. Perform nonstress test (NST), contraction stress test (CST), biophysical profile as required
   d. Determine fetal lung maturity (L/S ratio, Pg level) with fluid from an amniocentesis
   e. Examine mother taking note of weight (loss of >3 pounds may indicate postterm pregnancy) and condition of cervix
2. Management when cervix is not ripe but maternal-fetal unit is healthy—watchful waiting with close surveillance of the status of the maternal-fetal unit using appropriate antepartal tests

3. Management when cervix is not ripe but maternal-fetal unit is compromised by high risk factors (PIH, diabetes) or signs of postmaturity syndrome are present
    a. Ripen cervix with prostaglandin E_2 gel or laminaria and induce labor
    b. Perform a cesarean section
4. Management when cervix is ripe—induce labor
5. Amnioinfusion (instillation of warm sterile normal saline into uterine cavity)—may be used to treat or prevent variable decelerations when oligohydramnios is present

VI. Stimulation of the process of labor

A. Augmentation of labor

1. Purpose—used for hypotonic dysfunctional labor, protracted active phase, slowing of labor progress as a result of epidural anesthesia
2. Methods
    a. Breast stimulation—facilitates spontaneous release of oxytocin from the posterior pituitary gland by stimulating the nipple manually or with a breast pump
    b. Amniotomy (artificial rupture of the amniotic membranes)—enhances prostaglandin production and allows fetal head to act as cervical dilator
        (1) It is recommended that cervix be at least 4 cm dilated and fetal presenting part be engaged
        (2) Assessment and care measures before and after amniotomy are the same as for spontaneous rupture of the membranes
    c. Intravenous administration of Pitocin (Table 11-3)

B. Induction of labor—necessary when a valid medical reason exists, such as postmaturity, IUGR, fetal stress, PROM, chorioamnionitis, high risk pregnancy (such as PIH, diabetes), history of precipitous labor or birth

C. Assessment for readiness of the maternal-fetal unit for labor stimulation procedures

1. Criteria for stimulation are met
    a. Fetal lung maturity is established with an accurate gestational age and/or amniotic fluid testing
    b. Fetal size, presentation, and position are determined and fetus is capable of passage through the maternal pelvis
    c. Fetal presenting part is engaged

Table 11-3. Augmentation-Induction of Labor Using Pitocin—Administration and Nursing Implications

Principles of Administration	Nursing Implications
Pitocin Synthetic form of the posterior pituitary hormone, oxytocin Stimulates the uterine myometrium to contract by increasing prostaglandin production and formation of oxytocin receptors Dosage can be decreased as labor progresses since sensitivity to oxytocics increases and body production of prostaglandins and oxytocin is adequate to maintain labor	
Establish a primary line with an electrolyte solution such as Ringer's lactate, 5% dextrose in Ringer's lactate or ½ normal saline; an electrolyte based solution is used to prevent water intoxication related to the antidiuretic effect of Pitocin; the primary line provides a route for other IV meds that may be needed (use distal port) and a means to maintain access to the circulatory system if Pitocin is discontinued Add Pitocin to an IV solution and label the bag; the type and amount of the IV solution as well as the amount of Pitocin added will be determined by physician orders and hospital protocol; consideration is given to the hydration status of the patient ▼ 15 U Pitocin/250 ml = 60 mU/ml; 1 mU/min = 1 ml/hour ▼ 10 U Pitocin/1000 ml = 10 mU/ml; 1 mU/min = 6 ml/hour Never add any other medication to the Pitocin solution Insert tubing from Pitocin solution through infusion pump-controller Piggyback Pitocin solution to the primary line at the port closest to the IV insertion site (proximal port) Turn on the piggyback at the desired rate of infusion and follow protocol for advancement of rate	Assess status of maternal-fetal unit at intervals of at least 15 minutes when increasing dosage and 30 minutes when maintaining or decreasing dosage (see Box 11-1) Observe for signs of *intolerable side effects* requiring immediate action ▼ Hyperstimulation of the uterus—uterine contractions that meet the following criteria — Frequency < q 2 minutes — Duration >75 to 90 seconds — Minimal to no relaxation of uterus during resting phase and excessive intrauterine pressure during a contraction (>75 mm Hg) ▼ Nonreassuring-ominous FHR patterns ▼ Signs of water intoxication — Nausea and vomiting — Hypotension, tachycardia, arrhythmias — Decreased urinary output — CNS changes—headache, confusion, altered level of consciousness ▼ Pulmonary edema Take immediate action when *warning signs* are identified ▼ Discontinue Pitocin infusion but maintain primary infusion

Pitocin—cont'd

- ▼ Start at 0.5 mU to 1 mU/min (induction) or 0.5 mU/min (augmentation)
- ▼ Increase at 1 to 2 mU/min increments every 30 to 60 minutes; document maternal-fetal-labor status prior to each increment in chart or flow sheet and on monitor strip
- ▼ Usual maximum dosage required for induction is ≤20 mU/min and ≤10 mU/min for augmentation
- ▼ Rates >20 mU/min require physician assessment and order since side effects become more likely at the higher rates; *rate must never exceed* 40 mU/min
- ▼ Increments continue until contractions meet the following criteria
  - — Frequency q 2 to 3 minutes
  - — Duration 45 to 60 seconds
  - — Moderate to strong intensity (an average of 70 mm Hg with an intrauterine pressure catheter)
  - — 30-second rest period with adequate resting tone (<20 mm Hg with intrauterine pressure catheter)
  - — These requirements should be met within 8 to 12 hours of the start of the induction; if not the induction is discontinued and the patient is allowed to rest; may be resumed at a later time or a cesarean section is performed
- ▼ Once criteria for contractions are met the infusion is maintained at the rate attained until the cervix is 5 to 6 cm dilated; at that point a gradual decrease in oxytocin is begun in decrements of 1 to 2 mU/min every 30 to 60 minutes
- ▼ If signs of fetal distress are detected—turn on side, administer oxygen via mask at 6 to 10 L/min, increase rate of primary infusion if fluid overload is not present
- ▼ Notify physician
- ▼ Prepare to administer tocolytics, as ordered, for hyperstimulation of the uterus
- ▼ Document all data and actions taken

Maintain adequate hydration—IV infusion rate of 125 cc/hr

Provide comfort measures and emotional support

d. Uterine myometrium is capable of withstanding the demands of childbirth including absence of upper segment scarring, trauma, overdistention-overstretching as with multiple gestation or grandmultiparity

2. Current physical status of maternal-fetal unit is determined
   a. Baseline maternal vital signs
   b. General health status
   c. Presence of signs indicative of readiness for labor
      (1) Lightening
      (2) Passage of mucous plug
      (3) Noticeable Braxton-Hick's contractions—false labor
      (4) Cervical ripeness—use Bishop's scale (Table 11-4) to determine cervical readiness to respond to process of labor and need for pharmacological ripening
         (a) Score of <5 indicates a relatively unreceptive cervix with limited chance for successful stimulation of labor
         (b) Score of 5 to 8 has a 95% success rate
         (c) Score of ≥9 has little to no chance of failure
   d. Presence of signs of labor
   e. Fetal maturity and well being
      (1) Gestational age—ultrasound measurement, amniocentesis for lung maturity
      (2) Well being of the fetus—NST, biophysical profile, CST
      (3) Position, presentation, lie, size in relationship to the maternal pelvis
      (4) Baseline tracing of the FHR pattern for 15 to 20 minutes prior to the start of the Pitocin, taking note of nonreassuring patterns

D. Pharmacological measures used to ripen the cervix

1. Assess status of maternal-fetal unit (see Box 11-1) and Bishop's scale (see Table 11-4) prior to and after administration of ripening agent

Table 11-4. Bishop's Scale to Determine Cervical Ripeness

Cervical Factor	0	1	2	3
Dilatation	Closed	1-2	3-4	>4
Effacement	0-30%	40-50%	60-70%	80%
Station	−3	−2	−1, 0	+1, +2
Consistency	Firm	Medium	Soft	—
Cervical position	Posterior	Midposition	Anterior	—

2. Determine that criteria for stimulation of labor have been met
3. Prostaglandin E_2 gel applied to the cervix to ripen—softens and thins the cervix
   a. Determine if contraindications are present such as asthma, pelvic infection, vaginal bleeding, cardiopulmonary, hepatic or renal disease, allergy, nonreassuring FHR patterns
   b. Intracervical route—most effective route for a cervix with a Bishop's scale <3
      (1) Insert 0.5 mg in 2 to 5 ml of gel just below internal cervical os
      (2) Repeat at 6 hour intervals no more than 3 times or 1.5 mg in 24 hours
      (3) Do not use if membranes are ruptured
   c. Intravaginal route—effective route for a cervix with a Bishop's scale of 4 to 5
      (1) Insert 1 to 5 mg in 2 to 10 ml of gel into vagina so it touches outside of cervix
      (2) Repeat in 4 to 6 hours
      (3) May use if membranes are ruptured
   d. Client position—place client in dorsal lithotomy position for insertion and instruct her to remain in bed in a lateral position for 30 to 60 minutes after the insertion; may ambulate if condition is stable
   e. Induction can usually begin in 6 to 12 hours
   f. Side effects include uterine hyperstimulation, nonreassuring FHR patterns, nausea or vomiting, diarrhea
4. Laminaria (desiccated seaweed) or synthetic (Dilapan or Lamicel) cervical dilators are inserted into the cervical canal where they absorb fluid, swell, and thereby slowly dilate and ripen the cervix
   a. Determine if contraindications are present such as pelvic infection, rupture of membranes, nonreassuring FHR patterns
   b. 4 to 9 dilators (tents) are inserted and held in place with sponges placed in the vagina
   c. Risks or side effects include infection, premature rupture of the membranes, cervical trauma, bleeding, nonreassuring FHR patterns, cramping, urinary retention due to pressure of expanding dilator on the bladder

E. Administration of Pitocin to augment or induce labor—Table 11-3 describes principles of Pitocin administration during labor and nursing implications related to its use

VII. Cesarean section birth—necessary when a sound medical-obstetrical reason exists, other measures to secure safe delivery have failed, and/or the health of the maternal-fetal unit is in jeopardy

A. Incisions—most common approaches

1. Abdominal—transverse, suprapubic
2. Uterine—transverse into lower uterine segment

B. Types

1. Emergency—unexpected cesarean birth related to changes in the status of the maternal-fetal unit
   a. Fetal distress or stress
   b. Failure of descent related to cephalopelvic disproportion
   c. Prolapse of umbilical cord
   d. Maternal hemorrhage (placental previa, abruptio placenta), worsening of PIH
2. Elective—planned cesarean birth related to such factors as
   a. Scarring of upper uterine segment associated with previous classic (vertical uterine incision) cesarean birth or uterine surgery or trauma
   b. Active genital tract infections such as herpes
   c. Fetal factors including hydrocephalus, spina bifida, breech or shoulder presentation, multiple gestation

C. Preoperative care measures

1. Physical measures
   a. Establish IV infusion using 18-gauge catheter
   b. Insert indwelling urinary catheter
   c. Prepare surgical site as required by agency policy (shave site, cleanse site with antiseptic soap)
   d. Administer medications such as
      (1) Anticholinergics to dry respiratory secretions if general anesthesia will be used
      (2) Antacids such as Bicitra to neutralize gastrointestinal secretions if an emergency cesarean section is to be performed under general anesthesia; helps to prevent aspiration pneumonia
      (3) Tocolytics, usually terbutaline subcutaneously, if strong uterine contractions are present
   e. Obtain specimens for CBC, type and cross match, urinalysis
2. Psychosocial measures—especially important if surgery is unexpected and is the result of an emergency situation

a. Explain clearly and simply the reason for cesarean birth, purpose for the prepatory measures, what to expect in the operating room
b. Verify informed consent forms are complete
c. Approach the woman and her family in a calm, assured manner—limit environmental stimuli as much as possible
d. Encourage a family centered approach as much as is possible. Example: father in operating room, immediate interaction with newborn at time of birth.

D. Postoperative care measures

1. Physical measures—typical postoperative procedures are required as well as postpartum precautions
   a. Ongoing assessment of maternal status
      (1) Vital signs, heart and breath sounds
      (2) Condition of breasts, fundus, abdominal incision
      (3) Characteristics of lochia
      (4) Level of comfort
      (5) Elimination patterns of bowel and bladder including presence of bowel sounds, passage of flatus, characteristics of urine
      (6) Circulatory status of extremities including signs of thrombophlebitis
   b. IV fluid intake and limited oral intake (ice chips, clear liquids) until peristalsis returns and flatus is passed
   c. Pain relief measures
   d. Administration of oxytocics to enhance contraction of uterus—Pitocin is often added to first one or two liters of IV fluid
   e. Measures to prevent postoperative complications—including coughing and deep breathing, position changes every 2 hours, TED stockings, leg exercises, early ambulation
2. Psychosocial measures
   a. Encourage expression of feelings concerning inability to delivery vaginally, childbirth events
   b. Assist with parental attachment to newborn, breast-feeding, and newborn care—may be inhibited as a result of maternal pain, fatigue, and limited mobility
   c. Prepare woman and family for requirements of a longer recovery period—make referrals as needed

E. Vaginal birth after cesarean (VBAC)

1. Should be encouraged for subsequent pregnancies since low segment incisions are unlikely to rupture making labor and vaginal birth following a cesarean nearly as safe as labor and birth following a previous vaginal delivery
2. Trial of labor (TOL)—4 to 6 hours of labor to determine how labor will progress and if VBAC is possible and safe
   a. Also used when there are questions regarding adequacy of maternal pelvis
   b. Ongoing assessment and complete documentation of maternal-fetal-labor status are critical to ensure a positive outcome

REVIEW QUESTIONS

1. Uterine dystocia may be associated with a pattern of hypotonic uterine contractions. Nurses should realize that
   a. Hypotonic contractions typically occur during the active phase of the first stage of labor
   b. Nulliparous women are most likely to exhibit this type of contraction pattern
   c. Hypotonic contractions are characteristically regular, of low intensity, and occur at a frequency of 4 or fewer in a 10-minute period
   d. Management often involves therapeutic rest using sedatives

2. A nulliparous woman in labor has been diagnosed with a prolonged latent phase of the first stage of labor. Which is true regarding this dysfunctional labor pattern?
   a. Diagnosis for this woman would have been made once the duration of the latent phase exceeded 14 hours
   b. Hypotonic uterine contractions are typically associated with this labor pattern
   c. Management often involves therapeutic rest
   d. Cephalopelvic disproportion (CPD) with failure of the fetal head to stimulate the cervix is often the underlying cause of this pattern

3. Which is a criteria used to diagnose an arrested active phase?
   a. Rate of dilatation less than 1.2 cm/hour for the nullipara
   b. Rate of dilatation less than 1.5 cm/hour for the multipara
   c. Absence of progress in dilatation for more than 2 hours
   d. Absence of fetal descent for 30 minutes or more

4. The fetal presentation of a multiparous woman is breech. Which is *not* typically associated with the birth of a fetus from a breech presentation?
   a. Hypoxia related to cord prolapse and compression
   b. Difficult passage of fetal head related to limited time to mold and to accomplish the cardinal movements of labor
   c. Aspiration of amniotic fluid containing meconium
   d. Precipitous labor and birth

5. A sign that a pregnant woman is in preterm labor would be
   a. Cervical ripening with effacement up to 80% and dilatation up to 2 cm
   b. Uterine contractions that occur at a frequency of 4 contractions in one hour
   c. Uterine contractions with a duration of at least 20 seconds
   d. Pain associated with uterine contractions is intense, constant, and located in the upper abdomen over the fundus

6. A pregnant woman at 27 weeks' gestation calls the nurse stating that she thinks that her labor has begun. She describes uterine contractions of increasing frequency and duration accompanied by discomfort in her lower back. The nurse should instruct this woman to
   a. Report to the hospital immediately
   b. Empty her bladder and drink 3 to 4 eight ounce glasses of water
   c. Rest in a lateral position and count her contractions for 4 hours
   d. Ambulate for 20 minutes to determine if the contractions will diminish in intensity

7. The labor of a pregnant woman at 43 weeks' gestation is being induced. The nurse caring for this woman must be alert for which of the following complications associated with postterm labor and postmaturity syndrome
   a. Polyhydramnios
   b. Precipitous labor
   c. Increased baseline variability and tachycardia
   d. Late and variable deceleration of FHR patterns

8. When caring for a postmature newborn, the nurse should be alert for signs indicative of
   a. Hyperbilirubinemia
   b. Cranial damage associated with severe molding
   c. Hyperglycemia
   d. Cardiac dysfunction

9. A nulliparous woman in labor received an epidural block during the active phase of her labor. Shortly afterwards the progress of her labor slowed. Based on physician's order, the nurse could expect to use which action to augment the progress of this woman's labor?
   a. Administer 10 U of oxytocin (Pitocin) over 2 minutes directly into her vein (IV push)
   b. Assist with amnioinfusion
   c. Stimulate one nipple for short periods between contractions
   d. Apply prostaglandin E_2 gel to her cervix

ANSWERS, RATIONALES, AND TEST-TAKING TIPS

Rationales	Test-Taking Tips
1. Correct answer: a	
Hypotonic contractions typically follow a normal latent phase in multiparous women. These contractions do not develop a regular pattern and occur at a frequency of <3 in 10 minutes. Typical management involves augmentation of labor once cephalopelvic disproportion (CPD) is ruled out.	Recall that the uterus is a muscle and in multiparous women the muscle may be stretched from use and may result in hypotonic contractions. Thus, nulliparous women tend to have stronger uterine function in relation to strength of contraction. Eliminate response *b*. Eliminate response *c* since hypofunction of most anything typically results in irregular function, not regular. Eliminate response d since sedatives may further contribute to the hypotonicity.
2. Correct answer: c	
For a nulliparous woman, the latent phase must exceed 20 hours for a diagnosis of prolonged latent phase to be made. CPD is associated with a protracted or arrested active phase. Hypertonic, not hypotonic, contractions are associated with this dysfunctional labor pattern.	Go with what you know for this question. If you are not sure of options *a, b,* or *d,* option *c* sounds reasonable especially with the clue in the stem of a prolongued labor. Select option *c.*
3. Correct answer: c	
Responses *a* and *b* are criteria for diagnosis of a protracted active phase. Fetal descent must be absent for more than 1 hour to be a criteria for arrested active phase.	Note key word "arrested" active phase which means *stopped*—think cardiac arrest—the heart stops. With this in mind, look at the given responses and narrow to responses *c* or *d* with the word "absence." Then use an educated guess in that appropriate fetal descent probably needs at least an hour, so response *c* is probably the best answer.

4. Correct answer: d

Breech labors tend to be prolonged since the soft buttocks are not effective as a cervical dilator. Responses *a, b,* and *c* are all associated with a breech birth, thereby increasing the risk for fetal injury.

Remember the word "breech" has two e's and so does the word "feet"; thus, this is the fetal breech approach to expulsion. Did the word "precipitous" cause confusion? Then look at the other responses and with a common sense approach think that if the feet come out first then the head has to be inside longer and the cord can slip out. Thus, any of the situations in responses *a, b,* and *c* could happen; so the best response is *d.* Remember to go with the choice based on what you know! Precipitous means *quick.*

5. Correct answer: a

Uterine contractions must occur at a rate of 1 contraction every 10 minutes or less and must last at least 30 seconds. Discomfort is often minimal, vague, and variable; it may be dismissed as GI upset or even go unnoticed.

If you have no idea which response is the correct answer, cluster the responses. Responses *b, c,* and *d* present findings related to contractions; eliminate these and select response *a* which is different.

6. Correct answer: b

Conservative measures should be tried for 1 hour first to see if labor can be suppressed. Activity involved in coming to the hospital or ambulation can stimulate labor further. Ambulation is used later in pregnancy to help to distinguish between false and true contractions. Ambulation will cause false labor contractions to subside.

The number of weeks' gestation is important—27 weeks—is quite early. Eliminate response *c* since it suggests to wait for 4 hours, much too long in this situation. Eliminate response *d* since activity may further the labor which would be detrimental at 27 weeks. Of the two remaining responses *b* seems the best choice since the given data do not indicate an emergency to get to the hospital immediately.

7. Correct answer: d

Late decelerations occur related to placental aging which reduces uteroplacental perfusion. Variable decelerations occur related to drying of the umbilical cord from meconium and compression of the cord from oligohydramnios. Decreased variability is likely related to the factors described above. Labor is usually prolonged since the fetus is often large and the head is more calcified thereby decreasing its ability to mold.

Remember that postterm is late and results in late decelerations. This information may be enough to answer a question correctly as it is in this question.

8. Correct answer: a

Increased RBC production related to hypoxia leads to hyperbilirubinemia as excess RBCs are broken down after birth. Cranial damage is unlikely since the head is more calcified and unlikely to mold significantly. Hypoglycemia occurs because glucose stores are depleted as a result of the stress of a prolonged pregnancy and a difficult birth. Cardiac dysfunction is not a common finding but respiratory distress may occur if meconium was aspirated.

Eliminate response *b*—molding is minimal since skull is more calcified. Think if the fetus had to stay longer and then reserves of energy and glucose would have a tendency to be used up; eliminate response *c*. With responses *a* and *d* left there is little reason to suspect cardiac dysfunctions and recall that it is more common that the bilirubin levels elevate; select response *a*.

9. Correct answer: c

Amniotomy is used to enhance labor since rupture of membranes increases prostaglandin production and allows fetal presenting part to act as dilator. Amnioinfusion is used for oligohydramnios to prevent cord compression. During labor, Pitocin is always mixed in an IV solution and administered using a carefully controlled drip rate. Prostaglandin E_2 gel is used to ripen the cervix in preparation for an induction.

Key rule: Pitocin is not given IV push; it is given in a drip. If you had no idea if the other responses were correct or not, try this approach: responses *a* and *c* would be invasive and response *c* is noninvasive; select the noninvasive to do first; select response *c*. Note that responses *b* and *d* are incorrect actions as explained in rationale.

CHAPTER 12

The Process of Physical Recovery Following Birth

STUDY OUTCOMES

After completing this chapter, the reader will be able to do the following:

- Define the key terms listed.
- Describe the anatomic and physiologic basis for the changes that occur during the process of recovery following birth.
- Identify the expected assessment findings indicative of successful recovery and the warning signs indicative of ineffective recovery for
  - the reproductive system
  - oxygenation-circulation
  - nutrition and fluid-electrolytes
  - bowel and urinary elimination
  - physical activity and rest
  - the integument

KEY TERMS

Fourth stage of labor	The period of physiologic stabilization immediately following birth; lasts approximately 1 to 2 hours.
Fourth trimester	The 3-month period of adjustment the postpartum woman and her family undergo as a result of the process of pregnancy and birth, and the impact of newborn care responsibilities.
Involution	Process whereby the reproductive organs including the uterus return to their approximate prepregnant state.
Postpartum (postnatal) period	The 6- to 8-week period of maternal recovery following birth; also called the puerperium.

CONTENT REVIEW

I. The changes during the puerperium

A. **Anatomic and physiologic adaptations to pregnancy are reversed following birth from**
   1. Decreased hormonal levels especially estrogen and progesterone following the separation and delivery of the placenta
   2. Decreased uterine size following birth of the fetus and removal of the placenta and amniotic fluid and membranes

B. **Process of recovery involves**
   1. Retrogressive changes—return of body systems to a nonpregnant state
   2. Progressive changes—continued adaptation required to care for and nurture the newborn
      a. Lactation—initiation of milk production
      b. Parenting—taking on the role of caregiver

C. **Puerperium is a period of vulnerability for the woman and her family**
   1. Physically at risk for such problems as
      a. Hemorrhage
      b. Infection of breasts, uterus, bladder, episiotomy or lacerations
      c. Thrombophlebitis
      d. Constipation
   2. Psychosocially at risk for problems
      a. Depression
      b. Altered family processes

c. Disturbance in body-image and self-esteem
d. Role conflict
e. Altered sexuality patterns

D. Successful recovery is a gradual process influenced by

1. Maternal physical status including
   a. Maternal health habits including nutrition, hygiene
   b. Level of energy—activity and rest balance
   c. Level of comfort
   d. Presence of health problems
2. Maternal emotional status including reaction to the newborn and the responsibilities of the newborn's care
3. Health status of the newborn
4. Quality of care, support, encouragement from family and support system, including healthcare providers
5. Maternal knowledge concerning recovery, self-care measures, newborn characteristics and care

E. The recovery process of the mother after giving birth includes three areas (Table 12-1)

1. Anatomic and psychologic changes
   a. The reproductive system
   b. Oxygenation—circulation
   c. Nutrition and fluid—electrolytes
   d. Elimination
   e. Physical activity and rest
   f. The integument
2. Expected assessment findings
3. Warning signs—ineffective recovery

Table 12-1. Recovery Process of Mother After Giving Birth

Anatomic and Physiologic Changes	Expected Assessment Findings	Warning Signs—Ineffective Recovery
A. Reproductive System		
Breasts		
Initiation of the lactation cycle ▼ Decreased estrogen and progesterone levels with delivery of placenta leading to suppression of prolactin (lactogenic hormone) activity; pituitary continues to increase prolactin secretion stimulating alveolar cells to secrete milk ▼ Increased blood-lymph flow to breasts ▼ Milk ducts distend with milk Breast-feeding woman—lactation cycle continues as a result of ongoing secretion of prolactin due to ▼ Sucking of infant ▼ Emptying of breasts	Postpartum day 1 to 3 ▼ Essentially no change ▼ Soft, nontender ▼ Secretion of colostrum—yellowish liquid precursor to milk Postpartum day 3 or 4 ▼ Primary engorgement (increased blood and lymph flow) may progress to secondary engorgement (distention of breasts with milk—bluish, white liquid) — Swollen, firm or hard — Warm, prominent venous network — Tender and painful — Leakage of milk	Palpation of a persistent lump that does not disappear after feeding, application of warm packs, or massage Cracks, blisters, bruises, redness on areola Inversion of the nipples Signs of mastitis ▼ Chills, fever ▼ Malaise, nausea ▼ Unilateral breast tenderness with localized redness and swelling

Nonbreast-feeding woman—lactation cycle ceases as a result of ▼ Natural suppression: absence of sucking stimulus and emptying of breasts leads to milk accumulation and negative feedback which suppresses prolactin secretion OR ▼ Pharmacologic suppression: administration of lactation suppressants—estrogen (Tace) or prolactin inhibitors (Parlodel) Natural suppression is recommended more frequently as a means of avoiding medication side effects.	During period of lactation ▼ Breasts—full, nontender ▼ Areolae—intact without bruising, blisters, cracking, redness ▼ Nipples—prominent, erectile ▼ Blocked milk sac or duct may be palpated as a lump; disappears when sac or duct empties Recovery to nonpregnant status about 1 month after cessation of lactation	
Uterus Involution—return of uterus to approximate nonpregnant size and condition (remains slightly larger) ▼ Decreased estrogen-progesterone level leads to autolysis—myometrial cells decrease in size with the breakdown of excess cellular protein	Involution reflected in progressive descent of the fundus ▼ End of third stage of labor with expulsion of the placenta — Midway between the umbilicus and symphysis pubis or slightly higher — Midline — 16 week gestation size	Subinvolution—delay in or failure of uterus and placental site to fully heal as noted by ▼ Persistence of lochia that does not progress as expected ▼ Periods of heavy bleeding ▼ Reversal of lochial stages, i.e., return to rubra after progressing to serosa

Continued.

Table 12-1. Recovery Process of Mother After Giving Birth—cont'd

Anatomic and Physiologic Changes	Expected Assessment Findings	Warning Signs—Ineffective Recovery
▼ Decrease in uterine volume with birth from uterus contracting while blood vessels are compressed to prevent hemorrhage	▼ During the first 12 hours following birth the fundus rises to — Level of the umbilicus or 1 cm above it — Midline ▼ After approximately 24 to 48 hours there is a gradual descent of the fundus — Rate of 1 to 2 cm/day with more rapid progress in breast-feeding women or women receiving oxytocics (medications that stimulate the uterus to contract) — Midline position	Position of fundus above umbilicus and deviated from midline—indicative of bladder distension
Regeneration of endometrium and placental site ▼ Vascular constriction leads to thrombus formation at placental site and destruction of outer layer of decidua ▼ Exfoliation—sloughing off of necrotic uterine tissue (outer decidual layer) and inner layer of endometrium regenerates without scar formation so that implantation in future pregnancies can occur ▼ Lochia—uterine discharge composed of varying amounts of decidual tissue and cellular debris, blood and lymph, bacteria ▼ Progress of endometrial regeneration is reflected in the pattern of changes in lochial characteristics: stage, amount, duration	Muscular contraction of the uterus results in ▼ Firm fundal consistency upon palpation ▼ Afterpains—cramping caused by periodic relaxation and contraction of the uterus; most common in — Women with a more stretched or enlarged uterus: multiparous, large fetus, multiple fetuses	Boggy or soft fundus—uterine contractions ineffective; danger of hemorrhage ▼ Fundus should become firm and remain contracted following massage or administration of oxytocic medications ▼ Failure to remain contracted could indicate problems such as retained placental fragments ▼ Failure of uterus to contract is reflected in — Passage of large clots — Heavy or excessive amount of lochia—pad saturated in 30 to 60 minutes (1 g weight = 1 ml blood) Signs of uterine infection noted ▼ Offensive, foul lochial odor ▼ Persistence of lochia serosa-alba ▼ Uterine tenderness ▼ Fever, malaise

- Breast-feeding women (release of oxytocin during feeding)
- Gradually diminish in intensity over the first few postpartum days

Progressive changes in lochia

- ▼ Lochia rubra—1 to 3 days postpartum; red, thick, small clots, trickles from vagina

Temporary increase or a sudden gush may be noted with a contraction, breast-feeding, fundal massage, ambulation

- ▼ Lochia serosa—3 to 10 days postpartum; light pink to brown, thinner in consistency
- ▼ Lochia alba—10 to 14 days postpartum but can last as long as 3 weeks; yellowish-white
- ▼ Amount decreases as stages progress (see Figure 9-2, p. 234)
  - Scant— <1" on pad/1 hour
  - Light— <4" on pad/1 hour
  - Moderate— <6" on pad/1 hour
- ▼ Odor—fleshy or musty; similar to menses

Continued.

Table 12-1. Recovery Process of Mother After Giving Birth—cont'd

Anatomic and Physiologic Changes	Expected Assessment Findings	Warning Signs—Ineffective Recovery
Cervix, Vagina, Perineum		
Cervix ▼ Loose, thin, fragile, soft ▼ Gradual return to firm consistency—easily distensible for about 4 to 6 days after delivery ▼ Internal os closes by 2 weeks ▼ Resumption of mucous secretion is slow especially for breast-feeding women since estrogen secretion is suppressed	Cervix appears edematous, ecchymotic External cervical os—changes from the circular appearance of a nulliparous woman to a jagged, slitlike appearance	Presence of nonlochial type bleeding could indicate unrepaired or poorly repaired lacerations of cervix, vagina, or perineum and/or poorly repaired episiotomy ▼ Spurting of bright red blood from vagina, perineum ▼ Continuous bright red, heavy bleeding with a firmly contracted fundus ▼ Persistent pelvic-perineal pain, pressure, swelling—hematoma formation
Vagina ▼ Thin, absence of rugae—rugae reappear in 4 weeks ▼ Regains approximate nonpregnant size in 6 to 8 weeks ▼ Return of secretory activity depends upon resumption of ovulation and secretion of estrogen	Flattened appearance of rugae is typical of multiparous women Vaginal dryness Dyspareunia (painful intercourse) may occur due to lack of vaginal secretions	
Labia—decreased tone	Labia appear flabby	
Perineum ▼ Decreased muscle tone ▼ Episiotomy—surgical wound heals in 2 to 3 weeks	Some redness, swelling, and bruising may be present for first day or two	Signs of infection ▼ Persistent redness and swelling ▼ Separation of wound edges ▼ Purulent drainage ▼ Persistent pain

▼ Lacerations—tearing of perineum; heals in 2 to 3 weeks — First degree—through skin and superficial tissues — Second degree—through perineal muscle — Third degree—additionally involves anal sphincter — Fourth degree—additionally involves anterior rectal wall	Wound edges—approximated No drainage Pain present but relieved with local or systemic relief measures	
Menstrual Cycle Delivery of the placenta results in a reduction in estrogen and progesterone levels that had suppressed the menstrual cycle Interdependent feedback mechanism of the hypothalamic-pituitary-ovarian axis gradually returns First few cycles following birth are usually anovulatory ▼ Lactating women—80% ▼ Nonlactating women—50%	Resumption of menstruation ▼ Nonlactating women — 6 to 8 weeks—40 to 45% of women — 12 weeks—65 to 75% of women — 24 weeks—90 to 100% of women ▼ Lactating women — 6 weeks—15% of women — 12 weeks—45% of women — 4 to 8 months for women who practice complete breast feeding (no supplementation) First few menstrual flows may be heavier than usual	Inadequate knowledge concerning return of ovulation and menstruation can result in pregnancy before the woman is physically or emotionally recovered or ready

Continued.

Table 12-1. Recovery Process of Mother After Giving Birth—cont'd

Anatomic and Physiologic Changes	Expected Assessment Findings	Warning Signs—Ineffective Recovery
B. Oxygenation-Circulation		
Blood Volume Reduction to nonpregnant levels in about 3 to 4 weeks Average blood loss with birth ▼ Vaginal—300 to 400 ml ▼ Cesarian—600 to 800 ml Reduction in physiologic edema—extravascular water retained during pregnancy enters the circulatory system and excreted via the kidneys; until excreted with diuresis and diaphoresis, increased fluid volume places stress on the heart and can lead to cardiac decompensation especially in women with cardiac disorders	Blood pressure ▼ Slight decrease related to analgesics, sedatives ▼ Slight increase related to change in vascular network/blood volume, physical exertion of labor, excitement after birth, pain ▼ Postural hypotension, especially after spinal block anesthesia, may occur when first rising to an upright position	Blood pressure ▼ Increase in diastolic with narrowing pulse pressure—early sign of hemorrhagic shock ▼ Continuing decrease in systolic pressure—worsening hemorrhagic shock ▼ Steady increase especially with headache—pregnancy induced hypertension (PIH)
Vascular Network Loss of uteroplacental circulatory network Loss of hormonal stimulation of vasodilation Cardiac output remains elevated for 1 to 2 days then declines returning to nonpregnant levels in 2 to 3 weeks	Pulse ▼ Puerperal bradycardia—slowing of pulse (50 to 70 BPM) due to hemodynamic changes following birth ▼ Slight increase in pulse may occur as a result of exhaustion, pain, excitement, dehydration Respirations—normal baseline range with return to nonpregnant pulmonary function in 6 to 8 weeks	Pulse—steady increase in rate and decrease in strength; hemorrhagic shock Respirations—signs of pulmonary edema associated with cardiac decompensation

Position of diaphragm and heart—non-pregnant position is regained when uterus is emptied and organs return to usual positions Hypercoagulability of blood—reduced over 4 to 5 weeks Varicosities of legs, anus, vulva regress as pelvic pressure is reduced with birth	Hematocrit and hemoglobin—change from baseline level during pregnancy ▼ Decrease day 1 to 2 related to hemodilution with blood loss and reabsorption of extracellular fluid ▼ Increases day 3 to 7 with diuresis and diaphoresis ▼ Reaches nonpregnant levels in 4 to 6 weeks	Signs of thrombophlebitis as a result of venous stasis associated with limited activity and clot formation associated with hypercoagulability Hct/Hgb—below expected ranges for pregnant women may be indicative of excessive and/or continuing blood loss
	White blood cell count ▼ Increased for first 10 days ▼ Average range 14,000 to 16,000 per mm^3 but can be as high as 20,000 to 25,000 per mm^3	WBC—increase of >30% within 6 hours is strongly suggestive of infection
C. Nutrition and Fluid-Electrolytes		
Appetite		
Returns to normal following recovery from anesthesia and fatigue Good appetite essential to stimulate appropriate nutritional intake to support healing and lactation	Presence of hunger and thirst following birth; request for larger portions of food, snacks Nausea and vomiting may be present during fourth stage of labor especially if general anesthesia was used	Poor appetite with limited intake Expressions of ▼ Excessive concern with body image and weight gained during pregnancy ▼ Determination to regain "shape" quickly

Continued.

Table 12-1. Recovery Process of Mother After Giving Birth—cont'd

Anatomic and Physiologic Changes	Expected Assessment Findings	Warning Signs—Ineffective Recovery
Weight Loss		
Early loss results from ▼ Delivery of fetus, placenta, amniotic membranes and fluid ▼ Fluid loss with diuresis and diaphoresis Continuing weight loss results from ▼ Sensible dietary modifications ▼ Sensible exercise and activity program ▼ Utilization of fat stores during lactation	Weight loss pattern ▼ 11 to 13 pounds immediately after birth with loss of uterine contents ▼ 9 pounds—fluid loss with diuresis and diaphoresis ▼ Continuing loss with return to prepregnant weight in 2 to 3 months	
Dehydration—may be present especially after long, difficult labors Lactation—production of milk requires energy gained through ▼ Increased caloric intake reflected in a nutritious diet ▼ Use of fat stores accumulated during pregnancy ▼ Physical and emotional rest	Signs of dehydration ▼ Elevated temperature up to 100.4° F in first 24 hours ▼ Concentrated urine ▼ Thirst	Temperature of ≥100.4° F after the first 24 hours strongly suggests infection especially if accompanied by chills, malaise, signs of infection in breasts or genitourinary tract

D. Elimination		
Bowel		
Flatus accumulates due to increased intestinal space following birth; peristalsis begins to increase as progesterone level decreases and flatus is passsed First bowel elimination may be delayed due to ▼ Decreased tone and peristalsis of intestines related to progesterone level ▼ Tenderness or pain related to episiotomy, lacerations, hemorrhoids—fear of further pain and "ripping stitches" with bowel movement ▼ Decreased abdominal muscle tone resulting from stretching during pregnancy ▼ Decreased activity level ▼ Effects of labor: enema (if given), diarrhea, decreased intake of food and fluids Hemorrhoids—may appear or enlarge with pressure of fetal part and vigorous pushing during labor; gradually decrease in size during the puerperium	Stronger, more frequent bowel sounds Passage of flatus Elimination of soft, formed feces by day 2 or 3 postpartum Hemorrhoids enlarged, edematous Hemorrhoidal discomfort	Holding back on passing feces due to excessive fear of pain and injury ▼ Constipation—no bowel movement by day 3 or 4 ▼ Straining with passage of feces increases pain experienced and may disrupt healing ▼ Excessively large and/or bleeding hemorrhoids

Continued.

Table 12-1. Recovery Process of Mother After Giving Birth—cont'd

Anatomic and Physiologic Changes	Expected Assessment Findings	Warning Signs—Ineffective Recovery
Bladder		
Reversal of renal adaptations takes 2 to 8 weeks By products of metabolic and regressive changes during recovery are excreted into blood and urine Postpartum diuresis—increased production of urine to rid body of fluid retained during pregnancy; bladder fills more rapidly High risk for urinary retention ▼ Edema and decreased sensitivity of bladder and urethra due to effects of labor, birth, and regional anesthetics ▼ Discomfort of lacerations and episiotomy ▼ Restoration of nonpregnant bladder tone and function, and usual elimination patterns occurs within one week	Voiding patterns ▼ Voids within 4 to 8 hours of birth ▼ Amount of each voiding should be at least 100 ml ▼ Total urine produced—about 3000 ml/24 hours Absence of bladder distension Common complaints during first few days include ▼ Delay in initiation of stream ▼ Slower stream ▼ Burning when urine comes in contact with episiotomy or lacerations Urine may contain protein (+1) due to autolysis, lactose with lactation, and blood due to hemorrhagic areas in bladder from labor and birth as well as contamination with lochia BUN increased due to autolysis	Signs of urinary retention and bladder distension ▼ Frequent voidings of less than 100 ml each—suggests overflow ▼ Continued feeling of urgency even after voiding ▼ Bladder palpable above symphysis pubis—manual pressure on bladder produces urgency ▼ Dullness upon percussion of bladder ▼ Displacement of uterus upward above umbilicus and/or laterally ▼ Displacement of uterus can result in loss of uterine contraction (boggy fundus) and increase in lochial flow (bright red bleeding) ▼ Repeated and prolonged retention and distention can lead to —Urinary tract infection (UTI) —Delay in return of normal bladder function and elimination patterns —Decrease in bladder tone

E. Physical Activity/Rest		
Abdominal Muscle Tone Returns gradually over 6 weeks Depends on prepregnant muscle tone, degree of stretching with pregnancy, and amount of adipose tissue Facilitated by postpartum exercises Offers limited support to abdominal contents and enlarged uterus	Abdominal muscles appear loose and flabby—soft and doughlike upon palpation Abdominal protrusion when upright—soft distended appearance Diastasis recti—separation of abdominal wall muscles—separation noted upon palpation and by contour of abdomen	Expressions of excessive disturbance with appearance—still "looks pregnant"; may have negative influence on nutrition and exercise during the postpartum period to rush return to prepregnant appearance Limited social support may inhibit ability to achieve a healthy balance of activity and rest
Movement and Activity Level May Be Affected by Muscle strain and soreness due to muscular efforts of labor and birth Perineal pain aggravated by movement Loss of sensation and ability to move lower limbs related to use of epidural or spinal anesthesia	Posture slightly bent, gait slow to reduce perineal pain when moving Muscle aching in arms, neck, shoulders, lower back, and pelvis	
Joints Stabilize within 6 to 8 weeks Joints in feet may not fully return to prepregnant position—feet remain slightly larger	Change in shoe size	

Continued.

Table 12-1. Recovery Process of Mother After Giving Birth—cont'd

Anatomic and Physiologic Changes	Expected Assessment Findings	Warning Signs—Ineffective Recovery
Fatigue is often present related to Sleep disturbances during later part of pregnancy Hormonal changes Work of labor and excitement of birth Altered rest-sleep patterns after birth ▼ Hospital environment ▼ Pain and discomfort ▼ Responsibilities of caring for self, newborn, and family Continuing fatigue negatively affects healing, lactation, and emotions		
F. The Integument		
Postpartum diaphoresis—reversal of physiologic edema of pregnancy results in profuse sweating during first week after birth Decrease in melanocyte stimulating hormone Peripheral vasodilation subsides as estrogen level decreases Elasticity of skin is regained	Night sweats Disappearance of melasma Complete or partial fading of ▼ Areola-nipple darkening ▼ Linea nigra Regression of palmar erythema and epulis; spider nevi may remain Loss of fine hair that grew during pregnancy Resumption of fingernail strength and consistency—firmer and stronger Fading of striae gravidarum from bright reddish-pink to silvery-white	

REVIEW QUESTIONS

1. As part of the postpartum assessment, the nurse examines the breasts of a primiparous breast-feeding woman who is one day postpartum. An expected finding would be
   a. Soft, nontender
   b. Leakage of milk
   c. Swollen, tender
   d. A few small blisters or bruises on the areola

2. The onset of the lactation cycle is initially dependent upon
   a. Increased secretion of prolactin
   b. Increased circulation to the breasts
   c. Sucking of newborn which empties the breasts
   d. Decreased levels of estrogen and progesterone with the delivery of the placenta

3. A postpartum bottle-feeding woman asks the nurse how long it will take before "my breasts are back to normal?" The nurse should tell the woman that the process of breast recovery after pregnancy, called involution, takes about
   a. 2 weeks
   b. 4 weeks
   c. 6 weeks
   d. 12 weeks

4. Palpation of the fundus 18 hours after birth reveals that it is firm, 2 fingerbreaths above the umbilicus, and deviated to the left of midline. The nurse should
   a. Massage the fundus
   b. Administer methergine 0.2 mg, PO that has been ordered PRN
   c. Assist the woman to empty her bladder
   d. Recognize this as an expected assessment finding

5. Which of the following women is *least* likely to experience afterpains?
   a. Primiparous, bottle-feeding woman who delivered a 7 pound baby at 40 weeks' gestation
   b. Multiparous woman who delivered twin boys at 27 weeks' gestation
   c. Primiparous, breast-feeding woman who delivered an 8 pound baby at 42 weeks' gestation
   d. Multiparous, gestational diabetic woman who delivered an 11 pound macrosomic baby at 38 weeks' gestation

6. When assessing a multiparous woman on her first day postpartum, the nurse would expect to find
  a. Fundus two fingerbreaths below the umbilicus, firm
  b. Lochia serosa, moderate, no clots or foul odor
  c. Full, tender breasts
  d. Painful, intact episiotomy with some erythema, edema, and bruising

7. Dyspareunia during the postpartum period is most likely the result of
  a. Inadequate secretion of vaginal mucus
  b. Flattened vaginal rugae
  c. Tenderness of cervix
  d. Pressure on uterus

8. During the early postpartum period, excessive blood loss can occur from a laceration or the episiotomy. Which finding is reflective of blood loss from this source?
  a. Trickle of thick, deep red blood from the vagina
  b. Boggy fundus
  c. Passage of large clots
  d. Persistent pelvic-perineal pain, pressure, and swelling

9. A postpartum woman who is breast-feeding asks the nurse about the return of ovulation and menstruation. The nurse should tell this woman that
  a. Ovulation does not resume until lactation ceases
  b. Menstruation resumes for the majority of breast-feeding women within 6 weeks of birth
  c. The first few cycles are usually anovulatory, especially for the breast-feeding women
  d. Complete breast-feeding is a reliable method of birth control

10. Which finding would be a source of concern if noted during the assessment of a woman who is 12 hours postpartum?
  a. Postural hypotension
  b. Temperature 100.4° F
  c. Bradycardia—pulse rate of 55 beats per minute
  d. Positive Homan's sign

ANSWERS, RATIONALES, AND TEST-TAKING TIPS

Rationales	Test-Taking Tips
1. Correct answer: a Breasts are essentially unchanged for the first 1 to 3 days after birth. Colostrum is present and may leak from the nipples. On day 3 to 4 primary engorgement begins, which can progress to secondary engorgement with *b* and *c* as characteristic findings during this time. Response *d* indicates problems with breast-feeding technique.	The important focus of this question is the time "one day postpartum." For an expected finding response *a* is more likely than the abnormals in the other responses.
2. Correct answer: d While responses *a, b,* and *c* are all important in the process of lactation especially in the continuation of the cycle, estrogen and progesterone levels must decrease to remove the suppression on prolactin activity and allow the lactation process to begin.	The important word in the stem is "initially" so this leads to thinking that after reading the responses you should establish the sequence of possible events. The first event is response *d* and therefore matches with the time framework of the question.
3. Correct answer: b Involution of the breast takes about 1 month (4 weeks) after birth for the bottle-feeding mother and 1 month after cessation of lactation for the breast-feeding mother.	Use the number strategy if you have no idea what is the correct answer. Eliminate the extremes—responses *a* and *d*. Make a conservative guess which is response *b,* the correct answer.

4. Correct answer: c

The findings indicate a full bladder which pushes the uterus up and to the right or left of midline. The course of action would therefore be to empty the bladder. A firm fundus should not be massaged. Methergine is not required since the fundus is firm.

Recall that a "fundal deviation" is typically derived from a "full bladder."

5. Correct answer: a

Afterpains are most common when uterus is overstretched as with a multiparous woman, a large fetus, multiple gestation. Additionally, breast-feeding stimulates the release of oxytocin which causes the uterus to contract.

First establish that the uterine stretch is least in a primiparous woman and eliminate responses *b* and *d* with the multiparous woman. Less stretch = less afterpains. Then eliminate response *d* with an educated guess that a more natural feeding method might release hormones to contract the uterus as compared to bottle-feeding.

6. Correct answer: d

Episiotomies often exhibit the findings described as a result of the pressure of birth, local anesthesia, and the inflammatory process essential for healing. Fundus should be 1 finger below and midline. Lochia should be rubra, moderate, with no clots or foul odor. Breasts should be soft and nontender.

The key factor in the stem is "time"—one day postpartum.

7. Correct answer: a

Until resumption of ovulation and the secretion of estrogen, vaginal dryness

Think of what you know in general about dyspareunia—a common cause is a dry vaginal mucosa

will be present related to limited production of lubricating mucus. Rugae do not affect intercourse. Responses *c* and *d* while possible are unlikely to be problematic once intercourse resumes a few weeks after birth.

especially in the older woman with hormonal changes with menopause. Then associate the changes in hormonal production after pregnancy to make an educated guess, response *a*.

8. Correct answer: d

Response *d* describes hematoma formation from accumulation of blood and clot formation in the tissue related to incompletely repaired lacerations or episiotomies as well as other types of pelvic injuries. Response *a* is an expected characteristic of moderate lochia rubra. Apparent blood loss from lacerations and episiotomies would be spurting of bright red blood. Responses *b* and *c* are characteristic of blood loss related to uterine atony.

Think anatomy—responses *a, b,* and *c* do not really point to the perineal area where an episiotomy or laceration is typically found.

9. Correct answer: c

The menstrual cycle resumes even while the woman is breast-feeding, though it is delayed for as long as 4 to 8 months in women who practice complete breast-feeding. Most breast-feeding women experience return of menstruation after 12 weeks. Breast-feeding is never to be used as a method of birth control.

Note that response *c* addresses both ovulation and menstration— "first few cycles . . . anovulatory." The other responses give statements related to only one of the two topics asked by the client.

10. Correct answer: d

Responses *a* and *c* are expected related to circulatory changes after birth. Temperature of 100.4° F in the first 24 hours is highly reflective of dehydration which is easily corrected by increasing oral fluid intake. Positive Homan's sign is suggestive of thrombophlebitis.

In given situation of a post procedure client response *d* is of greatest concern. Eliminate the other responses by reviewing what are the expected findings.

CHAPTER 13

Psychosocial Adjustment to the Newborn

STUDY OUTCOMES

After completing this chapter, the reader will be able to do the following:

- Define the key terms listed.
- Identify factors which influence the process of parental and family attachment and adjustment to the newborn.
- Describe behaviors indicative of effective and ineffective parental attachment to the newborn.
- Discuss nursing measures effective in promoting parental and family attachment and adjustment to the newborn.
- Describe the stages of maternal psychosocial recovery and adjustment following pregnancy and birth.

KEY TERMS

Attachment	A reciprocal process whereby an enduring bond is established between the infant and its parents and family.
Engrossment	Intense paternal interest and involvement with his newborn.
Letting-go (interdependence stage)	Last stage of the maternal psychosocial recovery process characterized by the giving up of the role as a pregnant woman for the role of mother and the reestablishment of other roles such as that of partner-spouse.
Postpartum blues (baby blues)	Mild, transient letdown feeling or depression that occurs approximately 3 days after birth and again 1 month later; typically lasts from 3 days to 1 week.
Postpartum depression (psychosis)	Severe mood disorder that is prolonged in nature and requires professional intervention.
Taking hold	Stage of maternal psychosocial recovery beginning about 3 days after birth that is characterized by vacillation between the need for nurturing and the need to take charge of self and newborn.
Taking in	Stage of maternal psychosocial recovery during the first 1 to 2 days following birth when maternal dependency needs predominate.

CONTENT REVIEW

I. Overview of psychosocial adjustment with an application of the nursing process

A. The postpartum period is a time of role transition for

1. Parents of first or parents of more than one child
2. Brother or sister
3. Grandparents

B. All family members need to make emotional adjustments as family processes, roles, and relationships change

C. Nurses must develop awareness of cultural variations regarding postpartal and newborn care practices and beliefs

D. A potential for crisis exists during this period of transition and adjustment—influencing factors include

1. Perception of the event—degree to which addition of a new family member is viewed realistically in terms of

   a. Recognizing that parenthood requires additional responsibilities and commitment
   b. Anticipating that sibling jealousy and regression is a normal occurrence as children adjust to a new baby
   c. Accepting that temporary role conflict can occur during the process of adjusting family, parenting, and career roles
2. Coping mechanisms—degree to which they are utilized and the level of their effectiveness
   a. Attending classes to learn about newborn care
   b. Reading appropriate literature related to parenting
   c. Seeking guidance and accepting help from available resource persons such as nurses, lactation consultants, physicians, family members, and friends
3. Situational supports—degree to which these supports are available *and* supportive
   a. Plan of support—mutually determined and agreed upon during pregnancy. Example: parent, grandparent roles and responsibilities identified and accepted.
   b. Willing to accept assistance from community agencies. Examples: WIC, well baby clinics, parenting support groups.

E. Nurses need to develop an awareness of required family adjustments and to utilize the nursing process to support family efforts to incorporate the newborn into their lives

1. Assessment should take note of
   a. Presence of factors influencing adjustment
   b. Cultural influences including beliefs, rituals, and assigned family responsibilities related to the care of the mother and newborn after birth
   c. Level of parental knowledge and experience
   d. Effectiveness of each family member's transition to incorporate the newborn into their lives—sibling and grandparent visitation, telephone follow-up, and home visitation are ideal times for observation
   e. Family-newborn interactions and progress in parental-newborn attachment (Table 13-1)
2. Typical nursing diagnoses related to maternal-family recovery and adjustment
   a. Ineffective individual coping related to conflicting demands of family, newborn care, and career responsibilities
   b. Situational low self-esteem related to perceived difficulty in meeting the needs of newborn

Table 13-1. Behavioral Indicators of Effective and Ineffective Attachment

Effective Attachment Behaviors	Ineffective Attachment Behaviors
Utilization of Touch	*Utilization of Touch*
Caresses with fingertips—uses hands to explore newborn's body	Touches limited to essential contact—feeding, changing diaper
Cuddles newborn close to body	Handles with carelessness, indifference
Kisses newborn	Shows little sign of affection
Gently handles and administers care	
Utilization of Visual Contact	*Utilization of Visual Contact*
Gazes at newborn	Looks away from newborn
Makes eye contact	Avoids eye contact
Inspects newborn's characteristics	
Verbalization	*Verbalization*
Chooses name with care	Makes persistent negative statements regarding newborn's appearance and behavior
Uses name or affectionate nickname when talking to or speaking about newborn	Uses derogatory nicknames when talking to or speaking about newborn
Expresses pleasure regarding newborn, its appearance and behavior	Expresses continued disappointment regarding gender of newborn
Identifies newborn characteristics that resemble family members	
Expressions of Interest in Newborn	*Expressions of Interest in Newborn*
Displays eagerness to learn about the proper care of newborn	Ignores or does not recognize newborn's cues such as hunger, discomfort
Seeks feedback concerning care efforts	Expresses limited interest in learning about or caring for newborn
Asks questions about newborn and its condition	Demonstrates eagerness to send newborn back to nursery
Expresses disappointment when newborn must return to nursery	Asks few questions regarding status of newborn
Identifies and responds to newborn's cues such as for hunger and discomfort	

▼ *Caution* regarding parental interaction with a newborn, behavioral indicators of ineffective attachment should be evaluated carefully, over time and in the context of situational factors such as history of dysfunctional labor, fatigue, pain, inexperience, fear, and cultural beliefs. *Never rush to judge!*

c. Potential for family growth related to birth of healthy newborn
d. Alteration in family processes related to addition of new family member
e. Risk for altered parenting related to inexperience and inadequate family support

3. Nursing support is a critical factor in the process of maternal-family adjustment; nursing measures include
   a. Encouraging family members to openly express their feelings, concerns, and questions
   b. Working with the mother to develop approaches that will help her to balance and prioritize personal and family needs
   c. Providing information through health teaching
   d. Creating opportunities for the family to interact with and practice caring for the newborn
   e. Making referrals to community agencies as indicated by the needs of the family
      ▼ Nursing interventions must be sensitive to the cultural variations determined during the assessment process
4. Evaluation of the effectiveness of the interventions needs to be accomplished; evaluation criteria can include
   a. Client reports during telephone follow-up that she feels more confident in caring for newborn and has even found a little time to participate in activities with her friends
   b. Family members interact in a positive manner with their newborn
   c. Parents demonstrate skill as they bathe and feed newborn
   d. Parents apply appropriate safety principles when caring for the newborn and altering their home environment
   e. Parents used the sibling visitation opportunity to acquaint other children with the new baby

II. Process of parental-family attachment to the newborn

A. Attachment

1. *Attachment* and *bonding* describe the development of the parent-family-newborn relationship
2. Bonding—the early stage of attachment; parents experience attraction to their newborn as they make eye contact, touch and stroke, and experience the newborn's grasp and suck

3. Attachment—a reciprocal process; represents development of feelings of loyalty and affection that tend to grow and strengthen over time
   a. The process begins during pregnancy and can be facilitated by such activities as
      (1) Hearing the fetal heart beat
      (2) Seeing its image on ultrasound
      (3) Perceiving fetal movements and activity responses to extrauterine stimuli such as voices, music, emotions
   b. The process continues following birth and is enhanced by activities and policies that facilitate early, close, frequent contact, interaction, and communication between the newborn and its family (Box 13-1)

B. Six factors influencing the process of attachment

1. Nature of the relationship of the father and the mother with each other and with their own parents since it is within these relationships that parents learn how to love and care for others including their new baby and other children
   a. Emotional health and ability of each person to form strong positive relationships, to give and receive affection

Box 13-1. Nursing Measures Designed to Facilitate Attachment

Provide parents interaction time with their newborn as soon as possible after birth

Create family centered birthing practices that include birthing rooms, presence of family members at the birth, and celebratory activities (champagne, photographs, cakes)

Introduce newborn to parents, teaching them about newborn characteristics, behaviors, and sensory capabilities

Show parents how to communicate with their newborn by using touch, eye contact, and speech

Facilitate parent participation in the care of the newborn by providing
- ▼ Classes, demonstrations, supervised practice related to infant care
- ▼ Positive feedback regarding skill attainment
- ▼ Rooming-in with newborn and mother-baby/couplet care
- ▼ Unlimited paternal visiting hours

Demonstrate newborn's ability to respond to parental care and communication

Foster family interaction with newborn by providing siblings and grandparents with opportunities to communicate with the newborn and participate in its care

   b. Stability and quality of the relationships in terms of openness of communication, mutual respect, affection, and concern for each other, and loyalty
   c. Supportive social network within which these relationships exist, such as other family members (aunts, uncles, cousins), friends
   d. Cultural expectations and influences with regard to family role relationships and responsibilities
2. Pregnancy experience—attachment is facilitated by a positive pregnancy experience
   a. Physical and emotional health of the mother
   b. Adequacy and nature of support received from family, friends, and healthcare providers
   c. Parental and family attitudes toward the pregnancy—wanted, planned, unplanned, unwanted
3. Childbirth events
   a. Labor and delivery progress
      (1) Met and followed expectations
      (2) Problems developed requiring unexpected medical intervention, operative procedures, separation of family members from each other and newborn
   b. Measures employed by the birthing agency (hospital, birthing center) to initiate the process of attachment following birth
4. Postpartum condition of mother and newborn are conducive to the initiation of attachment fostering activities that allow for close, frequent contact with the newborn
5. Newborn characteristics
   a. Appearance
      (1) Reflective of expectations
      (2) Identifiable resemblance to family members
      (3) Presence of external anomalies or injuries
   b. Gender
      (1) Desired gender
      (2) Importance of the gender of the newborn to parents and family—cultural implications
   c. Ability to respond to parents and family
      (1) Makes eye contact
      (2) Grasps strongly
      (3) Responds to voices by alerting or quieting behaviors
      (4) Responds to caregiving efforts—latches on strongly to the breast, falls asleep after feeding

d. General temperament
   (1) Consolability—ability to console self and to respond to consoling and soothing efforts of family
   (2) Cuddliness
   (3) Difficult to arouse or console, irritable
e. Presence of physical anomalies or illnesses requiring follow-up and causing concern

6. Parental characteristics
   a. Age and maturation level
      (1) Adolescent parents may lack maturity to cope with the responsibilities and frustration of newborn care until they have completed the tasks of adolescence—their own needs and that of their infants often conflict
      (2) Older parents may encounter conflict between parenting and career demands
   b. Experience and knowledge regarding newborn care and characteristics-behaviors including access to information, role models, guidance
   c. Ability to recognize the needs of the newborn and meet these needs with confidence
   d. Cultural expectations and beliefs regarding the role responsibilities and behaviors of a mother and of a father

III. Maternal psychosocial recovery-adjustment following pregnancy and birth and maternal role attainment

A. Process of recovery is reflected in progress through a set of stages (Rubin, 1975) as described in Table 13-2

1. Progress through the stages and achievement of competence and comfort with the role of mother is highly individualized and influenced by
   a. Maternal factors
      (1) Accomplishment of the developmental tasks of pregnancy
      (2) Events during pregnancy and childbirth and mother's perception of them—Did she do a good job? Did she reach her goals and expectations?
      (3) Maternal health status
      (4) Stability of relationship with family members especially the father of the baby
      (5) Level of confidence and self-esteem

Table 13-2. Stages of Maternal Psychosocial Recovery Following Pregnancy and Birth

Factor	Taking In Stage Dependent	Taking Hold Stage Dependent-Independent	Letting Go Stage Interdependence
Typical duration (highly individualized)	First 1 to 2 days following birth	Follows taking in stage and lasts 4 to 5 weeks	Follows taking hold stage and indicates psychosocial recovery is completed
Behaviors Emotions	▼ Dependency needs predominate ▼ Physical needs for rest, food, pain relief must be met ▼ Wants to be cared for ▼ Expresses need to reflect on events and behavior during labor and birth ▼ Reduced attention span related to pain and fatigue limits learning readiness ▼ Asks questions and expresses concern regarding status of self/newborn	▼ Vacillates between her need for nurturing and her need to take charge of self-newborn ▼ Begins to focus on meeting needs of newborn ▼ Progresses in her ability to care for self and newborn ▼ Responsive to practice and learning opportunities ▼ Fatigue occurs related to recovery and caregiving demands ▼ Baby blues may occur ▼ Daily routines and patterns are established	▼ Gives up role as pregnant woman for role as mother ▼ Reestablishes role as spouse-partner and resumes career role ▼ Views newborn as a separate being from herself ▼ More willing to involve others in care of newborn so she can take time for self ▼ Family patterns and roles are adjusted

Continued.

Table 13-2. Stages of Maternal Psychosocial Recovery Following Pregnancy and Birth—cont'd

Factor	Taking In Stage Dependent	Taking Hold Stage Dependent-Independent	Letting Go Stage Interdependence
Implications for Nursing	▼ Nurturing of the mother helps her to progressively nurture her baby and care for herself ▼ Meet needs for pain relief, nutrition, and periods of uninterrupted rest ▼ Assist with care of newborn so mother can rest ▼ Encourage participation in a childbirth review, helping her to analyze and to accept the experience as it occurred; videotapes of the birth can be used for this review when the mother feels ready and has someone to watch it with her and discuss her concerns and questions ▼ Provide short health teaching sessions that focus on essential information required for safe discharge ▼ Incorporate practice, reinforcement, review, and written materials as appropriate	▼ Help mother to plan realistically for tasks ahead including time for meeting own needs ▼ Provide opportunity for and encourage rooming-in or mother-baby care—helpful for learning and getting to know the newborn ▼ Identify family members and friends who will assist her with newborn care and family demands—help her to realize it is okay to ask for and accept help ▼ Provide teaching sessions and demonstrations that include family ▼ Help her to learn how to prioritize—what is essential and what can wait	▼ Prepare mother for feelings such as sadness and guilt that she may experience when separating self from newborn to resume career role ▼ Discuss changes that may occur in relationship with spouse-partner including issues of sexuality, feelings of jealousy and competition with newborn for attention ▼ Evaluate family recovery and make referrals if signs of ineffective recovery are present and persistent

(6) Maternal age
(a) Younger mother may lack the knowledge, life experiences, socioeconomic resources, and family support needed to develop as a parent
(b) Older mothers may have sufficient knowledge, life experiences, economic and social support required for parenting yet may also experience career demands and a need to be a perfect parent
(7) Level of stress and role strain-conflict

b. Newborn factors
(1) Newborn health status
(2) Newborn temperament—responsiveness to caregiving and affection

2. Maternal behaviors indicate readiness to progress to the next stage of recovery
a. Early discharge limits the nurse's ability to observe behaviors and facilitate progress
b. Inform mother and her family of the behaviors characteristic of each stage and the supportive activities that facilitate progress
c. Telephone follow-up and home visits are helpful in determining degree of progress

3. Referral to community agencies that provide home visitation may be helpful in situations where mothers are at risk as a result of
a. Early discharge
b. Limited support including family, financial, emotional
c. Lack of experience and knowledge
d. Inadequate attachment behaviors and disinterest in caring for the newborn

▼ Adolescent or single mothers often exhibit these risk factors and require support in their parenting efforts

B. Self-esteem influences confidence in and performance of the maternal role

1. Personal evaluation of her behavior during pregnancy and childbirth
2. Personal evaluation of her success as a mother influenced by
a. "Ideal mother" myth—a woman is born knowing how to care for her baby and her baby will be immediately responsive to her care
b. Role of mother she defined for herself when meeting the developmental tasks of pregnancy

c. Reactions of others (family, friends, healthcare providers) to her performance
d. Response of newborn to her care efforts
e. Skill of others in care of newborn—may be discouraged if she determines that her skill is inadequate when compared to others such as the father of the baby, her mother, mother-in-law, sister

C. Alterations in maternal mood, emotions

1. Fluctuations in mood occur as a result of many interrelated factors
   a. Changes in hormonal levels with delivery of the placenta
   b. Presence of fatigue, pain, and discomfort
   c. Transitions in relationships for self and family
   d. Responsibilities of newborn care, concerns about health status of newborn, adequacy of breast-feeding, and anxiety regarding effectiveness as a mother
   e. Role strain and conflicts as other demands compete with demands of newborn
2. Postpartum blues (baby blues)
   a. Majority of postpartum women experience the blues approximately 3 days after birth and again at approximately 1 month postpartum
   b. The blues are a normal occurrence, mild and transient in nature, and typically last 3 days to 1 week
   c. May progress to a mild, self-limiting depression
   d. Especially vulnerable are
      (1) Career women who wait until later in life to have their first child and have developed an idealistic view of motherhood
      (2) Adolescent mothers
      (3) First-time mothers
      (4) Mothers with a limited support system of family and friends with which to share concerns and experiences
   e. Characteristic blues behaviors include irritability, moodiness, restlessness, crying spells, sleeplessness, anger, anxiety, withdrawal with decreasing interest in surroundings
   f. Effective therapeutic measures
      (1) Anticipatory guidance-preparation of the woman and her family regarding stressors of the postpartum

period and healthy coping mechanisms to deal with stress of this period
- (2) Involve family in a therapeutic approach that includes identification of characteristic blues behaviors and implementation of supportive measures
- (3) Supportive measures to suggest
  - (a) Take time out to rest, sleep, do things for self or with friends
  - (b) Share responsibilities of newborn care with family—asking for and accepting help is okay
  - (c) Family and friends to provide positive reinforcement for mothering efforts

3. Postpartum depression (psychosis)—characteristic behaviors
   - a. Exaggeration of behaviors associated with the blues
   - b. Hostility and inappropriate responses directed toward herself, newborn, and family
   - c. Emotional lability
   - d. Difficulty coping
   - e. Behavior that is psychotic (out of touch with reality)
   - f. Capability of doing harm to herself or her newborn

IV. Adolescent mothers

A. Require support in their work to attain the role of mother—recognition that they do have the potential for parenting

B. Efforts as mothers must be evaluated

1. Progress of attachment
2. Progress in development of parenting skills that will meet their newborn's physical, emotional, and developmental needs
3. Expression of feelings regarding the newborn and their skills as mothers
4. Ability to
   - a. Evaluate their parenting skills
   - b. Seek and accept help and guidance
   - c. Identify newborn cues and needs

C. Level of self-esteem and confidence must be fostered by

1. Teaching and demonstrating appropriate parenting skills and responses
2. Opportunities for supervised practice
3. Provision of praise and positive reinforcement when successful

V. Paternal adjustment

A. Paternal role behaviors following birth are influenced by the father role he defined as he adapted to his partner's pregnancy and the expectations of his culture

1. Fathers of today often take on a more active, nurturing parent role than their own fathers
   a. View relationship with mother as partnership
   b. Attend parenting classes
   c. Dual income and career families are becoming the norm
2. Paternal role behaviors may emphasize socialization and play activites rather than caregiving behaviors
3. Parental role responsibilities should be mutually defined by both parents and result in a satisfying experience for both
4. Paternal participation in active caregiving should be fostered by including him in newborn care classes and providing opportunities for him to participate in the care of the newborn

B. Engrossment—facilitated by touch, eye to eye contact, awareness of newborn similarities to himself, and positive newborn responses to his voice and care

C. Fathers are an important source of maternal support—often identified by the mother as her most significant support person

1. Parental relationship and their ability to support and encourage one another should be assessed
2. Father should be provided with information regarding
   a. Maternal recovery following birth including her physical and emotional needs
   b. Supportive or care measures he can implement to facilitate her recovery

D. Fathers are an important source of support and guidance for their children by providing

1. The care and attention siblings need to facilitate their adjustment to the new baby
2. A role model for male behavior needed by their children as they determine their concept of what is male and develop relationships with men
3. Note: The importance of fathers is under intense research. There is great concern regarding the societal impact of the growing number of single parent households with mother as the primary caregiver and with limited to no male influence.

VI. Sibling adjustment

A. **Siblings must now deal with the**
   1. Reality of the newborn and the impact it has on their position in the family
   2. Need to share their parents' love, time, and attention
   3. Increased responsibilities and loss of free time as they are required to participate in the care of the newborn and help with household tasks
   4. Loss of immediate gratification of their needs as the newborn takes precedence

B. **Influencing factors**
   1. Age and level of maturation—the younger child may have greater difficulty waiting for needs to be met and sharing of parents while the older child may resent the demands of added responsibilities
   2. Nature of their preparation for the birth and the degree they were allowed to participate in the events of pregnancy and birth
   3. Security of their relationship with their parents
   4. Level of self-esteem they have developed
   5. Nature of previous experiences they have had with newborns including interaction with friends who have had newborns in their families
   6. Characteristics of the newborn and the degree to which it meets the sibling's expectations—small and helpless, not a playmate as promised; a brother, not a sister as they had hoped

C. **Typical sibling reactions to the arrival of a newborn**
   1. Enthusiastic, excited, eager to help care for newborn, express concern for newborn and use gentle touch and kisses to communicate
   2. Anger and rejection directed toward the newborn and even parents—"If you loved me so much why did you need another baby?"
      a. Initial anger, resentment, and impatience are to be expected as normal reactions
      b. Continuing anger accompanied by physical expressions against newborn and disturbances in life activities such as eating, sleeping, and school require professional evaluation
   3. Relationship with mother may undergo a transitory change
      a. May reject mother upon her arrival home as they react to the feeling of abandonment and separation anxiety they experienced when she left them to give birth
      b. May cling to mother afraid she will leave them again

4. Regression may occur in younger children
    a. The adjustment required with the birth of a baby is a stressor
    b. May be used to gain attention for themselves and the same loving care they see given to the baby
    c. Children may ask to be breast or bottle fed, wear diapers, sleep in parents' room with baby
    d. Regression is usually self-limiting and resolved in a few days to a few weeks; continuing regression may be an indicator of adjustment problems

D. Siblings must be supported in their process of attachment and adjustment to the newborn (Box 13-2)

1. Parents play the major role in this process assisted by grandparents, other family members, friends, and healthcare providers
2. Nurses have a responsibility to inform parents about typical sibling reactions and practical measures that can facilitate their adjustment
3. Family centered activities during and following birth should be encouraged

Box 13-2. Parental Activities that Facilitate Sibling Adjustment to Newborn

Participate in sibling visitation
Involve other children in preparations made for the homecoming of mother and newborn
Help other children to choose and/or make a special gift to give to mother and newborn
Consider feelings of other children upon arrival home with newborn—father should carry baby into the home leaving mother free to interact and hug the other children
Provide special gifts to give to the other children upon arrival home and when visitors bring gifts for the baby
Set aside special time of affection and attention just for the other children without interruption from the new baby
Pay attention to the activities and events occurring in the lives of the other children
Involve other children in the care of the new baby according to their ability and with recognition of their need for their own time and space
Encourage younger children to take care of their doll while mommy takes care of the baby

VII. Grandparent adjustment

A. Grandparents are affected by the childbirth experience of their children and often play an integral role in family adaptation to a new baby; they usually

1. Serve as role models for parenting skills
2. Facilitate maternal physical and emotional recovery by providing comfort, care, and emotional support in an accepting, nonjudgmental manner
3. Assist parents in helping siblings to adjust to newborn by providing them with loving care and attention
4. Care for grandchildren while parents work or go to school

B. Grandparent adjustment following birth is influenced by

1. Relationship established with their children
2. Attitude and views regarding being a grandparent and what it entails
3. Groundwork laid during pregnancy in terms of
   a. Degree of involvement in the pregnancy
   b. Their children's view of the grandparent role
   c. Ability to develop, with their children, a plan for their involvement in the care and nurturing of the grandchild
4. Ability to accept new approaches to child rearing adopted by their children
   a. Blend old with the new in a mutually satisfying way
   b. Attend classes to learn how to help and what to do, such as with breast-feeding
5. Cultural expectations and beliefs regarding the role of grandparents following birth of a grandchild

C. Grandparents may be placed in a more active caregiver role when the parents are adolescents

1. Immaturity and inexperience of an adolescent parent may compel grandparents to take over, blurring the role boundaries between grandparent and parent and creating the problem of who is the major caregiver
2. Resumption of primary parent role by the adolescent may lead to conflict not only for the grandparent but for the child as well—"who is my mommy?"
3. Adolescent parent role should be nurtured and supported

REVIEW QUESTIONS

1. Which family is most likely to experience a maturational crisis related to the birth of a new baby?

a. Father wishes to participate in the physical care of the baby while the mother has expressed the belief that baby care is a woman's work

b. Parents have planned special activities that are designed to give attention to their older children without the new baby present

c. First time parents have enrolled in parenting classes designed for new parents even though they have the help and support of their extended family

d. Prior to discharge, first time parents have asked the nurse for the name of a lactation consultant and the location of a La Leche group since the mother does not feel confident with breast-feeding

2. The nurse should understand that the parent-newborn attachment process

a. Begins after the baby is born

b. Requires that parents and newborn interact with each other immediately after birth

c. Is enhanced by early, close, frequent contact and interaction of parents with newborn

d. Is affected by the health status of the mother during the postpartum period but not during pregnancy

3. When making a visit to the home of a postpartum woman 1 week after birth, the nurse should recognize that the woman would characteristically

a. Express a strong need to review events and her behavior during the process of labor and birth

b. Exhibit a reduced attention span, limiting readiness to learn

c. Vacillate between the desire to have her own nurturing needs met and the need to take charge of her own care and that of her newborn

d. Have reestablished her role as a spouse-partner

4. Which of the following women is least likely to exhibit postpartum blues?

a. Multiparous woman (G3 P3003) whose husband took his 2 week vacation from work to help care for the older children while she takes care of the new baby

b. Primiparous woman who gave birth to a healthy full-term baby boy whom she will be breast-feeding

c. Adolescent primipara, whose family is embarrassed by her pregnancy, will be living in her parents' home with her new baby until she graduates from high school in 1 year
d. Primiparous woman, aged 39, who plans to continue her career as a lawyer and take care of her new baby girl

5. Paternal role behaviors and degree of involvement in infant care
a. Should be determined by the mother as the primary caregiver
b. Is fostered by encouraging the father to participate in newborn care classes
c. Should be limited to the areas of discipline, play, and modeling of the male role
d. Are primarily influenced by the father's culture

6. Four hours after a difficult labor and birth, a primiparous woman refuses to feed her baby, stating that she is too tired and just wants to sleep. The nurse should
a. Tell the woman she can rest after she feeds her baby
b. Recognize this as a behavior of the taking hold stage
c. Record the behavior as ineffective maternal-newborn attachment
d. Take the baby back to the nursery, reassuring the woman that her rest is a priority at this time

7. Parents can facilitate the adjustment of their other children to a new baby by
a. Having the children choose or make a gift to give to the new baby upon its arrival home
b. Emphasizing activities that keep the new baby and other children together
c. Having the mother carry the new baby into the home so she can show the other children the new baby
d. Reducing stress on other children by limiting their involvement in the care of the new baby

8. When caring for a postpartum family, the nurse should foster attachment to their newborn. In order to fulfill this goal the nurse should
a. Limit visiting hours so the mother can rest
b. Use videos to teach parents about newborn care
c. Insist that parents participate in the rooming-in with the newborn option offered by the hospital
d. Introduce parents and family members to the newborn, teaching them about typical newborn characteristics, behaviors, and sensory capabilities

ANSWERS, RATIONALES, AND TEST-TAKING TIPS

Rationales | **Test-Taking Tips**

1. Correct answer: a

In response *a* parents have not developed mutually acceptable parental role responsibilities. Responses *b, c,* and *d* all reflect a realistic view of postpartum stressors and appropriate coping mechanisms to deal with the stressors.

Cluster the responses *b, c,* and *d* in that they present information about both working as a team. Response *a* presents information that each parent has a different view; this will contribute to a crisis.

2. Correct answer: c

Attachment begins during pregnancy as the fetal heart beat is heard, fetal image is viewed in a sonogram, and fetal movement is perceived. It is affected by events and well being during all stages of pregnancy. Attachment is progressive and ongoing, therefore failure to have immediate contact because of maternal or newborn health problems will not have serious long-term effects as long as opportunities for close, frequent contact is provided.

Remember that attachment is a "process" and not a reaction from one event. Thus, responses *a, b,* and *d* are too narrow to be the best response.

3. Correct answer: c

One week after birth the woman should exhibit behaviors characteristic of the taking hold stage. Responses *a* and *b* are characteristic of the taking in stage, while *d* reflects the letting go stage.

Note that time, one week after birth, is an important factor to reading the question and selecting the correct response.

4. Correct answer: a

Response *a* reflects present experience and support both of which help to reduce the incidence of the blues. Responses *b*, *c*, and *d* describe women who exhibit one or more risk factors associated with the blues and depression, namely adolescent mothers with limited support, older mothers with a career, or primiparous women.

If you have no idea of the correct response, try clustering responses *b, c,* and *d* with the "primipara"; the multipara in response *a* is likely the best answer. Another strategy is to identify that the situation in response *a* provides a support system and repeat experience; as with anything in life if a person has had some experience with an event and has support systems in place the emotional reaction will be minimized. Compare first semester to third semester nursing students' emotional reactions to course clinical work.

5. Correct answer: b

Paternal behaviors and degree of involvement in infant care should be determined by both parents to their mutual satisfaction. Paternal role responsibilities are unlimited especially today as many fathers want to play a more active role in the care of their children. Many factors, in addition to culture, influence the father role, such as relationship with own father, education, lifestyle.

Look at some restrictive words in responses *a, c,* and *d* to eliminate them as the best response. In response *a* "determined by the mother" is too one-sided; in response *c* "be limited to" is too narrow of an approach; and in response *d* "primarily culture" is too restrictive.

6. Correct answer: d

Response *a* does not take into consideration the need for the new mother to be nurtured and have her needs met during the taking in stage. The behavior described is typical of this

Note the key words in the stem "four hours difficult labor primiparous." Common sense helps to identify that this is a first and exhausting experience for the mother; she needs her rest at this time.

stage and not a reflection of ineffective attachment unless the behavior persists. Mothers need to reestablish their own well being in order to effectively care for their baby.

7. Correct answer: a

Special time should be set aside just for the other children without interruption from the newborn. Someone other than the mother should carry the baby into the home, so she can give full attention to the other children. Children should be actively involved in the care of the baby according to their ability without overwhelming them.

Apply a general concept for acceptance of a given situation: active involvement facilitates acceptance of new situations whether it be related to clients, families, or yourself.

8. Correct answer: d

Visiting hours should be unlimited for the father so he can be there as a source of support and to learn how to care for their newborn. Demonstrations and hands-on care are more effective than videos. Parents should be encouraged but not forced to participate in rooming-in with their newborn if it is available.

The need as stated in the stem is to "foster attachment." Eliminate responses *a* and *c* since the actions to "limit" and "insist" do not facilitate involvement. In narrowing the responses to either *b* or *d,* response *d* is the best answer since it is more comprehensive and recall teaching-learning theory: for psychomotor skills live demonstration and return demonstration is the best, not videos.

CHAPTER 14

Application of the Nursing Process during the Postpartum Period

STUDY OUTCOMES:

After completing this chapter, the reader will be able to do the following:

- Define the key terms listed.
- Describe the impact of early discharge on the application of the nursing process during the postpartum period.
- Identify factors that should be assessed when determining the progress of recovery following birth.
- Identify nursing diagnoses typical of the postpartal period.
- Describe measures found to be effective during the postpartum period to
  - prevent excessive blood loss and enhance healing
  - prevent infection
  - relieve discomfort
  - facilitate bowel and bladder elimination
  - lose weight gained during pregnancy and restore abdominal muscle tone

KEY TERMS

Early discharge	Discharge of mother and newborn within 12 to 24 hours following an uncomplicated vaginal birth.
Perineal care	Methods used to cleanse and soothe the vulva and episiotomy following birth for the purpose of preventing infection, enhancing healing, and reducing maternal discomfort.
Postpartum check	Systematic approach used for the assessment of essential factors (breasts, fundus, lochia, perineum) indicative of maternal physical recovery following birth.
Sitz bath	Sitting in warm water for 15 to 20 minutes at least twice a day to enhance healing and comfort and facilitate cleansing of the perineum.

CONTENT REVIEW

I. Postpartum Period—Overview of Guidelines

A. A holistic approach that considers the mother's physical recovery as well as the psychosocial adjustment of herself and her family to the reality of a newborn and the responsibilities of its care, should be used when planning for care

B. Early discharge—is increasing in popularity as a means to facilitate maternal recovery and family adjustment and to reduce healthcare costs

C. A comprehensive, coordinated maternal-newborn healthcare program that begins during pregnancy is needed to support early discharge since the physical status of the mother and time limitations following birth interfere with her learning readiness, her ability, and the nurse's capability to fully prepare the woman and her family for the care requirements of the postpartum period

1. Critical care pathways, as a method of case management, can facilitate the provision of health care in early discharge programs
   a. Patient outcomes and care tasks are outlined and assigned a time for completion
   b. The time frame is comprised of the prenatal period, the hours from admission to discharge during parturition and the early postpartum period, and the postdischarge period

2. New and innovative care delivery systems have been designed to facilitate administration of care in a short period of time
    a. Women *l*abor, *d*eliver, *r*ecover, and spend the *p*ostpartum period until discharge in one room (the LDRP room) being cared for by a limited number of nurses in order to facilitate completion of all care requirements without duplication or omission
    b. Mother-baby or couplet care coordinate the health care of the postpartum woman and her newborn

D. A comprehensive, coordinated maternal-newborn healthcare program should include

1. Prenatal education services that provide information regarding
    a. Prepared childbirth techniques
    b. Maternal assessment and care during the prenatal, parturition, and postpartum periods
    c. Newborn care and parenting basics
    d. Breast-feeding preparation
2. Healthcare agencies that provide childbirth services
    a. Facilitate spontaneous vaginal births that are family centered
    b. Support the recovery process following birth
    c. Determine readiness for discharge on the basis of an individualized assessment of maternal-newborn health status
3. Discharge planning that provides essential health care and teaching related to the prevention, early detection, and prompt treatment of
    a. Maternal problems
        (1) Hemorrhage
        (2) Infection
        (3) Thrombophlebitis
        (4) Constipation or urinary retention
        (5) Postpartum depression
    b. Neonatal problems
        (1) Respiratory distress
        (2) Inadequate nutrient and fluid intake—dehydration
        (3) Infection
        (4) Hyperbilirubinemia
4. Postpartum programs that provide continuing assessment and care during the 6-week period of recovery following birth
    a. Telephone follow-up as a cost effective method for determining the status of the mother, her newborn, and family and identifying problems which require health teaching, counseling, home visitation or referral to community agencies (Box 14-1)

Box 14-1. Postpartum Telephone Follow-Up

Suggested Format for Assessment of Maternal-Newborn and Family Status
Describe how you are feeling today
What have you been doing to take care of yourself?
How does the baby seem to you?
Describe how the baby has been eating and sleeping
What has been the greatest source of happiness for you since coming home?
What has been the greatest source of stress for you since coming home?
What are your concerns?
How are the other members of your family doing since you and the baby came home?
How can I help to make things easier for you?

Modified from NAACOG (1986). *Postpartum follow-up—a nursing practice guide. OGN Nursing Practice Resource.* Washington, DC: (AWHONN) Association of Women's Health, Obstetric, and Neonatal Nurses (formerly NAACOG).

b. Home visitation especially for primiparous women and women-newborns-families experiencing problems (Box 14-2)
c. Community services such as parenting support groups, lactation consultants, day care

II. Assessment process during the postpartal period

A. Review prenatal history and assessment—to determine

1. Obstetrical history in terms of
   a. Previous pregnancies or births and their outcomes—*gravida, para*
   b. History of postpartum complications such as hemorrhage, infection, depression
2. Nature of prenatal care
   a. Gestational week at entry into care
   b. Consistency of visits
   c. Woman's impression of care received—important for follow-through with health care during the current postpartal period and for future pregnancies
3. Health status during pregnancy
   a. Estimated date of birth (EDB)
   b. Adaptations to physical and psychosocial changes of pregnancy including the development of complications of pregnancy such as gestational diabetes, pregnancy induced hypertension (PIH), bleeding, thrombophlebitis
   c. Presence of health problems such as diabetes, heart disease, asthma, infection

Box 14-2. Home Visitation Guidelines Following Early Postpartum Discharge

Assessment

Maternal recovery following pregnancy and birth
Newborn adaptation to extrauterine life
Family adaptation to birth and the newborn
Environmental adequacy—cleanliness, warmth, and safety
Knowledge of postpartum recovery and utilization of measures designed to enhance the health of mother, newborn, and family
Need for community support services

Interventions

Review:	signs of effective and ineffective recovery for mother and infant, action to take if signs of ineffective recovery are noted, self-care and infant care measures, breast-feeding techniques, process of infant growth and development, measures to promote positive family adaptation to newborn, family planning methods
Discuss:	feelings and concerns regarding the birth experience, postpartum recovery, and infant care
Support:	parenting efforts by providing guidance, positive reinforcement, and encouragement
Utilize:	community agencies by making referrals as needed to such services as WIC, lactation consultants, well baby clinics, daycare centers, family planning clinics, parenting support groups
Involve:	family in the process of assessment and care

d. Medical interventions including medications, hospitalization, bedrest
e. Laboratory-diagnostic tests performed and their results
▼ Blood type and Rh factor is of special importance during the postpartum period so comparison can be made with newborn blood type and Rh factor to determine if further testing and Rhogam administration are required

4. Prenatal classes attended such as those related to childbirth preparation, breast-feeding techniques, parenting skills, sibling preparation

B. Review of parturition events

1. Onset of labor compared to EDB
2. Physical and emotional status of mother during labor
   a. Stability of vital signs
   b. Fluid balance in terms of intake (oral, IVs), output, signs of fluid deficit or excess
   c. Elimination—bladder (spontaneous, catheterization) and bowel (enema, diarrhea)

d. Blood loss
e. Pain experience and effectiveness of relief measures including prepared childbirth techniques
f. Presence of a support person or coach
g. Woman's impression of the experience and the quality of her performance

3. Status of the fetus
   a. FHR patterns
   b. Signs of distress or stress
   c. Presentation and position for birth
4. Progress of labor
   a. Onset of labor and its duration
   b. Labor patterns established—partogram
   c. Rupture of membranes—time, method (spontaneous or amniotomy), characteristics of the fluid
5. Birth
   a. Time and method of birth
      (1) Spontaneous vaginal
      (2) Vaginal with assistance of forceps, vacuum extraction
      (3) Cesarian birth, including reason
   b. Separation and expulsion of placenta
      (1) Spontaneous
      (2) Manual removal
      (3) Condition—intact, fragments retained, degree of aging, signs of infection
6. Pharmacologic interventions
   a. Oxytocics administered
      (1) Type and amount
      (2) Induction-augmentation
      (3) Stimulation of uterine contraction after birth
   b. Analgesics-anesthetics
      (1) Type and amount
      (2) Effectiveness
      (3) Side effects experienced
7. Current status of the newborn

C. Assessment of physical recovery following birth

1. Assessment of physical recovery must be thorough, accurate, and communicated or documented since discharge decisions are made based on analysis of this data
2. Frequency of assessment is determined by status of the woman, presence of risk factors, and the time elapsed since birth—a recommended minimum frequency would be

a. Fourth stage of labor every 15 minutes during the first hour and every 30 minutes during the second hour
b. Following the fourth stage of labor
   (1) First 24 hours—every 4 hours
   (2) After first 24 hours—every 8 hours
3. Postpartum check (Box 14-3)—method of providing the woman with essential information related to postpartum healing; signs of effective or ineffective healing and measures that enhance or disrupt the healing process
   ▼ The postpartum check can be adapted for utilization as a self-assessment method by the woman following discharge
4. Assessment of reproductive recovery
   a. Breasts
      (1) Consistency in terms of lactation—soft, full, engorged
      (2) Type of nipples—flat, everted, inverted
      (3) Integrity of nipples and areola—intact, cracked, bruised, blistered, reddened
      (4) Discomfort—breast tenderness, nipple soreness
      (5) Signs of infection
      (6) Leakage
   b. Fundus
      (1) Position—height, location
      (2) Consistency
      (3) Afterpains
   c. Bleeding
      (1) Type—lochia, nonlochial (episiotomy or laceration)
      (2) Amount
      (3) Stage, color
      (4) Presence of clots or odor
5. Assessment of the status of oxygenation and circulation
   a. Vital signs—compare with values obtained during pregnancy and childbirth
      (1) Blood pressure
      (2) Pulse—apical and radial
      (3) Respirations and breath sounds
   b. Status of lower extremities
      (1) Circulation
      (2) Edema
      (3) Signs of thrombophlebitis
6. Assessment of nutrition and fluid and/or electrolyte balance
   a. Appetite including intake of food and fluid since birth
   b. Presence of nausea and vomiting

Box 14-3. The Postpartum Check

Timing: Choose a time when the mother is comfortable and you will not be interrupted; this will facilitate health teaching and discussion

Client Preparation

Fully explain the procedure in terms the client understands

Instruct the client to empty her bladder and to save her perineal pad, by placing it in a paper bag

Position the client in a supine position with a pillow under her head and arms at her sides

Maintain privacy throughout the procedure by pulling the curtain, closing the door, and exposing only the part of the body being examined

Include client's partner if they desire

Asepsis

Wash your hands

Obtain a pair of clean gloves for use when assessing perineum and perineal pad

Examine by proceeding from breasts to legs—cleanest area first

Examine the Breasts

Consistency of the breasts (soft, firm, engorged) and the progress of lactation

Degree of tenderness or discomfort and its location, i.e., generalized or localized, unilateral, nipples especially during latch on

Condition of the nipples and areolas—intact, cracking, bruising, blisters, redness

Leakage (characteristics)

Care measures utilized such as cleansing, use of creams (vitamin E, Masse), type of bra worn

Examine the Abdomen

▼ Abdominal muscles will be more relaxed and palpation easier if the client bends her knees slightly (pillows underneath knees may also help) and keeps her arms at her sides

Fundus—consistency (firm, boggy), height (finger breaths or cm at, above, or below the umbilicus), location (midline, deviated to right or to left); presence of afterpains

Abdomen—muscle tone, distention, striae, linea nigra, bowel sounds, bowel elimination patterns

Bladder—distention; voiding patterns

Examine the Perineal Area

▼ Perineum is more easily visualized if the client assumes a lateral position with upper leg slightly flexed forward

Box 14-3. The Postpartum Check—cont'd

Put on a Clean Pair of Gloves and Loosen Pad

Condition of the episiotomy or laceration—REEDA: redness, edema, ecchymosis, drainage, approximation of wound edges
Presence of hemorrhoids
Presence of perineal discomfort
Hygienic status of the perineal area
Care measures utilized such as washing of perineal area and use of peribottle, topical preparations, and sitz bath
Examine perineal pad (current pad and pad saved) for lochia—stage, odor, clots, amount

Remove Gloves and Wash Hands

Examine the Legs

Circulatory status—color, warmth, capillary refill, pedal pulses, presence of varicosities
Edema of feet, ankles, calves
Signs of thrombophlebitis—erythema, swelling, tenderness, Homan's sign positive
Deep tendon reflexes (DTR) especially for women with pregnancy induced hypertension (PIH)
Return of movement and sensation following epidural or spinal anesthesia
▼ Throughout the postpartum check the nurse should teach the client how to assess herself, describe her current status and explain signs indicative of effective and ineffective healing

c. Weight—comparison of current weight with prepregnant weight and weight at the end of pregnancy
d. Temperature
e. Hydration status—signs of dehydration or fluid excess

7. Assessment of elimination patterns
   a. Bowel
      (1) Bowel sounds
      (2) Passage of flatus, stool
      (3) Hemorrhoids—size, condition, soreness
   b. Bladder
      (1) Frequency and ease of urination
      (2) Characteristics of urine including amount, color, clarity, odor—measure first few voidings
      (3) Presence of signs indicative of urinary tract infection
8. Assessment of physical activity and rest patterns
   a. Ambulation including gait, posture

b. Muscle tone especially abdominal
c. Return of movement and sensation following administration of epidural or spinal anesthesia
   (1) Instruct woman to move legs up and down, side to side, flex knees, and dorsiflex-plantarflex feet
   (2) Touch parts of legs and ask woman to identify location
d. Muscular and joint pain related to the process of childbirth
e. Activity or energy level
f. Sleep patterns—presence of fatigue

9. Assessment of the status of the integument
   a. Appearance and condition of the skin, mucous membranes, nails, hair including changes related to pregnancy
   b. Hygienic status and practices
   c. Condition of wounds—episiotomy, abdominal incision
      (1) REEDA—redness, edema, ecchymosis, drainage, approximation of wound edges
      (2) Pain related to the wound
10. Common laboratory testing—compare current findings with those obtained prenatally
   a. CBC—taking note of hematocrit-hemoglobin, RBCs, platelets, and WBCs
   b. Indirect coombs and Rh testing to determine if Rh sensitization has occurred when an Rh-negative woman has an Rh-positive newborn and if the woman is a candidate to receive Rhogam which must be administered within 72 hours of birth
   c. Urinalysis using a clean catch, midstream specimen (prevents lochia and other secretions from contaminating the urine sample)

D. Assessment of psychosocial recovery following birth

1. Maternal self-concept
   a. Perceptions of physical self
      (1) Feelings expressed regarding current body-image and how her body feels
      (2) Description of current health status
   b. Perceptions of personal self
      (1) Evaluation of her pregnancy experience and the effectiveness of her performance during childbirth
      (2) Self-ideal regarding being a mother compared to reality
   c. Behaviors indicative of progress through the stages of recovery

d. Knowledge level concerning
  (1) Self-assessment measures to determine status in terms of effective or ineffective recovery
  (2) Measures to enhance healing including
    (a) Nutritional and fluid requirements
    (b) Appropriate activity and exercises
    (c) Hygienic practices
    (d) Relief measures for pain and discomfort
    (e) Rest requirements
    (f) Stress reduction techniques

2. Role function
  a. Current roles and potential for role conflict
  b. Parenting role
    (1) Beliefs and values related to the maternal, paternal, and grandparent roles
    (2) Personal evaluation of effectiveness as a mother
    (3) Role mastery behaviors exhibited
    (4) Responses of others to her parenting skills
3. Interdependence
  a. Progress of attachment—parents and family to newborn
  b. Parental expectations regarding the response of other children to the newborn
    (1) Nature of prenatal preparation for the addition of newborn to the family
    (2) Activities planned to facilitate their adjustment to the newborn
  c. Status of family and support system
    (1) Availability and composition of the woman's family and support system
    (2) Stability of the relationships
    (3) Degree and quality of support offered by family and support system
    (4) Willingness of the woman to ask for and accept help
  d. Home environment in terms of its adequacy in meeting newborn's needs for cleanliness, warmth, safety, stimulation
  e. Need for referral to community agencies such as WIC, well baby clinics, lactation consultants, parenting support groups

III. Nursing diagnoses related to the common problems and risks encountered by the postpartal woman

A. Risk for fluid volume deficit

B. Risk for infection

C. Altered patterns of urinary elimination
D. Constipation
E. Alteration in nutrition—more or less than body requirements
F. Pain
G. Risk for alteration in parenting
H. Altered family processes
I. Parental role conflict

▼ Common nursing diagnoses (A to F above) encountered during the postpartum period, along with selected client outcomes, nursing interventions, and evaluation criteria are described in Table 14-1. Nursing diagnoses related to parenting and family processes (G-I above) are discussed in Chapter 13 and Chapter 17.

Table 14-1. Common Nursing Diagnoses Encountered During the Postpartum Period

A. Risk for Fluid Volume Deficit Related to Blood Loss with the Process of Childbirth and Recovery

Client Outcomes: Client will

Heal without excessive blood loss
Identify signs indicative of effective healing of the reproductive tract following birth
Identify measures to enhance healing
Incorporate measures to enhance healing into her living patterns after discharge

Nursing Interventions	Evaluation Checklist—Client
Assess progress of involution by checking vital signs, fundus, characteristics of lochia, episiotomy, laceration Massage fundus if boggy-flaccid by supporting the lower uterus, grasping the fundus through the abdominal wall, and massaging it until firm Administer oxytocics as ordered ▼ Oxytocin (Pitocin) in IV fluid or slowly IV push ▼ Methylergonovine maleate (Methergine) (IM or PO) assessing BP prior to and 5 to 10 minutes after administration—hold dose if BP ≥140/90 Encourage client to void every 2 hours to prevent bladder distention that can interfere with uterine contraction Teach and/or demonstrate ▼ Fundal check and massage ▼ Stages of lochia and its expected characteristics Discuss measures to enhance healing ▼ Get out of bed and begin ambulation slowly ▼ Activity restrictions such as lifting heavy objects >5 lbs, climbing stairs	Exhibited firm fundus, midline location, and descent of 1 cm each postpartum day Exhibited expected progress of lochia ▼ Rubra, serosa, alba ▼ Moderate to scant amount ▼ Small clots, no odor Exhibited stable vital signs Described expected fundal changes, and stages or characteristics of lochia Demonstrated fundal palpation and massage Developed a plan for recovery that included ▼ Balanced, nutritious meals ▼ Family support for heavy household chores ▼ Rest when baby naps and other children are in school ▼ Exercise program of approved postpartum exercises Discussed with partner the use of condom and spermicidal foam as method of birth control until diaphragm can be refitted Stated she would like to have another child but is going to wait until this baby is at least 2 years old

Continued.

Table 14-1. Common Nursing Diagnoses Encountered During the Postpartum Period—cont'd

Nursing Interventions	Evaluation Checklist—Client
A. Risk for Fluid Volume Deficit Related to Blood Loss with the Process of Childbirth and Recovery—cont'd	
Nursing Interventions—cont'd	
▼ Acceptable activities and postpartum exercises which enhance circulation and prevent thrombophlebitis ▼ Frequent rest periods ▼ Good nutrition that includes a balance of nutrients especially protein, vitamins, and iron ▼ Measures to prevent constipation ▼ Birth control measures to facilitate spacing of pregnancies—at least a 2-year interval between pregnancies is recommended	
B. Risk for Infection Related to the Effects of Vaginal Birth	
Client Outcomes: Client will Heal without infection Identify signs and symptoms indicative of infection Identify measures that will prevent infection Utilize appropriate measures to prevent infection	
Nursing Interventions	**Evaluation Checklist—Client**
Assess client for findings of infection by checking vital signs, breasts, characteristics of lochia, episiotomy or lacerations, urination patterns and characteristics of urine Utilize aseptic principles, scrupulous handwashing, and universal precautions when caring for client	Exhibited no signs of infection ▼ Stable vital signs ▼ Breasts intact without localized, warm, tender areas ▼ Episiotomy or lacerations—no redness, edema, drainage; wound edges approximated, perineum clean

B. Risk for Infection Related to the Effects of Vaginal Birth—cont'd

Nursing Interventions—cont'd

Teach client signs and symptoms of infection and how to check temperature, breasts, episiotomy or lacerations, lochia, and urine for their presence

Teach and/or demonstrate
- ▼ Breast care measures (Box 14-4)
- ▼ Perineal care measures (Box 14-5)

Teach measures to prevent bladder infection
- ▼ Increase fluid intake to 3 L/day including fluids that increase acidity of urine such as cranberry juice
- ▼ Empty bladder frequently—every two hours—to prevent stasis of urine

Teach measures to enhance healing and maintain resistance to infection
- ▼ Good nutrition—protein, fluids, vitamins
- ▼ Balance of rest and activity
- ▼ Stress reduction measures
- ▼ Avoid intercourse until healing has taken place—use principles of safer sex
- ▼ Good general hygiene

Evaluation Checklist—Client—cont'd

- ▼ Urinating moderate amounts clear urine without difficulty
- ▼ Lochia following expected progression without odor

Described findings indicative of breast, uterine, episiotomy or lacerations, and bladder infection

Wore clean bra that supported breasts; used only warm water when cleansing breasts; and applied breast milk to nipples and areola

Washed perineum with soap and water in morning and at bedtime; used peribottle and changed pad when voiding every 2 to 3 hours

Used sitz bath BID and applied topical anesthetic spray QID

Described lifestyle practices that included a balanced diet, 6 to 8 hours of sleep each night, and an occasional 30 minute nap in the afternoon when the baby was sleeping

Continued.

Table 14-1. Common Nursing Diagnoses Encountered During the Postpartum Period—cont'd

C. Altered Patterns of Urinary Elimination Related to Effects of Pregnancy/Childbirth on Renal System

Client Outcomes: Client will

Void within 4 to 6 hours of birth
Empty bladder at each voiding without difficulty
Will not exhibit bladder distension

Nursing Interventions	Evaluation Checklist—Client
Utilize measures to facilitate voiding ▼ Assist client into an upright position for voiding, sitting forward so urine does not touch episiotomy ▼ Provide privacy ▼ Stimulate urination by running water, placing hands in warm water, blowing bubbles in a glass of water using a straw, sitting in a sitz bath Measure first few voidings—assess amount and characteristics Palpate abdomen, above symphysis pubis, to check for distended bladder Encourage fluid intake of 3000 ml/day Perform straight catheterization (requires physician order) if bladder is distended and client is unable to void ▼ Explain what you are going to do ▼ Perform perineal care to remove lochia ▼ Use good lighting since edema may make urethra difficult to visualize ▼ Use gentle approach since area is very tender	Voided 350 ml of urine within 5 hours after birth Exhibited pattern of voiding moderate amounts of urine every few hours without difficulty Exhibited no bladder distension when abdomen was palpated during postpartum check

D. Constipation Related to Painful Hemorrhoids and Decreased Intestinal Motility Associated with Pregnancy

Client Outcomes: Client will

Have soft formed bowel movement by third postpartum day
Utilize appropriate measures to facilitate bowel elimination

Nursing Interventions

Assess client for bowel sounds, passage of flatus, usual elimination patterns

Teach client measures that are effective in safely stimulating bowel elimination

- ▼ Fluid intake of 3000 ml/day
- ▼ Roughage or bulk in diet including raw fruit and vegetables, bran cereals, whole wheat bread or muffins
- ▼ Periods of activity such as ambulation, postpartum exercises

Administer, as ordered, a stool softener or laxative such as docusate sodium (Peri-Colace) or a rectal suppository such as bisacodyl (Duculax)

Administer fleets enema as ordered if above measures are ineffective—may be contraindicated if a 3 or 4 degree laceration is present

Utilize local pain relief measures after a bowel movement—perineal care, sitz baths, topical applications

Evaluation Checklist—Client

Exhibited active bowel sounds in all four quadrants

Reported having a soft formed bowel movement on postpartum day two

Described daily intake of 2500 to 3000 ml of fluids including fruit juices such as prune juice

Included at least one source of roughage at each meal and ate fresh fruit as a snack

Ambulated frequently during each day and planned to begin participating in a postpartum exercise program within one week

Continued.

Table 14-1. Common Nursing Diagnoses Encountered During the Postpartum Period—cont'd

E. Alteration in Nutrition < Body Requirements Related to Knowledge Deficit Concerning Postpartum Nutrient Requirements and Weight Loss Patterns

Client Outcomes: Client will

State nutrient requirements of postpartum period
Maintain a nutrient intake reflective of the nutrient requirements of the postpartum period
Participate in an exercise program appropriate for postpartum women
Lose weight gained during pregnancy at a rate of ½ to 1 pound per week

Nursing Interventions

Weigh client
Discuss expected progress of weight loss during the postpartum period
Explain the importance of an approach to weight loss that combines good nutrition and appropriate exercise
Teach client the components of a postpartum diet that supports healing and lactation—the diet and prenatal vitamins recommended for pregnancy can be continued for the 6-week postpartum period

- ▼ Calories supply nutrient and energy requirements for healing—approximately 500 calories/day above requirements for the postpartum woman are needed for lactation (each ounce of milk produced requires 20 calories)
- ▼ Proteins, vitamin C, and Zinc are crucial for healing
- ▼ Fluid intake of 3 L/day are required with an additional 1 to 2 L required if breast-feeding

Evaluation Checklist—Client

Exhibited a loss of 12 of the 35 pounds gained during pregnancy when weighed on the first postpartum day
Reported a 24-hour dietary intake that reflected nutrient requirements for healing and lactation
Exhibited a weight loss of 5 pounds at her 6-week postpartum checkup
Expressed satisfaction with pace of weight loss and return of nonpregnant body contours
Performed postpartum exercises daily

E. Alteration in Nutrition < Body Requirements Related to Knowledge Deficit Concerning Postpartum Nutrient Requirements and Weight Loss Patterns—cont'd

Nursing Interventions—cont'd

- ▼ Complex carbohydrates (fruits, vegetables, whole grains) are excellent sources of nutrients and roughage
- ▼ Iron rich foods and/or iron supplements are required if HCT/HGB levels are low
- ▼ Avoid use of alcohol, tobacco
- ▼ Teach postpartum exercises that facilitate weight loss and restoration of abdominal muscle tone

F. Pain Related to Effects of Vaginal Birth

Client Outcomes: Client will

Request medication as needed for pain relief
Experience pain relief
Utilize appropriate pain relief measures

Nursing Interventions

Determine source, intensity, and duration of pain
Provide relief measures appropriate to the source and intensity of the pain
Provide local relief measures such as

- ▼ Breast care (see Box 14-4)
- ▼ Perineal care (see Box 14-5)
- ▼ Sims position for perineal pain
- ▼ Squeeze buttocks together before sitting down

Evaluation Checklist—Client

Requested ibuprofen (Motrin) for persistent, afterpains of moderate intensity
Reported relief within 30 minutes of administration of medication
Stated hemorrhoidal discomfort was relieved following use of sitz bath
Applied topical anesthetic gel every 6 hours to relieve episiotomy discomfort

Continued.

Table 14-1. Common Nursing Diagnoses Encountered During the Postpartum Period—cont'd

F. Pain Related to Effects of Vaginal Birth—cont'd
Nursing Interventions—cont'd
Instruct to request analgesic before pain becomes severe Provide analgesics as ordered such as ▼ Acetaminophen (Tylenol) with or without codeine ▼ Ibuprofen (Motrin) (especially effective for afterpains) ▼ Darvon, Compound-65, oxycodone HCl (Tylox) Encourage use of relaxation and breathing techniques taught in childbirth classes Provide comfort measures to enhance relaxation or rest and effectiveness of pain relief measures Explain to the client the importance and safety of pain relief measures even for breast-feeding mothers Assess effectiveness of pain relief measures

Box 14-4. Client Instructions for Breast Care During the Postpartum Period

Instructions for the Client Who Is Bottle-Feeding

Hygiene: wash breasts at least once a day, as the *first* part of shower or bath; use a mild soap; rinse well

Support: wear a clean bra that fully supports entire breast until breasts have returned to their nonpregnant status in about one month

Care of engorged breasts

- Wear snug supportive bra or breast binder
- Avoid exposure of breasts to hot water during the shower—have water run over shoulders not over breasts
- Apply cold packs to breasts to reduce tenderness
- *Never* express milk from breasts, since more milk will be produced
- Change absorbent pads used to collect leakage frequently and avoid use of plastic liners since keeping moisture against nipples and areolas can lead to excoriation or cracking and infection

Instructions for the Client Who Is Breast-feeding

Hygiene: wash nipple and areola of each breast with a clean cloth and warm water at the first part of shower or bath and before and after each breast-feeding session; allow to air dry thoroughly; avoid soap since it may dry and irritate the nipple and areola leading to cracking and infection

Support: wear a clean bra that fully supports the entire breast until breast-feeding is discontinued and breasts return to their nonpregnant status about one month later

Care of nipples and areola

- Use correct breast-feeding techniques related to latch on, removal from, and position at breast
- Apply colostrum or milk after breast-feeding as a safe, effective measure to maintain suppleness and integrity of the nipples and areola
- Use nipple creams (Masse, vitamin E, Mammol) if recommended by healthcare provider, sparingly and apply *after* breast-feeding, to nipple and areola that have been cleansed and dried; never apply over nipple opening or a cracked area; remove prior to breast-feeding using warm water
- Change absorbent pads used to collect leakage frequently and avoid use of plastic liners since keeping moisture against nipples and areolas can lead to excoriation or cracking and infection

Continued.

Box 14-4. Client Instructions for Breast Care During the Postpartum Period—cont'd

Care of engorged breasts

- ▼ Empty the breasts frequently using good breast-feeding technique to prevent or to limit the extent of engorgement
- ▼ Apply warmth (warm packs, shower) to breasts, massage breasts, express some milk to soften breasts and nipples; this practice facilitates latch on and stimulates the letdown reflex
- ▼ Apply cold packs to breasts after feeding to reduce tenderness and decrease swelling
- ▼ Wear supportive bra

Care of sore nipples and areola

- ▼ Initiate feeding on breast that is not sore or least sore
- ▼ Limit duration of sucking on sore breast
- ▼ Stimulate letdown reflex using breast massage before newborn latches on
- ▼ Keep nipples and areola dry
  - — Expose to air after feeding
  - — Use breast milk to soothe
  - — Use breast or nipple shells to allow for circulation of air and to prevent further irritation from rubbing of nipple and areola against bra

Box 14-5. Client Instructions for Perineal Care During the Postpartum Period

Hygiene

Wash perineal area from front to back using a clean washcloth, soap and water at least twice a day (A.M. and P.M.) and after a bowel movement

Use a different part of the cloth for each stroke and do not separate labia while washing

Rinse with a peribottle filled with warm water by directing the flow backward; never direct the flow upward into the vagina

Pat dry

Use a peribottle, filled with warm water, to cleanse the perineum after each urination and pad change

Change peri pads frequently (at least every 2 to 3 hours), putting them on and taking them off from front to back; during application of a new pad, never touch the side of the pad that comes in contact with the vulva and perineum

Application of Topical Preparations for Pain Relief

Apply ice packs intermittently (on for 20 to 30 minutes and off for 60 minutes) during the first 12 hours following birth

Use topical preparations (anesthetics-antiseptics) sparingly approximately QID

Apply directly to the episiotomy or lacerations after the perineum has been cleansed; never apply to the peri pad

Use preparations only as needed for discomfort

Utilization of Sitz Bath

Use sitz bath—sitting in warm water—at least BID to enhance healing and comfort, and facilitate cleansing

Use of cool to cold water can be effective in reducing discomfort in some women

Perform perineal care before taking a sitz bath

Use warm water and continue the bath for approximately 15 to 20 minutes

Wash the sitz bath basin with soap and water after use

▼ Wear clean gloves when assisting client with perineal care

REVIEW QUESTIONS

1. When performing a postpartum check, the nurse should
   a. Instruct the woman to empty her bladder prior to the check
   b. Place the woman in a supine position with her arms overhead for the examination of her breasts and fundus
   c. Perform the check as quickly as possible
   d. Wear sterile gloves when assessing the pad and perineum

2. The physician has ordered the administration of Rhogam to an Rh-negative postpartum woman. The nurse should administer the Rhogam no later than how many hours after birth?
   a. 12
   b. 24
   c. 48
   d. 72

3. A breast-feeding woman would demonstrate the need for further instruction regarding breast care if she
   a. Washes the nipple and areola of each breast with warm water
   b. Applies vitamin E cream to each nipple and areola just prior to breast-feeding her baby
   c. Avoids use of soap on nipples and areola
   d. Uses colostrum or milk to soothe and protect nipples and areola

4. The breasts of a bottle-feeding woman are engorged. The nurse should tell her to
   a. Wear a snug, supportive bra
   b. Allow warm water to soothe the breasts during a shower
   c. Express milk from breasts occasionally to relieve discomfort
   d. Place absorbent pads and plastic liners into her bra to absorb leakage and prevent staining of clothing

5. The breasts of a breast-feeding woman are engorged. Which of the following would *not* be recommended as a relief measure?
   a. Wear a supportive bra
   b. Limit frequency of feedings until engorgement subsides
   c. Apply warm packs prior to a feeding and then massage breasts to express some milk and stimulate the letdown reflex
   d. Apply cold packs to breasts after feeding

6. The right nipple and areola of a breast-feeding woman are sore. There is a crack present on the right areola along with a small bruise. The nurse should tell the woman to
   a. Apply vitamin E cream or lanolin to the crack
   b. Initiate feeding on the right breast
   c. Use a different feeding position for each breast-feeding session
   d. Limit duration and frequency of feedings

7. Perineal care is an important infection control measure. When evaluating a postpartum woman's perineal care technique, the nurse would recognize the need for further instruction if the woman
   a. Uses soap and warm water to wash the vulva and perineum
   b. Washes the vulva and perineum from symphysis pubis back to episiotomy, then over the episiotomy to the anus
   c. Changes her perineal pad every 2 to 3 hours
   d. Uses the peribottle to rinse upward into her vagina

8. Which measure would be *least* effective in preventing postpartum hemorrhage?
   a. Massage the fundus every ½ to 1 hour for the first postpartum day
   b. Encourage the woman to void every 2 hours
   c. Administer methergine 0.25 mg every 4 to 6 hours, PRN as ordered
   d. Teach the woman the importance of rest and nutrition to enhance healing

9. An appropriate relief measure that the nurse could recommend to a postpartum woman with a midline episiotomy would be
   a. Place ice packs against the episiotomy for a 1-hour period every 2 hours during the first 24 hours following birth
   b. Sit in a warm water sitz bath for 15 to 20 minutes
   c. Apply a topical anesthetic to the episiotomy at every pad change
   d. Put the topical preparation on the back of the perineal pad to make application easier

10. Postpartum women experience an increased risk for urinary tract infection. A prevention measure the nurse could teach the postpartum woman would be
   a. Acidify the urine by drinking 3 glasses of orange juice each day
   b. Maintain a fluid intake of 1 to 2 liters each day
   c. Empty bladder every 4 hours throughout the day
   d. Perform perineal care on a regular basis

ANSWERS, RATIONALES, AND TEST-TAKING TIPS

Rationales	Test-Taking Tips
1. Correct answer: a	
Palpation of the fundus is facilitated by a relaxed abdomen—place arms at sides and instruct woman to bend knees. Clean gloves are required to examine the perineum. Time should be taken to perform the examination since it is an ideal time to teach the woman about how the body heals, signs of effective or ineffective healing, and self-care measures.	Eliminate responses *c* and *d* from the words "quickly" and "sterile." There is no need to have the woman put her arms over her head.
2. Correct answer: d	
Although often given shortly after birth, 72 hours is the latest that Rhogam can be given effectively.	Remember: *t*hree days maximum for *t*herapeutic *t*reatment with Rhogam.
3. Correct answer: b	
Responses *a, c,* and *d* are all correct techniques. If creams are used they should be applied after a feeding once breasts have been cleansed with warm water and air dried. Colostrum or milk is a safer more effective alternative to creams.	The words "just prior to . . . feeding" in response *b* calls attention to the need for further teaching. Besides if the nipples are covered with creams which typically taste bad, the infant will not feed well.
4. Correct answer: a	
Cold packs reduce tenderness whereas warmth would increase circulation thereby	Recall warmth dilates to possibly result in further swelling; removal of breast milk stimulates more

increasing discomfort. Expressing milk results in continued milk production. Plastic liners keep nipples and areola moist leading to excoriation and cracking.

milk production; and plastic next to any skin will promote skin breakdown. The pressure of a snug, supportive bra minimizes milk production and irritation. It is also important to identify that the question is about a woman who is "bottle-feeding."

5. Correct answer: b

Responses *a, c,* and *d* are all effective relief measures for the breast-feeding mother. Frequent emptying of the breasts using good breast-feeding technique prevents or limits the extent of engorgement if it occurs.

Be alert that the situation is a woman who is breast-feeding. If you have no idea of the correct answer, try to cluster the responses *a, c,* and *d* under a positive approach without restriction. Note in response *b* the NOT recommended relief measure is different than the other responses since the action is "limit frequency."

6. Correct answer: c

Feeding should be initiated on the least sore breast first since the infant's suck is usually more vigorous at the beginning of a feeding. Never apply creams over a crack since it will inhibit healing. Use breast milk instead. Frequency of feeding is not limited but the duration of feeding on the sore breast may be decreased for a short period of time. Alternating positions applies pressure to different areas of the areola.

If you have no idea of the correct answer, cluster options *a, b,* and *d* to be of a more narrow nature. Select option *c* since it seems logical and associate that if a client gets reddened skin while in bed the action is to change the position, so in this situation maybe it is the better action of the given choices.

7. Correct answer: d

Responses *a*, *b*, and *c* are all appropriate measures. The peribottle should be used in a backward direction toward the perineum. The flow should NEVER be directed upward into the vagina.

Apply the basic principle of perineal care: go from front to back and do not direct flow "into" the vagina for prevention of infection. The peribottle is not to be used as a douche.

8. Correct answer: a

The fundus should be massaged only when boggy. Massaging a firm fundus could cause it to relax. Responses *b*, *c*, and *d* are all effective measures to enhance contraction of the uterus and to facilitate healing.

Recall that the fundus is a muscle. When firm and then massaged, like any muscle it can become relaxed. Also response *a* can be identified as incorrect in that an action is recommended for a client without assessment or evaluation of the effectiveness of the intervention; this negates the sequential steps in the nursing process.

9. Correct answer: b

Ice packs should be applied for only 20 to 30 minutes at a time and repeated after one hour. They are used during the first 12 hours following birth. Use topical preparations as needed but no more than 4 times a day. Apply topicals directly to the episiotomy for maximum effectiveness.

Use common sense to eliminate response *a;* ice to a site for more than 30 minutes potentiate the risk of skin breakdown and over an incision may prevent normal healing. The word in response *c* that eliminates it as a correct response is "every" pad change. The warm water of a sitz bath promotes comfort, cleansing, and circulation for healing.

10. Correct answer: d

Urine is acidified with cranberry juice. The woman should drink at least 3 liters of fluid a day and empty her bladder every 2 hours to prevent stasis of urine.

Key words in the stem that lead to the correct answer are "increased risk" for UTI and "prevention measure."

CHAPTER 15

Complications Associated with the Postpartum Period

STUDY OUTCOMES

fter completing this chapter, the reader will be able to do ie following:

- Define the key terms listed.
- Identify the major complications of the postpartum period.
- Discuss the factors that place the postpartum woman at risk for the development of complications.
- Describe the major assessment findings, nursing diagnoses, and treatment approaches for
  - postpartum hemorrhage
  - postpartum infection

KEY TERMS

Endometritis	Uterine infection usually at the placental site that can spread to the fallopian tubes and peritoneum creating a major threat to fertility and life.
Hematoma	Accumulation of blood within tissue of the pelvis or genitalia (labia, vagina, perineum) as a result of bleeding from a blood vessel damaged during the process of childbirth.
Mastitis	Infection of breast tissue.
Maternal mortality rate	Number of maternal deaths related to the complications of pregnancy, birth, and the postpartum (puerperium) per 100,000 live births.
Postpartum hemorrhage	Blood loss of ≥500 ml or a blood loss representing ≥1% of body weight following birth.
Uterine atony	Uterine hypotonia noted as a boggy or flaccid fundus.

CONTENT REVIEW

I. Overview of concerns with postpartum complications

A. **Major complications encountered as a part of postpartum recovery include**
   1. Hemorrhage
   2. Infection
   3. Postpartum depression or psychosis

B. **Complications occur as a result of ineffective recovery following pregnancy and birth and are more common among women whose**
   1. Pregnancy was considered to be high risk in terms of such factors as pregnancy induced hypertension (PIH), diabetes, multiple gestation, placental abnormalities
   2. Labor was dysfunctional and required medical or surgical intervention
   3. Postpartum lifestyle is inadequate in terms of rest, nutrition, hygiene, and social support

C. **Determination of risk factors associated with complications of the postpartal period assists the nurse in identifying clients who are most likely to develop these problems**

D. **Postpartum complications are a major cause of maternal mortality—hemorrhage, with postpartum hemorrhage as the most common type of excessive blood loss associated with pregnancy**

E. Early discharge following birth requires that women be instructed regarding

1. Prevention—self-care measures related to hygiene, nutrition, rest, activity, social support have been found to be effective in preventing major complications
2. Early detection—signs and symptoms indicative of ineffective recovery and the development of complications
3. Prompt treatment—actions to take if signs of complications are detected. Examples: massage fundus, when to call healthcare provider (physician, midwife).

F. Complications can interfere with

1. Maternal attachment to newborn and development of parenting skills; nurses should
   a. Provide short periods, within the tolerance level of the woman, for interaction with her newborn; gives her a chance to see, touch, and gradually care for newborn
   b. Encourage expression of feelings
2. Family coping as a result of delay in maternal recovery—nursing interventions include
   a. Encouragement of family members to express feelings
   b. Provision of opportunities for family members to be together
   c. Discussion of strategies that may be helpful in constructively readjusting family processes such as involvement of grandparents, other family members, and friends in care of other children; use of homemaker services

II. Postpartum hemorrhage

A. Blood loss of ≥500 ml or a blood loss representing ≥1% of body weight following birth

▼ Hypervolemic state of pregnancy provides initial protection and delays the onset of shock

1. Early postpartum hemorrhage—occurs within the first 24 hours following birth and is primarily the result of
   a. Uterine atony
   b. Lacerations of the labia, perineum, vagina, cervix
   c. Hematoma—use of forceps or vacuum extraction and pressure from presenting part are common causes for this damage
   d. Clotting disorders
      (1) Disseminated intravascular coagulation (DIC)—abnormal, diffuse clotting pattern that depletes clotting factors and results in massive bleeding

(2) Decreased platelets as can occur with severe PIH and the HELLP syndrome

2. Late postpartum hemorrhage—occurs from the 2nd postpartum day until the 28th postpartum day, most often during the first week or two and is primarily the result of
   a. Subinvolution especially at the placental site—delayed return of the uterus to its nonpregnant size and function
   b. Retained placental fragments
   c. Infection

B. Risk factors associated with postpartum hemorrhage

1. Dystocia
   a. Prolonged or precipitous labor patterns
   b. Interventions such as external version, forceps, vacuum extraction, birth by cesarean section
   c. Stimulation of labor with oxytocin (Pitocin)
2. Overstretching of the uterus—inhibits uterine ability to contract and leads to atony
   a. Macrosomia
   b. Hydramnios
   c. Multiple gestation
   d. Grand multiparity—five or more pregnancies and births
3. Placental abnormalities
   a. Abruptio placenta—bleeding can use up clotting factors leading to DIC and can force blood into myometrium limiting the ability of the fundus to contract
   b. Placenta previa—decreased contractility of lower uterine segment
   c. Placental adherence to uterine wall—manual removal, retention of fragments which limit ability of uterus to contract
4. Administration of magnesium sulfate in the treatment of preterm labor or PIH; ability of uterus to contract is inhibited by an elevated Mg level
5. Uterine infection such as chorioamnionitis associated with prolonged rupture of the membranes

C. Nursing diagnoses and major assessment findings related to hemorrhage—goal is early detection leading to prompt intervention with prevention of hemorrhagic shock and major life threatening complications (shock lung, DIC, renal necrosis)

1. Alteration in cardiac output related to uterine atony with blood loss from lack of muscle constriction

2. Fluid deficit related to blood loss—assess amount (pad counts and pad weight 1 g = 1 ml), character, and source of blood loss
   a. Uterine
      (1) Profuse, bright red blood with clots
      (2) Fundus boggy
   b. Laceration or episiotomy
      (1) Bright red blood in steady stream or trickle
      (2) Fundus firm
   c. Hematoma
      (1) Concealed bleeding
      (2) Increasingly severe pelvic pain or pressure and vaginal fullness; complaints of urge to defecate
      (3) Tissue bulging or swelling
      (4) Urinary retention as a result of pressure on bladder or urethra
      (5) Fundus firm
3. Alteration in vital signs reflecting fluid deficit—hypovolemia
   a. Blood pressure
      (1) Initially a widening of the pulse pressure as a result of a decrease in systolic pressure and a compensatory increase in diastolic pressure associated with peripheral vasoconstriction
      (2) Progressing to hypotension
   b. Pulse—rapid progressing to rapid, weak, and irregular
   c. Respirations—rapid, deep progressing to rapid, shallow, and irregular
   d. Temperature decreases
4. Alteration in renal tissue perfusion related to hypovolemia associated with hemorrhage—decreasing urine formation progressing from oliguria (< 30 ml/hr) to anuria
5. Alteration in peripheral tissue perfusion related to compensatory vasoconstriction associated with hypovolemia
   a. Pallor
   b. Cool progressing to cold
   c. Dry progressing to moist, clammy
   d. Delayed capillary refill
6. Alteration in cerebral tissue perfusion related to hypovolemia associated with hemorrhage
   a. Restlessness, anxiety
   b. Lightheadedness, faintness, dizziness, vertigo

c. Diminishing level of consciousness and responsiveness, lethargy
d. Mental cloudiness, confusion

D. Interventions relate to source and degree of blood loss

▼ Women who are hemorrhaging and in shock need one-on-one care. They should never be left alone.

1. Measures to reduce blood loss
   a. Uterine atony—stimulate uterine contraction
      (1) Massage uterus until firm
      (2) Stimulate nipples manually or with breast-feeding—increases endogenous secretion of oxytocin by the pituitary gland
      (3) Administration of oxytocics (listed in order of use)
         (a) Oxytocin (Pitocin) infusion, adding 20 to 40 U to 1000 ml of an IV solution—administer at a recommended rate of 10 to 15 ml/min
         (b) Methylergonorine maleate (Methergine) 0.2 mg IM
            ▼ Assess BP prior to and 5 to 10 minutes after administration since hypertension is a dangerous side effect—hold dose if BP is ≥140/90
         (c) Prostaglandin F_{2a} (Carboprost Tromethamine) 0.25 mg IM
            (i) Used if uterine atony-hemorrhage is unresponsive to other drugs and interventions
            (ii) Repeated every 1½ to 3½ hours as determined by firmness of fundus but not to exceed 12 mg in 24 hours
            (iii) Should not be given if pelvic inflammatory disease or cardiac, pulmonary, renal, or hepatic disorders are present
            (iv) Should be used with caution if the woman is an asthmatic
            (v) Administer with an antiemetic and antidiarrheal
      (4) Insert catheter to prevent bladder distension and to monitor renal perfusion by noting urinary output per hour
   b. Surgical intervention to evacuate a hematoma, remove placental fragments, or repair lacerations or episiotomy

2. Replace fluid losses—carefully monitor response to treatment by measuring I&O and assessing for signs of fluid excess
   a. Infusion of crystalloid or colloid solutions
   b. Blood transfusion
3. Enhance circulation to heart and lungs by facilitating venous return
   a. Position client with small pillow under head and legs elevated from the hips to an angle of 20 degrees
   b. Alternate position every 2 hours
4. Strict asepsis for care measures since there is an increased risk for infection with hemorrhage
5. Reduce fear and anxiety and enhance rest
   a. Provide explanations and keep client and family informed
   b. Consolidate or plan care to provide periods of uninterrupted rest
   c. Povide comfort measures to enhance relaxation

      ▼ Interventions related to advancing hemorrhage and shock are beyond the scope of this textbook. The reader is referred to a medical-surgical text for a comprehensive discussion of hemorrhagic shock.

III. Postpartum infection

A. Four major sites for infection during the postpartum period

1. Reproductive tract
   a. Endometritis
   b. Cervix, vagina, perineum, vulva
2. Urinary tract
3. Incisional
   a. Episiotomy, laceration
   b. Abdominal incision of cesarean birth
4. Breasts—mastitis

B. Six risk factors associated with postpartum infection

1. Dystocia
   a. Prolonged labor process—duration >24 hours
   b. Multiple invasive procedures especially if associated with break in aseptic technique
      (1) Repeated vaginal examinations especially after membranes have ruptured
      (2) Catheterization
      (3) Interventions such as forceps, vacuum extraction, cesarean birth
      (4) Internal fetal monitoring

c. Prolonged rupture of membranes—>24 hours before birth
d. Retained placental fragments
2. Inadequate hygienic practices—general hygiene as well as breast and perineal care
3. History of health problems such as repeated genitourinary infections, diabetes, anemia, poor nutrition
4. Postpartum hemorrhage
5. Ineffective breast-feeding techniques leading to cracking and breakdown of nipples and areola
6. Poor nutritional status

C. Nursing diagnoses and major assessment findings related to postpartum infection—goal is early detection leading to prompt intervention and prevention of complications that can permanently effect reproductive functioning

1. Alteration in body temperature related to the effects of the infection process
   a. Body temperature ≥100.4° F
   b. Present on 2 consecutive days following the first 24 hours after birth
   c. Accompanied by tachycardia and tachypnea
   d. Dehydration and breast engorgement must be ruled out as a basis for temperature elevation
2. General findings related to infection
   a. Risk for fluid deficit related to
      (1) Diaphoresis
      (2) Anorexia
      (3) Nausea and vomiting
   b. Alteration in comfort related to
      (1) Malaise, fatigue, lethargy
      (2) Chills
      (3) Headache
   c. Elevation in white blood cell count
3. Specific findings related to infection site—alteration in comfort related to
   a. Reproductive tract
      (1) Foul smelling lochia
      (2) Uterine tenderness—may be enlarged
      (3) Low backache
      (4) Pelvic pain
      (5) Dysuria
   b. Incisional infection
      (1) Redness—erythema
      (2) Edema

(3) Drainage—purulent with foul odor
(4) Separation of wound edges
(5) Alteration in comfort

c. Urinary tract
(1) Frequency, urgency
(2) Alteration in comfort—dysuria
(3) Cloudy urine, odor, hematuria

d. Breasts
(1) Infected nipple and areola fissure or crack
(2) Edema and engorgement as infection spreads to breast tissue
(3) Hard, red, tender mass or abscess
(4) Most often findings involve one breast (unilateral)

D. Interventions relate to the severity of the infection as well as the site of involvement

▼ Consideration of universal precautions and aseptic principles is critical to prevent the spread of infection to other sites and persons

1. Interventions for alteration in body temperature
   a. Monitor temperature, vital signs, fluid balance
   b. Administer antibiotics to destroy causative organism
      (1) Obtain specimen of drainage, urine for culture prior to the initiation of antibiotic treatment
      (2) Intravenous (IV piggyback) and oral are the most commonly used routes of administration
      (3) Utilize appropriate principles to obtain maximum antibiotic effect
   c. Remove causative organism by incision and drainage of abscesses
   d. Administer antipyretics when fever is elevated >102° F and is accompanied by discomfort such as headache, joint pain
      (1) Fever is therapeutic since it enhances the action of the immunological system and the effectiveness of antibiotics
      (2) Tylenol is preferred since it is not associated with clotting disorders or gastrointestinal distress
   e. Encourage nutrient and fluid intake to prevent dehydration and energy depletion
      (1) Small, frequent meals of easily digested foods
      (2) Fluid intake of at least 3000 ml/day
   f. Administer fluids intravenously if oral intake is insufficient to balance fluid loss and energy depletion

g. Measures to cool the body and cleanse the skin
   (1) Cool environment
   (2) Dry, cotton linen and clothes
   (3) Cool cloth on forehead
   (4) Shower, sponge bath

2. Interventions for alteration in comfort
   a. Local applications of heat or cold using packs, pads, sitz bath
   b. If mother is breast-feeding, keep breasts empty and preserve lactation process by pumping breasts and discarding milk until infection is resolved and antibiotics are discontinued
   c. Cleanse skin and mucous membranes of irritating, foul smelling drainage
3. Interventions for fatigue and anxiety
   a. Organize care—provide uninterrupted rest periods
   b. Provide explanations and keep the client and family informed of progress since fear regarding future reproduction and ability to continue breast-feeding may be present

REVIEW QUESTIONS

1. The nurse should evaluate each postpartum woman for factors that increase her risk for hemorrhage. Which of the following postpartum women is at low risk for postpartum hemorrhage?
   a. Multiparous woman who experienced a precipitous labor and birth
   b. Primiparous woman who gave birth to an 8 pound newborn
   c. Multiparous woman who gave birth to her sixth child
   d. Primiparous woman who continues to receive an infusion of magnesium sulfate for preeclampsia

2. Early postpartum hemorrhage—hemorrhage that occurs within the first 24 hours after birth—is *least* likely to occur as a result of
   a. Subinvolution of the uterus, especially the placental site
   b. Uterine atony
   c. Lacerations of the labia, perineum, vagina, or cervix
   d. Hematoma formation within the tissue of the pelvis and genitalia

3. A postpartum woman is bleeding profusely, fully saturating her perineal pad in 1 hour. The saturated pad weighs 50 g. This would represent a blood loss of approximately how many ml?
   a. 25
   b. 50
   c. 75
   d. 100

4. An early sign of hypovolemia associated with excessive blood loss would be
   a. Urinary output <25 ml/hour
   b. Widening of the pulse pressure
   c. Irregular apical heart beat
   d. Cold, clammy skin

5. When caring for a postpartum woman who is hemorrhaging the nurse would NOT expect to administer
   a. Prostaglandin E_2
   b. Pitocin
   c. Methergine
   d. Prostaglandin F_{2a}

6. Which of the following factors presents the lowest risk for postpartum infection?

a. 14 hour labor followed by a spontaneous vaginal birth
b. Membranes ruptured for 28 hours prior to birth
c. Vacuum extractor used to assist with internal rotation and birth of the fetal head
d. Internal monitors applied to assess FHR patterns and intrauterine pressure

7. A woman diagnosed with mastitis and receiving antibiotics should

a. Feed her baby from the uninfected breast
b. Discontinue breast-feeding
c. Begin feeding on the uninfected breast first
d. Maintain lactation by pumping both breasts and discarding the milk

ANSWERS, RATIONALES, AND TEST-TAKING TIPS

Rationales	Test-Taking Tips
1. Correct answer: b	
Women described in *a, c,* and *d* all exhibit risk factors associated with postpartum hemorrhage, since each factor interferes with ability of the uterus to contract.	Key words in the question are "low risk." Cluster the responses multiparous, think stretched uterus from multiple births, and primiparous with a complication of higher risks.
2. Correct answer: a	
Subinvolution is most closely associated with late postpartum hemorrhage (2nd day until the 28th day) along with retained placental fragments and infection.	Think logically—hemorrhage with lacerations and hematoma—eliminate two of the responses. Recall that atony means loss of tone of the given parameter, in this case the uterus; this situation would promote the presence of a boggy uterus. Thus, the only response left is *a;* subinvolution think of a slow involution.
3. Correct answer: b	
1 g of weight equals approximately 1 ml of blood.	If you have no idea of the correct response, match the number in the stem with the answer or use the number technique: eliminate the highest and lowest numbers—25 and 100—and then use a conservative approach to select 50.
4. Correct answer: b	
Responses *a, c,* and *d* all reflect worsening hypovolemic shock and are later appearing signs.	The most important word in the stem is "early" sign. Note an increasing heart rate would also be a first sign; however it is not one of the given responses.

5. Correct answer: a

Prostaglandin E_2 is primarily used in gel form to stimulate cervical ripening.

Remember that Prostaglandin $_{E2}$ is used in *E*arly labor not postpartum.

6. Correct answer: a

Of the four options listed, response *a* represents the lowest risk because 14 hours is an average duration for labor and a spontaneous birth, without the use of forceps or vacuum extractor, is the expected outcome. Response *b* is a risk factor because the rate of infection increases dramatically once 24 hours have passed since the membranes have ruptured; responses *c* and *d* increase risk because they are invasive procedures.

First identify that responses *c* and *d* are invasive—think infection risk increased—and eliminate. With responses *a* and *b* left, note that the time in response *b* is longer therefore infection risk is higher. Select response *a* as correct.

7. Correct answer: d

Infants should not receive breast milk as long as infection is present and the mother is being treated. Lactation should be maintained since breast-feeding may be resumed once the problem is resolved.

Note that responses *a, b,* and *c* are less comprehensive; for example response *a* doesn't say what to do with the infected breast.

CHAPTER 16

Physiologic Adaptations to Extrauterine Life

STUDY OUTCOMES

After completing this chapter, the reader will be able to do the following:

- Define the key terms listed.
- Describe the full-term neonate's anatomic and physiologic adaptation to extrauterine life.
- Identify expected assessment findings and variations and warning signs of ineffective adaptation or deviations from the norm related to

  respiration
  circulation
  nutrition-fluid and electrolytes
  temperature regulation
  elimination—bowel and bladder
  neurologic function
  muscular activity and rest
  sensation
  endocrine-reproductive function
  integument

KEY TERMS

Acrocyanosis Bluish tinge to hands and feet of newborn especially when exposed.

Erythema toxicum Newborn rash characterized by round, erythematous areas with small, raised yellowish centers; often a response to the environment.

Habituation Newborn's ability to shut out environmental stimuli.

Lanugo Fine, downy hair found on the shoulders, back, pinna of ears, and forehead of the newborn.

Milia Plugged sebacious glands that look like pimples; found on face, especially the chin and nose.

Moro reflex Immediate extension and abduction of newborn's arms with fingers fanning out as thumb and forefinger form a *C* as a result of a sudden, intense stimulus; adduction and flexion of the arms into an embrace type position follows the initial response.

Neonatal period First 28 days of life.

Periods of reactivity Periods comprising the transition to extrauterine life; the transition lasts approximately the first 6 to 8 hours of life and is characterized by instability of newborn's behavioral states and physiologic function.

Rooting reflex Newborn will turn head and open mouth when side of cheek, lips, or mouth are stimulated with a finger or nipple.

Vernix caseosa White, odorless, cheesy substance that covers the newborn's integument at birth.

CONTENT REVIEW

I. Overview of physiologic adaptations

A. Neonatal period—one of rapid growth and development

1. Deviations from the norm, if left undetected and untreated, may result in irreversible damage to the newborn and its well being. Example: oxygen deprivation associated with ineffective breathing patterns can have an adverse effect on the neurological system.
2. The healthy full-term newborn requires close and ongoing observation to distinguish expected assessment findings and variations from warning signs of ineffective adaptations or deviations from the norm that require intervention from a healthcare provider

3. The newborn's parents must receive support, guidance, and instruction in the observation and care of their new baby
4. Early discharge programs must ensure follow-up of the newborn and its parents by competent healthcare providers

B. The full-term healthy neonate typically experiences less mature function of its body systems than an adult, which can result in

1. Limited reserves in times of stress. Example: cold stress or chilling of the newborn can compromise the respiratory system and deplete glucose stores.
2. A risk for infection, hypothermia-hyperthermia, fluid imbalances, injury, and hyperbilirubinemia

II. The anatomic and physiologic adaptations of the full-term neonate to extrauterine life are described in Table 16-1

Table 16-1. Anatomic and Physiologic Adaptations of the Full-Term Neonate to Extrauterine Life

Anatomic-Physiologic Adaptations	Expected Assessment Findings and Variations	Warning Signs of Ineffective Adaptation Deviations from the Norm
I. Oxygenation		
▼ Effective function of both the respiratory and circulatory system is critical if the newborn is to receive adequate oxygen for survival—both systems function in an interdependent manner		
A. Respiration		
First Breath Stimulated by	*First Breath Occurs Immediately Upon Birth—Progresses to Lusty, Rhythmic Cry*	*Persistent*
Brief period of hypoxia at birth—carbon dioxide retained—respiratory center stimulated	*Respirations Reflect the Following Characteristics*	Bradypnea (≤15 breaths per minute)
Recoil of chest following compression during passage through birth canal	Rate: average of 40 with a range of 30 to 60 per minute	Tachypnea (≥60 breaths per minute)
Exposure to environmental stimuli—light, cool air, touch	Quiet and effortless without sternal retraction or nasal flaring	Crackles
Lungs Expand Easily as a Result of	Rate, depth, and rhythm vary according to activity level	*Episodes of Apnea ≥15 Seconds Accompanied by Cyanosis and Signs of Respiratory Distress*
Surfactant—reduces surface tension of alveoli—facilitates alveolar expansion and contraction with breathing	Brief periods of apnea without evidence of respiratory distress or cyanosis	*Signs of Respiratory Distress*
Fluid fills lungs while in utero—lungs are maintained in partial expansion	Diaphragmatic in nature—abdomen moves more noticeably with breathing than the chest	Nasal flaring
Fetal breathing movements occur in utero		Expiratory grunting
		Persistent sternal-intercostal retractions even at rest
		Chin tug
		Persistent and Copious Watery Drainage from Nose
		Bulging or Malformations of the Chest

Lung Fluid Must be Removed in Order to Facilitate Newborn Respiration One-third is squeezed out with chest compression at birth Remaining fluid is reabsorbed into circulatory and lymphatic systems within 12 hours of birth	*Auscultation of Lungs* Generally clear without presence of adventitious sounds ▼ Crackles may be noted until lung fluid clears; however usually no signs of distress are exhibited *Nose* Symmetrical, intact, broad nose with midline placement on face Patent—small amount of mucus may be present Sneezes to clear nasal passages No flaring of nares with breathing ▼ Nasal patency must be maintained since newborns are nasal breathers *Chest* Circular, barrel shape Expands and contracts symmetrically with breathing Chest and abdomen expand and contract in synchrony with breathing *Crying—Strong, Lusty, of Moderate Tone and Pitch, with Episodes Lasting About 3 to 7 Minutes Following Consoling Measures*	*Asymmetrical Chest Expansion* *Seesaw Respirations—Asynchronous Expansion and Constriction of Chest and Abdomen with Breathing* *Crying That Is High Pitched or Shrill, Weak, or Absent*

Continued.

Table 16-1. Anatomic and Physiologic Adaptations of the Full-Term Neonate to Extrauterine Life—cont'd

Anatomic-Physiologic Adaptations	Expected Assessment Findings and Variations	Warning Signs of Ineffective Adaptation Deviations from the Norm
B. Circulation		
With Birth, Circulation Changes From a Fetal to Adult Pattern	*Blood Pressure*	*Hypotension or Hypertension*
Loss of placental circulatory network with cutting of cord	Average 75/42 mm Hg at birth	*Systolic Pressure in Lower Extremities 6 to 8 mm Hg Less Than Upper Extremities*
▼ Decreased venous return leads to increased pressure in right side of heart	Range of 60 to 80/40 to 50 mm Hg	*Apical Beat Auscultated on the Right Side of the Chest*
▼ Increased arterial flow with increase in systemic vascular resistance leads to increased pressure in left side of heart	Approximately the same in upper and lower extremities	*Persistent*
▼ Foramen ovale (fetal shunt between right and left atria) closes as a result of the atrial pressure changes	*Apical Pulse*	Tachycardia ≥160 at rest
▼ Ductus venosus (fetal shunt which acts as a liver bypass) closes	Located on the left side, 4th intercostal space—pulsations may be visible and palpable	Bradycardia ≤120 per minute or resting rate <80 to 100 per minute
	Rate 120 to 140 per minute varies with activity level of newborn	Dysrhythmias
	▼ Sleep—as low as 100 per minute	Murmurs
	▼ Activity-crying episode—as high as 160 per minute with transient irregularity	*Femoral Pulses—Weak, Absent, or Asymmetrical*
	▼ Transient tachycardia after birth as high as 180 per minute	*Temperature of Extremities Asymmetrical With One Side Warmer or Cooler Than the Other*

Lungs fill with air at the first breath ▼ Decreased pulmonary vascular resistance ▼ Decreased pressure in right side of heart ▼ Increased pulmonary circulation leads to increased blood return to left side of heart and increased pressure in left side of heart ▼ Ductus arteriosus (fetal shunt that bypasses lungs) closes to allow full pulmonary circulation and blood gas exchange ▼ Ineffective respiratory patterns can lead to hypoxia with reopening of fetal shunts since permanent anatomic closure does not take place until infancy	Regular, strong, sharp, clear sounds *Transient, Minor Murmur May Be Auscultated Until Shunt Fully Heals Over* *Femoral Pulses—Bilaterally Equal and Strong* *Pulses are Palpated Simultaneously with Tips of Fingers Along Inguinal Ligament About Midway Between the Iliac Crest and Pubic Symphysis* *Temperature of Extremities—Bilaterally Warm with Cooler Hands and Feet Especially Upon Exposure*	

Continued.

Table 16-1. Anatomic and Physiologic Adaptations of the Full-Term Neonate to Extrauterine Life—cont'd

Anatomic-Physiologic Adaptations	Expected Assessment Findings and Variations	Warning Signs of Ineffective Adaptation Deviations from the Norm
Color of Newborn Is Influenced by Adequacy of respiratory-circulatory functioning Sluggish peripheral circulation results in color variations related to position and environmental temperature Elevated RBC count Blood vessels closer to the surface of the body as a result of a limited amount of subcutaneous fat	*Pink Color with Ruddy (Deep Red Color) Appearance Following Activity and Crying Episodes* *Acrocyanosis—Bluish Tinge to Hands and Feet Especially When Exposed; Hands and Feet May Also Feel Cooler to the Touch* *Mottling (Cutis Mamorata) Marbled, Irregular Coloration of the Skin When Exposed to Decreased Environmental Temperature* *Harlequin Sign—Difference in Color of Skin Related to Position of Newborn, i.e., When Lying on Side, Lower Half of Body Becomes Pinker While Upper Half of Body Becomes Pale Pink*	*Cyanosis—Circumoral, Generalized Pallor or Grayness* *Plethora—Very Dark Red Color*
Fetus Produces a Large Number of RBCs to Ensure Adequate Oxygen Transport during Intrauterine Life	*Hemoglobin: 14 to 29 g/dL with a Mean of 17* *Hematocrit: 43 to 69% with a Mean of 55%* *RBC Count: 5.7 to 5.8/mm*	*Hemoglobin and Hematocrit Levels Are Less Than or Greater Than Expected*

Hyperbilirubinemia (Elevated Bilirubin Levels, Primarily Unconjugated Bilirubin) Can Occur Since	*Physiologic Jaundice*	*Jaundice Appears in the First 24 Hours or Does Not Meet the Criteria Listed for Physiologic Jaundice*
Neonatal breathing supplies sufficient oxygen Excessive RBCs are destroyed causing bilirubin level to rise Breakdown and excretion of bilirubin are limited by ▼ Immaturity of the liver and its ability to breakdown bilirubin ▼ Limited milk intake inhibits subsequent stooling and reduces excretion of bilirubin which leads to bilirubin reabsorption into the circulatory system	Develops after first 24 hours of life and disappears by the 9th to 10th day of life Serum (unconjugated or indirect) bilirubin levels neither exceed 12 mg/100 ml nor is there an increase of more than 5 mg in one day Conjugated or direct bilirubin levels do not exceed 1 to 1.5 mg/100 ml Jaundice tends to progress in a cephalocaudal and proximodistal (see sequence of list below) direction, with extent of jaundice exhibited in dermal zones approximating bilirubin level, for example ▼ Nose: 3 mg/dL ▼ Face: 5 mg/dL ▼ Chest: 7 mg/dL ▼ Abdomen: 10 mg/dL ▼ Thighs: 12 mg/dL ▼ Knees to ankles, elbows to wrists: 15 mg/dL ▼ Feet, hands: >15mg/dL Jaundice fades uniformly	

Continued.

Table 16-1. Anatomic and Physiologic Adaptations of the Full-Term Neonate to Extrauterine Life—cont'd

Anatomic-Physiologic Adaptations	Expected Assessment Findings and Variations	Warning Signs of Ineffective Adaptation Deviations from the Norm
Postnatal Bleeding Tendency Occurs as a Result of Inability to synthesize vitamin K until intestinal flora develops as part of the digestion process Immaturity of the liver in terms of producing prothrombin and other clotting factors	*Petechiae—Red Pinpoint Hemorrhagic Areas Usually Appearing on the Presenting Part of Fetus during Delivery*	*Petechiae and Ecchymosis—Generalized or Over Areas of Body Unrelated to Pressure of Birth Especially if Persistent in Nature*
Hemorrhagic Areas Occur as a Result of Pressure and Trauma as Part of the Birth Process	*Hemorrhagic Area Noted in Sclera or Conjunctiva* *Ecchymosis (Bruising) May Occur* Facial from pressure of forceps use Occipital from pressure of vacuum extractor Buttocks and sacrum with a breech birth	

II. Nutrition/fluid and electrolytes

Adequacy of Intrauterine Nutrition and Fetal Growth is Reflected In	*Measurements*	*Measurements*
Neonatal body size and weight as compared to gestational age	Fall within the 10th to 90th percentile AND are appropriate for the estimated gestational age	Are <10th percentile or >90th percentile
Presence and amount of subcutaneous fat or adipose tissue	Measurements are consistent within the same percentile	Are inconsistent—fall in different percentiles, i.e., head circumference is in a larger percentile than weight
Limited Oral Intake Coupled with Fluid Loss Through Bowel and Bladder Elimination, during the First Few Days of Life, Results in a Loss of Weight and a Tendency Toward Dehydration	Comparisons should be made with parental or family body builds and history of other newborn birth weights	
	Weight ▼ Average range of 2500 to 4000 g (5 lb 8 oz to 8 lb 13 oz) ▼ Represents expected weight for gestational age (appropriate for gestational age (AGA)) ▼ Expected weight loss of 5 to 10% of birth weight during the first week of life and regained within 2 weeks	Weight ▼ <2500 g is considered to be a low birth weight (LBW) as a result of: — Intrauterine growth retardation—small for gestational age (SGA) — Preterm birth ▼ >4000 g is considered to be macrosomia or large for gestational age (LGA) ▼ Weight loss of >10% or delay in returning to birth weight may reflect dehydration or inadequate feeding patterns
	Head circumference ▼ Average range of 32 to 37 cm (12½" to 14½")	Head circumference ▼ <32 cm

Continued.

Table 16-1. Anatomic and Physiologic Adaptations of the Full-Term Neonate to Extrauterine Life—cont'd

Anatomic-Physiologic Adaptations	Expected Assessment Findings and Variations	Warning Signs of Ineffective Adaptation Deviations from the Norm
	▼ Usually 2 to 3 cm (1") larger than the chest circumference	▼ ≥4 cm larger than chest
	▼ Molding may result in a head circumference that is slightly smaller or equal to chest circumference for the first day or two after birth	
	▼ Head length represents ¼ of body length	
	Chest circumference ranges from 30 to 33 cm (12" to 13")	
	Abdominal circumference approximately the same as the chest, but increases after a feeding	
	Length 45 to 55 cm (18" to 22")	
	Fat Deposits Present	*Fat Deposits—Limited as Noted by*
	Sucking pads—fat deposits in the cheeks that give them a rounded or full appearance	Loose, baggy, wrinkled skin
	Integument—full with few wrinkles	Prominent clavicles and ribs
	Buttocks—rounded or full	Small or absent sucking pads
	Hydration Status Indicated by	*Hydration Status—Indicators of Dehydration or Inadequate Nutrient Intake*
	Weight gain or loss follows expected patterns	Weight loss
		Decreased amount and frequency of urination

	Turgor—resilience or hydration of integument determined by pinching skin over abdomen or thigh; skin should return to original state immediately upon release	Poor turgor—skin remains tented and is slow to return to original position
	Anterior fontanel flat	Depressed anterior fontanel
	Temperature within normal range	Temperature elevation may occur
	Voiding—6 to 10 voidings of pale yellow urine each day	
Digestion and Utilization of Nutrients	*Liver—Palpable in the Upper Right Quadrant about 2 cm Below the Costal Margin (Sharp Edge)*	*Liver—Enlarged with Rounded Edge*
Adequate for protein and simple carbohydrates	*Hyperbilirubinemia with Resultant Physiologic Jaundice after First 24 Hours*	*Glucose Level Fails to Stabilize within the Expected Range*
Limited with regard to complex carbohydrates and fats	*Slight Peripheral Edema at Birth Especially at Body Areas Experiencing Pressure during the Birth Process*	*Signs of Hypoglycemia Are Exhibited*
Liver Functions on an Immature Level with Limited Ability to	*Postnatal Bleeding Tendency*	Irritability or jitteriness
Conjugate bilirubin including that formed as a by-product of RBC breakdown	*Increased Tendency to Hypoglycemia*	Tremors
Produce plasma proteins, prothrombin, and other coagulation factors	Glucose levels fall after birth as a result of limited stores and utilization of glucose for energy	Lethargy
Store glycogen	Stabilize at 50 to 60 mg/dL during the transition period following birth	Poor feeding behavior
		Cyanosis

Continued.

Table 16-1. Anatomic and Physiologic Adaptations of the Full-Term Neonate to Extrauterine Life—cont'd

Anatomic-Physiologic Adaptations	Expected Assessment Findings and Variations	Warning Signs of Ineffective Adaptation Deviations from the Norm
Effective Feeding Behaviors Must be Present in Order to Supply the Required Fluids and Nutrients for Optimum Growth, Development, and Well Being	*Feeding Reflexes—Must be Present and Effective for Adequate Intake during Feeding*	*Weak or Absent, Asymmetrical Rooting Reflex*
Stomach	Rooting reflex ▼ Stimulus—before feeding, stroke side of cheek, lips, mouth with finger or nipple ▼ Response turns head toward stimulus, opens mouth, takes hold, and starts to suck	*Weak Suck—Need for Continued Encouragement to Continue to Suck and Swallow*
Filled with mucus and amniotic fluid during intrauterine life; removed after birth via vomiting and regurgitation; feeding and digestion is facilitated once it is removed	Suck—strong and rhythmic Swallow—coordinates with suck	*Swallow Is Not Coordinated with Suck Leading to* Excessive regurgitation while feeding Gagging, coughing, vomiting *Projectile Vomiting* *Slow to Rouse, Sleepy or Lethargic, Needs to be Awakened to Feed*
Capacity is limited to approximately 90 ml with an emptying time of 2 to 4 hours	*Exhibits Hunger Every 3 to 4 Hours by an Eagerness to Feed as Demonstrated by Sucking Movements of Mouth, Active Rooting, and Crying*	
Cardiac sphincter at entrance into stomach from esophagus is immature making regurgitation possible, especially with rapid and/or overfeeding; high risk for aspiration when supine	*Exhibits Satisfaction Following a Feeding by Sleeping for 2 to 5 Hours* *Gains Weight at Rate of Approximately 5 to 7 Ounces Per Week*	
Gastric acidity is reduced after the first week of life; infant increases formation of gas and development of colic from gas pains	*Mother and Newborn Demonstrate Satisfaction and Comfort with Chosen Feeding Method* *Regurgitation of Small Amounts of Milk*	

III. Temperature regulation		
Temperature Regulation Is Immature and Places the Newborn at Risk for Hyperthermia and Hypothermia Limited subcutaneous fat to insulate body bringing blood vessels closer to surface of body; blood influenced by environmental conditions Larger body surface (heat loss) compared to body mass (heat production) Sweat glands ineffective for first month of life—unable to sweat to dissipate heat Inability to change body posture to reduce the amount of body surface exposed to cool temperatures Inability to shiver for heat production *Brown Fat—Specialized Fat Located in Several Areas of the Newborn's Body (i.e., Nape of Neck, Between Scapula, Around Kidneys) Is Capable of a High Metabolic Rate That Produces Heat and Blood Is Warmed as It Circulates Through It*	*Axillary Temperature: 36.5 to 37° C (97.6 to 98.6° F)* *Temperature Stabilizes within Approximately 8 to 10 Hours of Birth* *Transitory Dehydration Fever Can Occur at Approximately 2 to 4 Days Following Birth Until Fluid Intake Balances Fluid Losses; Easily Reversed by Increasing Fluid Intake*	*Temperature Does Not Stabilize by 10 Hours after Birth* *Hypothermia (Subnormal Temperature) or Hyperthermia (Elevated Temperature) May Occur as a Result of Such Factors as* Environment that is too cold or too hot Over or underdressed Infection Dehydration *Cold Stress—Exposure to Cold Temperatures Results in* Increased activity with crying, restlessness, muscular movement which causes an increase in BMR leading to heat production Increased respiratory rate to meet increased oxygen demand which leads to stress on respiratory system and respiratory depression Depletion of glucose stores to meet energy demands of increased BMR means increased risk of hypoglycemia Increased activity level means fatigue *Hyperthermia Can Result in Dehydration Which Can Lead to Cerebral Damage*

Continued.

Table 16-1. Anatomic and Physiologic Adaptations of the Full-Term Neonate to Extrauterine Life—cont'd

Anatomic-Physiologic Adaptations	Expected Assessment Findings and Variations	Warning Signs of Ineffective Adaptation Deviations from the Norm
IV. Elimination		
A. Bowel		
Abdominal Muscles Are Not Fully Developed Leading to a Limited Ability to Fully Support Abdominal Contents	*Abdomen—Rounded, Symmetrical, Protuberant, Dome-Shaped; Prominence of Abdomen Increases after Feeding*	*Abdomen* Flat or flabby Hard, distended Asymmetrical
Intestinal Capacity Is Small Which Leads to More Frequent Bowel Movements—Gastrocolic Reflex (Bowel Movement during or Just after a Feeding as a Result of Its Stimulation of Peristalsis)	*Bowel Sounds Present within 1 to 2 Hours of Birth; Intermittent, Soft, Tinkling Sounds at a Frequency of 10 to 20 Seconds* *Anus Patent (Open) with Active Wink Reflex (Anus Contracts When Touched)*	*Bowel Sounds—Absent or Hyperactive with Visible Peristaltic Waves* *Anus—Imperforate*
Fecal Characteristics Are Influenced by Nature of Oral Intake	*Bowel Movements (BM)* First bowel movement within 24 to 36 hours of birth—influenced by timing of first feeding Frequency of stools ▼ Approximately 5 to 6 each day during the first 2 weeks ▼ Develops individual elimination pattern that can vary from a BM every other day to as many as 3 to 6 per day	*Bowel Movements* No stool by 36 hours or more Meconium has strong, foul odor Passage of hard, formed constipated type stool Passage of green, watery, diarrhea type stool ▼ Newborns receiving phototherapy for hyperbilirubinemia normally exhibit frequent, loose green stools Presence of blood or mucus in stool

Type of stools

- ▼ Meconium—dark greenish-black sticky stool composed of amniotic fluid, intestinal secretions, bilirubin, cells, blood; passed during the first few bowel movements
- ▼ Transitional stool—thin, slimy, greenish-brown to yellow; passed from 3rd to 6th day
- ▼ Milk stool
  - — Breast-fed newborn—loose, golden-yellow, nonirritating, sour milk odor
  - — Bottle-fed newborn—soft, pale yellow to light brown, more offensive odor

Continued.

Table 16-1. Anatomic and Physiologic Adaptations of the Full-Term Neonate to Extrauterine Life—cont'd

Anatomic-Physiologic Adaptations	Expected Assessment Findings and Variations	Warning Signs of Ineffective Adaptation Deviations from the Norm
B. Bladder		
Kidneys Must Take Over Elimination and Filtration Function of Placenta	*Voiding*	*Failure to Void by 24 Hours after Birth*
Renal System Functions at an Immature Level with Limited Ability to	First urination within 24 hours of birth	*Distended Bladder*
Concentrate urine	Frequency is approximately	*Weak or Hesitant Stream*
Maintain fluid, electrolyte, and acid-base balance especially in times of stress, such as vomiting, diarrhea, infection, improper feeding with formula that is too concentrated or too dilute	▼ 2 to 6 for first 2 days then up to 20 per day	
Bladder Capacity Is Approximately 40 ml	▼ 6 to 10 times per day after the first week of life	
	Stream of urine—full	
	Urine	
	Pale yellow, dilute, nearly odorless	
	Rust stained as a result of uric acid crystals	
	Specific gravity of 1.005 to 1.015 once fluid intake is established	

V. Neurological function

Nervous System

Lacks complete integration and function

Characterized by primitive reflex activity

Stimuli are used to elicit a variety of reflexes as part of the assessment of the integrity of neurological function

When Testing Reflexes Keep in Mind

Responses should be bilaterally strong and symmetrical

Accuracy is facilitated when the newborn is in a quiet, alert state

Repeated stimulation of a reflex will result in a diminishing response as a result of the newborn's ability to shut out environmental stimuli—called habituation

Stimulation may be ineffective in eliciting reflexes when the newborn is in a deep sleep state

Reflexes disappear during infancy and are replaced by purposeful activity

Common Newborn Reflexes

Moro Reflex (Figure 16-1)

Stimulus—hold in semisitting position and allow head and trunk to fall backward to an angle of 30 degrees OR place in a supine position on a flat surface then strike surface or clap hand above newborn—any sudden, intense stimulus should elicit the response

Response—immediate extension and abduction of arms with fingers fanning out as thumb and forefinger form a *C;* followed by adduction and flexion of arms into an embrace type position; the legs may move into similar positions as the arms

Grasp (Palmar/Plantar) Reflex

Stimulus—place finger in palm of hand; place finger at base of toes

Response—finger curl firmly around finger (palmar) and toes curl downward (plantar)

Reflex Responses to Stimuli Exhibit

Asymmetry with one side of body responding in a different manner or with less strength

Absent or weak response despite application of a strong stimulus and newborn not in a deep sleep state

Persistence of reflex response beyond expected time of disappearance

Continued.

Table 16-1. Anatomic and Physiologic Adaptations of the Full-Term Neonate to Extrauterine Life—cont'd

Anatomic-Physiologic Adaptations	Expected Assessment Findings and Variations	Warning Signs of Ineffective Adaptation Deviations from the Norm
Neurological Development Follows a Predictable Sequence of Cephalocaudal (from head to foot)—able to support head before sitting, able to sit before standing or walking Proximodistal (from midline to peripheral)—able to control shoulder movement before movement of hands and fingers, masters gross movement before fine movement, i.e., able to walk before able to write	▼ Grasp reflex is an important reflex to facilitate formation of attachment *Tonic Neck (Fencing) Reflex (Figure 16-2)* Stimulus—place in a supine position then turn head to one side; repeat stimulus to other side; may occur spontaneously Response—extends arm and leg on side to which head is turned while opposite arm and leg flex *Step-Walk (Dance) Reflex* Stimulus—hold in an upright position and allow feet to touch flat surface Response—flexes and extends knees making steplike movements *Crawling Reflex* Stimulus—place in a prone position (on abdomen) Response—crawling movements are made with arms and legs *Babinski Reflex* Stimulus—stroke sole of foot upward beginning at heel along lateral aspect of sole then move across ball of foot to big toe	

Response—toes hyperextend (fan out) and big toe dorsiflexes; described as a Babinski positive

Pull to Sit Reflex

Stimulus—place in a supine position, grasp hands or wrists, and pull to a sitting position

Response—head lags initially until upright, then head is brought into alignment with chest and shoulders and neck maintains control for a brief period before head falls forward

Continued.

Table 16-1. Anatomic and Physiologic Adaptations of the Full-Term Neonate to Extrauterine Life—cont'd

Anatomic-Physiologic Adaptations	Expected Assessment Findings and Variations	Warning Signs of Ineffective Adaptation Deviations from the Norm
Skull Bones Are Slightly Separated to Allow for Expansion of Skull during Brain Growth	*Head—Symmetrical and Round Once Molding Subsides* *Palpate Sutures and Fontanelles with Distal Finger Pads When Infant Is Quiet* Sutures—space between skull bones ▼ Slightly separated or open ▼ Transitory override or overlap of skull bones can be noted as a result of head compression during passage through birth canal (molding) Fontanelles—spaces in skull where suture lines meet ▼ Flat, some bulging can occur when crying or stooling ▼ Flat when upright and quiet ▼ Measure widest part of fontanelle from bone to bone ▼ Anterior fontanelle—diamond shaped; average size: 2.5 (width) to 4 cm length (1 to 1¾") ▼ Posterior fontanelle: triangular shape; 0.5 to 1 cm (0.2 to 0.4"); may not be palpable when molding is present	*Head: Persistent Asymmetry or Irregularity in Shape; Depressions or Fractures* *Sutures-Fontanelles* Widely spaced or enlarged, closed or fused sutures or fontanelles Sunken or depressed fontanelles Bulging fontanelles at rest—may indicate increased intracranial pressure

Caput Succedaneum (Figure 16-3A)
Edema over Presenting Part of Head as a Result of Pressure during Birth

Cephalhematoma (Figure 16-3B)
Development of a Hematoma between Periosteum and Skull Bone as a Result of Trauma or Pressure at Time of Birth

Continued.

Table 16-1. Anatomic and Physiologic Adaptations of the Full-Term Neonate to Extrauterine Life—cont'd

Anatomic-Physiologic Adaptations	Expected Assessment Findings and Variations	Warning Signs of Ineffective Adaptation Deviations from the Norm
VI. Muscular activity and rest		
Posture: Following Birth the Newborn Tends to Assume Its Intrauterine Posture	*Posture—General Flexion*	*Posture*
Upper and Lower Extremities: Appearance and Function Are Influenced by Both the Maturity and Development of the Neuromuscular System and Intrauterine Position	Extremities moderately flexed and adducted	Hypotonia with relaxed, extended extremities and floppy, lethargic posture
	Fists clenched	Hypertonia, jitteriness, irritability
	Slight tremors with movement and crying; occasional spontaneous startles	*Face—Persistent Asymmetrical Appearance or Movement*
	Temporary Positional Variations Gradually Subside	*Neck*
	Facial asymmetry as a result of intrauterine pressure from shoulder or arm	Webbing
	Legs in extension and stiff as a result of a breech presentation	Masses, enlarged lymph nodes or thyroid, distended veins
	Face	Limited or absent range of motion of neck; head held at an angle
	Symmetrical appearance at rest and when crying or feeding	Fractures or crepitation of clavicle
	Bilateral symmetry in movement of facial features	*Spine*
	Neck	Presence of pilonidal cyst, sinus or dimple, tuft of hair along spine
	Short, thick with skin folds, flexible	Limited movement
	Limited ability to support head in upright position except for short periods (pull to sit reflex)	Asymmetry, lateral curvature
	Ability to lift head (momentarily) and turn it to side when in the prone position	Spina bifida—congenital neural tube defect resulting in a lack of union between the laminae of the vertebrae, primarily in the lumbar area; spinal cord, membranes, and fluid may herniate through the opening to the back leading to serious problems

Full range of motion of shoulders and neck Clavicles intact *Spine—Midline, Straight, Flexible, Intact* *Extremities—Bilaterally Symmetrical as to Size and Movement* 10 fingers and 10 toes with free range of motion and strong grasp Creases on palms of hands; intact nails to fingertips (sharp) Creases on ⅔ of soles; plantar fat pad creates a flat-footed appearance Arms slightly longer than legs Legs may appear to be bowed with feet turning in slightly Strong muscle tone of arms and legs offers resistance to extension by examiner; arms may offer more resistance than legs Full range of motion of all joints but movement is asynchronous—arms and legs move fully but not in the same way at the same time *Hips-Femur—Intact as Exhibited by* Symmetrical gluteal folds Absence of a click when Ortolani's maneuver is performed	*Extremities* Asymmetry of extremities as to appearance, size, movement Fingers and toes ▼ Syndactyly (fused or webbed digits) ▼ Missing digits ▼ Polydactyly (extra digits) ▼ Simian crease on palms of hands suggests Down Syndrome Club foot—foot positioned downward and inward; may be bilateral, unilateral, and present to varying degrees Limitation or lack of movement of an extremity Hip displacement as exhibited by ▼ Asymmetrical gluteal folds on side of displacement ▼ Presence of a click when performing Ortolani's maneuver

Continued.

Table 16-1. Anatomic and Physiologic Adaptations of the Full-Term Neonate to Extrauterine Life—cont'd

Anatomic-Physiologic Adaptations	Expected Assessment Findings and Variations	Warning Signs of Ineffective Adaptation Deviations from the Norm
Transitional Period Following Birth, Approximately the First 6 to 8 Hours of Life, Is Characterized by Instability and Occurrence of Periods of Reactivity *The Newborn's Behavioral States and Physiologic Function Fluctuate Widely* *Observation of Neonatal Behaviors during These Periods Provides Important Data Related to Its Health and Well Being* *Newborns Develop Individualized Patterns of Sleep and Activity States (Table 16-2)*	*First Period of Reactivity—First 15 to 30 Minutes after Birth* Tachycardia (160 to 180 heart rate) Irregular, rapid respirations (60 to 80 rate), with brief periods of apnea Transient rales or crackles, grunting, nasal flaring, and chest retractions Alert, cries, sucks, displays interest in the environment, makes eye contact Transient tremors, spontaneous startles Able to begin feeding and to interact with parents *Period of Inactivity or Rest—Next 2 to 4 Hours (Some Authorities Say 60 to 90 Minutes)* Heart rate slows to 100 to 120 Respirations slow to 50 to 60, becoming easy and quiet Activity level decreases, becomes drowsy and enters a deep sleep state Level of responsiveness decreases, difficult to arouse Bowel sounds can be auscultated	*Newborn's Behaviors Do Not Meet Expectations with Regard to Periods of Reactivity, Stability of Body Systems, or Sleep and Activity Patterns*

Second Period of Reactivity Lasts 10 Minutes to Several Hours (Some Authorities Say 4 to 6 Hours)

Heart and respiratory rates fluctuate with transitory periods of tachycardia, tachypnea, and brief periods of apnea

Awakens from sleep, becomes alert and responsive to feeding and environment; activity alternates with periods of sleep

Gastric and respiratory secretions increase; gagging and regurgitation can occur

Bowel sounds increase; passes meconium

Voids

Following this period the newborn begins to exhibit stability of body systems and a pattern of sleep and activity

Sleep-Activity Patterns—Typical Behaviors Are Described in Table 16-2

Continued.

Table 16-1. Anatomic and Physiologic Adaptations of the Full-Term Neonate to Extrauterine Life—cont'd

Anatomic-Physiologic Adaptations	Expected Assessment Findings and Variations	Warning Signs of Ineffective Adaptation Deviations from the Norm
VII. Endocrine-reproductive function		
Influence of Maternal Hormones, Primarily Estrogen, Effect the Appearance of Breasts, and Genitalia of Both Male and Female Newborns	*Breasts*	*Breasts*
Pressure during a Breech Birth May Result in Bruising and Increased Edema of the Genitalia	Symmetrically placed	Malpositioned or widely spaced
	Size: 3 to 10 mm of tissue	Erythema and firmness around nipples
	Slight swelling and secretion of a milky substance called witch's milk	Supernumerary nipples—extra nipples along nipple line; often associated with renal anomalies
	Nipples prominent, well formed	*Ambiguous Genitalia—Genitalia Do Not Exhibit Characteristics Typical of Either Sex; Not Clearly Male or Female*
	Areola may be pigmented	
	Female Genitalia	*Female Genitalia*
	Labia majora—edematous, pigmented, meet at midline and cover labia minora	Enlarged clitoris with meatus at the tip
	Clitoris—edematous-prominent	Fused labia
	Urinary meatus—located below clitoris	Absence of vaginal opening
	Vernix caseosa found between labia and at groin	Fecal discharge from vagina
	Pseudomenstruation—odorless, mucoid vaginal discharge that may be blood tinged	Inflammation of urethra
		Foul smelling discharge

	Male Genitalia	*Male Genitalia*
	Scrotum—edematous, pigmented, pendulous and covered with rugae (wrinkles) Testes bilaterally descended and palpable in scrotum Penis—slender; erection may occur when genitalia are touched Urinary meatus—slitlike and located at tip of penis Prepuce (foreskin) membrane that covers glans penis ▼ Not easily retracted ▼ Removed at circumcision ▼ Smegma—a white cheesy substance found under the foreskin Cremasteric reflex—retraction of testes when chilled	Absence of rugae Testes undescended Hydrocele—accumulation of fluid in the scrotal sac; may resolve spontaneously Adherent, tight prepuce Urinary meatus not at the tip of the penis ▼ Epispadias—urinary meatus is on the dorsum (upper side) of penis; urinary sphincter is defective ▼ Hypospadias—urinary meatus is on the underside of the penis; sphincter remains intact *Inguinal Hernia*

Continued.

Table 16-1. Anatomic and Physiologic Adaptations of the Full-Term Neonate to Extrauterine Life—cont'd

Anatomic-Physiologic Adaptations	Expected Assessment Findings and Variations	Warning Signs of Ineffective Adaptation Deviations from the Norm
VIII. Sensory function		
Sensory Functions Are Fairly Well Developed at Birth and Provide the Newborn with the Capability to Interact with Its Environment and the People within It. The Attachment Process Is Enhanced by the Newborn's Ability to Make Eye Contact, Attend to Voices, Respond to Touch, and Recognize Odors, Including Mother's Milk	*Eyes* Size, shape, and all structures are symmetrical Position—distance between the inner aspects of the eyes equals the length of the eye (2 to 3 cm) Eyebrows distinct Eyelids—equal, freely moveable, open adequately; slightly edematous related to pressure at birth; erythema may be present as a reaction to ophthalmic ointment used after birth to prevent infection Eyeballs—round and firm Pupils—round, equal, reactive to light Iris—intact; blue-gray or brown Sclera—clear, bluish-white (slightly yellowish in dark skinned races); hemorrhagic area(s) may be present related to pressure at birth Cornea and lenses—clear, intact Conjunctiva—pink, moist; clear drainage and erythema may be present as a result of medication used after birth	*Eyes* Size, shape, structures asymmetrical Closely or widely set eyes Opacities-cataracts or ulcerations of cornea and lenses Pink color of iris Purulent discharge; persistent erythema Epicanthal fold or mongolian slant in nonorientals Asymmetry of pupil size; limited or absent (fixed dilation or constriction) reaction to light Blue or yellow sclera Persistent strabismus Unable to follow to midline or fixate on objects

Tears—scant or absent since tear glands begin to function at 2 to 4 weeks of age

Movement of the eyes:

- ▼ Random, somewhat jerky movements
- ▼ Follows objects (about 8" away) to midline; fixates momentarily
- ▼ Makes eye contact and gazes intently
- ▼ Pseudostrabismus—transient occurrence of a cross-eyed appearance until eye muscles are fully developed at about 4 months of age
- ▼ Doll's eye phenomenon—as head is turned eye movement lags behind first 10 days of life

Blink-Glabellar reflex

- ▼ Stimulus—tap forehead at bridge of nose with finger
- ▼ Response—both eyes blink simultaneously with first 4 to 5 taps

Continued.

Table 16-1. Anatomic and Physiologic Adaptations of the Full-Term Neonate to Extrauterine Life—cont'd

Anatomic-Physiologic Adaptations	Expected Assessment Findings and Variations	Warning Signs of Ineffective Adaptation Deviations from the Norm
	Ears Symmetrical appearance and placement with upper part of pinna slightly above outer canthus of eye Well formed with curved pinna and firm resilient cartilage Responds to sounds ▼ Moves head in direction of sound ▼ Loud, sudden noise: Moro reflex, cries ▼ Low pitched sound: quiets, soothes ▼ High pitched sound: alerts ▼ Recognizes and responds to sounds heard while in utero, such as father's or mother's voice, heart beat	*Ears* Placement below outer canthus of eye Asymmetrical placement or appearance Overly prominent or protruding ears Limited amount of cartilage Presence of skin tags, sinuses Limited or absent response to sounds
	Smell—Responds to Various Odors in Different Ways Turns away from strong or foul odors Turns toward pleasant or familiar odors, such as mother's scent and her milk	

Taste—Responsive to Different Tastes
Tasteless: no response
Sweet or pleasant taste: eager sucking, satisfaction
Sour/bitter taste: puckering, anger, grimace, cry
Touch—Responsive to Touch
Gentle patting, rubbing, cuddling: soothes, calms
Painful stimulus: cries, anger, increased activity

Continued.

Table 16-1. Anatomic and Physiologic Adaptations of the Full-Term Neonate to Extrauterine Life—cont'd

Anatomic-Physiologic Adaptations	Expected Assessment Findings and Variations	Warning Signs of Ineffective Adaptation Deviations from the Norm
IX. Integument		
Integument (Skin) Delicate and easily damaged Sensitive to handling and exposure to environment and substances including clothing, linens, diapers, lotions and soaps, feces or urine Breaks in the integrity—umbilical cord, circumcision, rashes, and abrasions or cracks—increase the risk of infection *Integument Is Protected In Utero by Vernix Caseosa (White Cheesy Substance) and Lanugo (Hairy Growth) That Cover the Surface of The Body; Begin to Wear Away as Term Approaches* *Sweat and Sebaceous Glands Do Not Begin to Function Until the 2nd Month of Life*	*Skin* Color: generally pink with deepening pigmentation related to ethnic or racial origin begins after birth Transient hyperpigmentation may occur related to maternal hormones: areola, genitalia, linea nigra Soft, smooth or full with few wrinkles Resilient (turgor), well hydrated with dryness or cracking at ankles, feet, and wrists Reddened, irritated areas may occur where skin comes in contact with environmental substances Vernix caseosa—white, odorless; removed with first bath though some may remain in creases or folds (groin, axilla, labia) Lanugo—fine, downy hair found on shoulders, back, pinna of ears, forehead Milia—plugged sebaceous gland that looks like pimples (whiteheads) and found on face especially on chin and nose; disappear spontaneously	*Skin* Characteristics present associated with a preterm newborn: ▼ Deep, ruddy color ▼ Edema: hands, feet, labia ▼ Thin, smooth ▼ Abundant lanugo and vernix caseosa Characteristics present associated with a postmature newborn: ▼ Thick, dry skin ▼ Desquamation (peeling) ▼ Absence of lanugo and vernix caseosa Presence of pustules, blisters, rashes, lacerations, excoriations, ecchymoses (bruises) Cafe au lait spots—light brown spots over body; presence of >6 Vernix caseosa—yellow/green reflects intrauterine passage of meconium; odor may indicate infection Hemangioma—birth marks associated with capillary formations

	Erythema toxicum—newborn rash characterized by round, erythematous areas with small, raised, yellowish centers; often a response to the environment; resolves spontaneously Mongolian spots—hyperpigmented, ecchymoticlike areas usually over buttocks and sacrum; commonly occur among dark-skinned newborns; fade gradually Telangiectatic nevi (stork bite marks)—flat, pink, easily blanched localized areas of dilated blood vessels found on the eyelids, bridge of nose, occiput, and nape of neck; deepen in color with crying; fade gradually over 1 to 2 years	▼ Strawberry mark (nevus vasculosus)—raised, sharply demarcated, bright or dark red, rough surfaced lesion that resembles a strawberry ▼ Port-wine stain (nevus flammeus)—nonraised, red-purple lesion that varies as to size, shape, and location (most frequently the face); does not blanch or fade with pressure
	Hair Silky, single strands Lies flat, growing toward face and neck	*Hair* Coarse or brittle Fine or wooly (preterm) Unusual growing patterns
	Mouth/Oral Cavity Mucus membranes ▼ Pink, moist, intact ▼ No white patches	*Mouth/Oral Cavity* Thrush (candidiasis)—white, adherent patches or plaques on tongue, palate, and buccal membranes; bleed when touched Cleft lip and/or palate

Continued.

Table 16-1. Anatomic and Physiologic Adaptations of the Full-Term Neonate to Extrauterine Life—cont'd

Anatomic-Physiologic Adaptations	Expected Assessment Findings and Variations	Warning Signs of Ineffective Adaptation Deviations from the Norm
	▼ Epstein's pearls—whitish, hard epithelial cysts on hard palate and gums	Large, protruding tongue; limitation in movement
	Soft or hard palate intact	Profuse salivation or drooling
	Lips	
	▼ Symmetrical, midline, intact	
	▼ Sucking blisters	
	Tongue: nonprotruding, freely moveable, symmetrical	
	Saliva: scant to none	
	Umbilical Cord	*Umbilical Cord*
	Gelatinous, full at birth	Bleeding, oozing around cord
	Whitish-gray color	Yellow/green discoloration or odor
	Odorless	1 artery may indicate internal anomalies, such as renal
	2 arteries and 1 vein	Umbilical hernia—outpouching or protrusion of abdominal contents into area of cord
	Progressive drying with no signs of infection present	Signs of infection or inadequate healing
	Falls off after about 1 week, slight bleeding (a few drops) can occur	

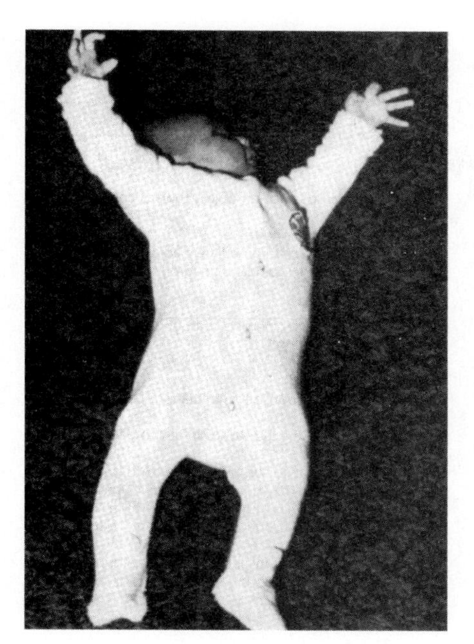

Figure 16-1. Moro reflex. (From Wong: *Whaley and Wong's nursing care of infants and children*, ed 5, St Louis, 1995, Mosby.)

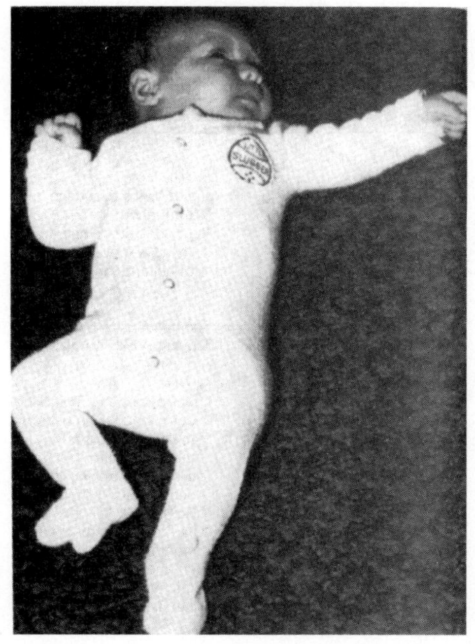

Figure 16-2. Tonic neck reflex. (From Wong: *Whaley and Wong's nursing care of infants and children*, ed 5, St Louis, 1995, Mosby.)

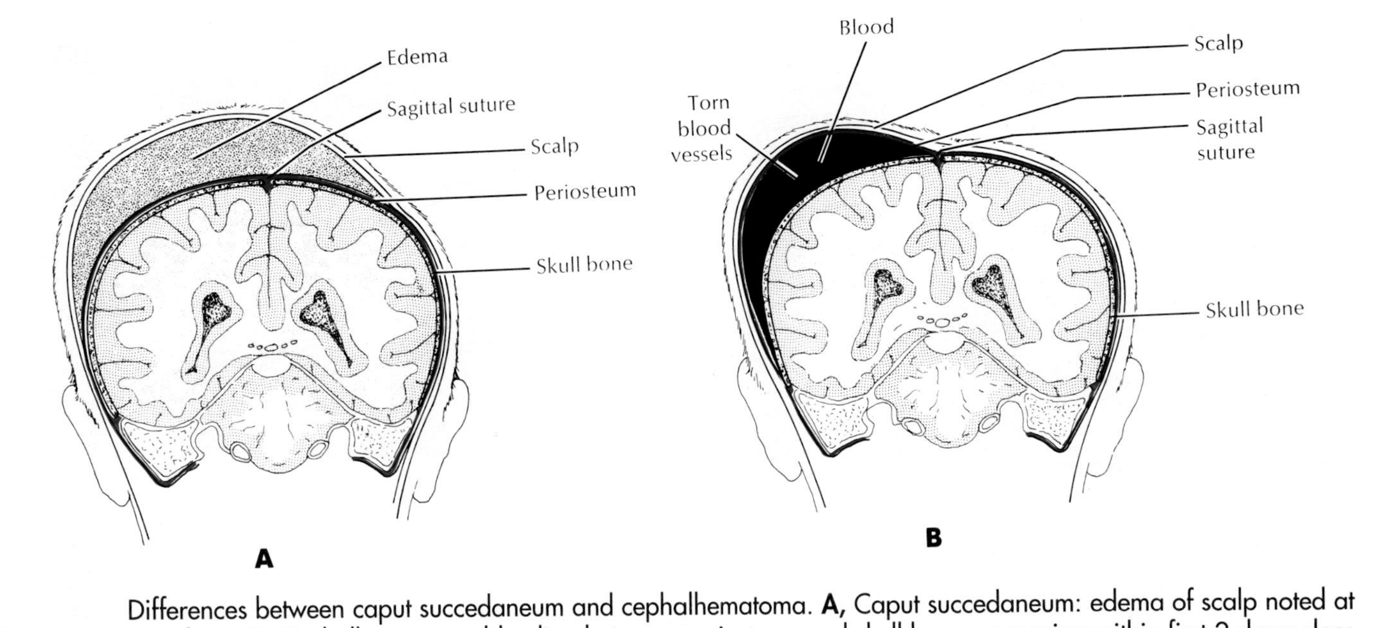

Figure 16-3. Differences between caput succedaneum and cephalhematoma. **A,** Caput succedaneum: edema of scalp noted at birth; crosses suture lines. **B,** Cephalhematoma: bleeding between periosteum and skull bone appearing within first 2 days; does not cross suture lines. (From Bobak IM et al: *Maternity and gynecologic care: the nurse and the family*, ed 5, St Louis, 1993, Mosby.)

Table 16-2. Behavioral States of the Infant

Behavioral State	Characteristic Behaviors
Sleep	
Deep Sleep Timing: approximately 4 to 5 hours/day; 10 to 20 minutes for each period of sleep	Respirations regular, deep, smooth Eyes closed, face relaxed Inactive except for spontaneous startles or jerks Little to no response to external stimuli, including loud noises Difficult to arouse even to feed
Light Sleep Timing: approximately 12 to 15 hours/day; 20 to 45 minutes for each period of sleep	Respirations irregular Eyes closed with rapid eye movements (REM) Low level of activity: random, smooth muscular movements and stretches, twitches, startles, sucking movements External stimuli can elicit startle responses or state changes, i.e., to deep sleep or drowsy
Awake	
Drowsy/Dozing Timing: variable	Respirations irregular Eyes open or closed, eyelids flutter, eyes do not make contact or focus Variable activity level with smooth movements and occasional startles External stimuli usually elicit a delayed response or state changes

Table 16-2. Behavioral States of the Infant—cont'd

Behavioral State	Characteristic Behaviors
Quiet Alert	
Timing: approximately 2 to 3 hours/day	Respirations regular Eyes open, alert, and bright Minimal motor activity Focuses on or attends to source of external stimuli (orientation) such as objects, faces, voices, and sounds; responds to the stimuli for an extended period of time Optimum state of arousal ideal for interaction with others
Active Alert	
Timing: approximately 1 to 4 hours/day along with the crying state	Respirations irregular Eyes open, looking around High level of motor activity with thrusting of extremities and occasional startles Strong response to external stimuli with startles and movements Increased sensitivity to discomfort, hunger, fatigue; fussiness can occur Typically noted prior to a feeding
Crying	
Timing: approximately 1 to 4 hours/day along with the active alert state	Loud, vigorous crying accompanied by active movement of extremities and color changes, such as ruddiness Limited response to external stimuli Prolonged efforts are usually required to console and calm infant

REVIEW QUESTIONS

1. Prior to discharging a 24-hour-old newborn, the nurse assesses its respiratory status. An expected finding at this time would be
   a. Respiratory rate 45, irregular
   b. Costal breathing pattern
   c. Nasal flaring with some sternal retraction
   d. Crackles upon auscultation

2. The parents of a newborn become concerned when they notice that their baby seems to stop breathing or hold its breath for a few seconds. After confirming the parent's findings by observing the newborn, the nurse should
   a. Notify the physician
   b. Assess newborn for additional signs of respiratory distress
   c. Explain to the parents that this is the expected pattern of breathing for a newborn
   d. Tell the parents not to worry since their newborn is healthy

3. The nurse would notify the pediatrician if which finding was noted when assessing the respiratory status of a newborn during the rest period between the first and second periods of reactivity?
   a. Crackles upon auscultation
   b. Easy and quiet respirations
   c. Periods of apnea of 5 seconds or less without cyanosis
   d. Average respiratory rate of 65 to 70 per minute

4. Measurement of the newborn provides data regarding the adequacy of intrauterine nutrition and fetal growth. An expected finding when measuring a full-term newborn would be
   a. Weight: 9 pounds 12 ounces or 4432 g
   b. Head circumference: 13 inches or 32.5 cm
   c. Chest circumference: 1 inch or 2.5 cm larger than the head circumference
   d. Abdominal circumference: approximates the circumference of the head

5. An assessment finding indicative of effective newborn feeding behavior would be
   a. Exhibits signs of hunger and eagerness to feed at least every 3 to 4 hours
   b. Sleeps for 1 hour after a feeding
   c. Gains approximately 2 to 4 ounces each week
   d. Sleeps through the night by 2 weeks of age

6. Nurses should recognize that newborns have a limited ability to regulate body temperature since they
   a. Have a smaller body surface compared to body mass
   b. Lose more body heat when they sweat than would an adult
   c. Have brown fat which has a higher metabolic rate thereby increasing the risk for hyperthermia
   d. Are unable to shiver effectively to increase heat production

7. When caring for a newborn the nurse must be alert for signs of cold stress which would include which of the following?
   a. Decreased activity level
   b. Increased respiratory rate
   c. Hyperglycemia
   d. Shivering

8. As the nurse helps a new mother change the diaper of her 16-hour-old newborn, the mother expresses concern that the bowel movement is almost black in color. She asks the nurse if something is wrong. The nurse should respond to this mother's concern by
   a. Asking the mother if she took iron during pregnancy
   b. Telling the mother that the stool is normal
   c. Testing the stool for occult blood
   d. Explaining to the mother that the stool is called meconium and is typical of a newborn's first few bowel stools

9. The milk stools of a breast-fed newborn should be
   a. Golden yellow
   b. Formed
   c. Slimy, greenish-brown to yellow
   d. Odorless

ANSWERS, RATIONALES, AND TEST-TAKING TIPS

Rationales	Test-Taking Tips

1. Correct answer: a

The expected respiratory rate range is 30 to 60 respirations per minute and are commonly irregular as to rate and depth. Newborns exhibit a diaphragmatic or abdominal breathing pattern. Response *c* reflects signs of distress along with grunting, chin tug, and seesaw respirations. By 24 hours of age lung fluid should have been absorbed into the circulatory and lymphatic systems.

Cluster responses *b, c,* and *d* into abnormal findings; think of adults as well as infants.

2. Correct answer: c

Newborns typically exhibit irregular respirations with periods of apnea. Periods of apnea should be <15 seconds and cyanosis should not occur. Since this newborn is exhibiting a normal breathing pattern *a* and *b* are not required; *d* does not give parents enough information regarding typical newborn breathing characteristics.

Response *a* is incorrect since enough data is not available. Response *d* has a phrase that typically makes a response incorrect: "not to worry." The wording of response *b* "assess . . . additional signs . . . distress" supports its elimination since the data given in the stem as described does not indicate "respiratory distress."

3. Correct answer: d

Responses *a, b,* and *c* are all expected findings during the rest period between periods of reactivity. The expected respiratory rate ranges between 50 and 60 respirations per minute during this period and becomes quiet and easy.

The rate of respirations is the clue for selection of the correct response.

4. Correct answer: b

Average weight range for a full-term newborn would be 2500 to 4000 gm or 5 lb 8 ounces to 8 lb 13 ounces. Chest circumference should be 2 to 3 cm or 1 inch smaller than the head circumference. Chest and abdominal circumferences should be approximately the same.

The approach here is to eliminate the wrong answers and end up with the correct response. Remember in the normal term newborn the chest = abdominal circumference. This is the one time in life when to say that a person, the newborn, has a "big head" is accurate since the head is larger than the chest. Remember that the maximum weight in pounds is a little over eight.

5 Correct answer: a

A newborn should sleep at least 2 hours after a feeding and gain 5 to 7 ounces per week. The newborn is not expected to sleep through the night.

Associate the maximum weight gain with the days of the week: 7 days, a maximum of 7 ounces. Note the important words in the question "effective . . . feeding behavior." Then make an educated guess based on what you know that every 3 to 4 hours babies are fed in the hospital and this continues at home.

6. Correct answer: d

The newborn has a larger body surface (heat loss) compared to body mass (heat production). Sweat glands are ineffective for the first few months of life. Brown fat is activated when the infant's temperature falls to increase heat production.

Refer to the rationale.

7. Correct answer: b

Additional signs of cold stress include increased activity level and crying (increase BMR and heat production),

If you have no idea of the correct response, use the ABCs and select the respiratory response.

hypoglycemia as glucose stores are depleted. Newborns are unable to shiver as a means to increase heat production; they increase their activity level instead.

8. Correct answer: d

The stool is meconium and its dark black-green color is unrelated to maternal intake of iron or the presence of blood. Response *b* does not provide the mother with enough information to reduce her anxiety.

If you have narrowed the responses to *b* or *d,* select the most comprehensive answer, response *d.*

9. Correct answer: a

Milk stools of a breast-fed baby are typically loose, golden yellow, nonirritating with a sour milk type odor. Transitional stools are typically greenish brown to yellow and slimy. Formed stools are more characteristic of the bottle-fed newborn.

Take an educated guess and use common sense to eliminate formed, slimy, and odorless; thus, response *a* is the only one left.

CHAPTER 17

Application of the Nursing Process during the Neonatal Period

STUDY OUTCOMES

After completing this chapter, the reader will be able to do the following:

- Define the key terms listed.
- Discuss infant mortality statistics in terms of implications for health care.
- Identify predictors of and leading causes for infant mortality.
- Identify measures that have been found to be effective in reducing the infant mortality rate and improving the health of infants.
- State the guidelines that should be followed when assessing the newborn.
- Describe the process of gestational age assessment and determination of the adequacy of intrauterine growth.
- Identify the common laboratory tests performed during the neonatal period.
- State the components of a psychosocial assessment of the newborn and its family.
- Identify the common nursing diagnoses of the neonatal period.
- Describe measures that are effective during the neonatal period related to facilitating respiration, thermoregulation, preventing infection, nutrition, and preventing accidental injury

KEY TERMS

Appropriate for gestational age (AGA)	Designation given to a newborn whose birth weight meets the growth expectations for gestational age; weight falls between the 10th and 90th percentiles or within 2 standard deviations of the mean for gestational age.
Infant mortality rate	Number of deaths in the first year of life per 1000 live births.
Large for gestational age (LGA)	Designation given to a newborn whose birth weight exceeds the growth expectations for gestational age; weight is above the 90th percentile or 2 standard deviations above the mean for gestational age.
Low birth weight (LBW)	Weight at birth is less than 2500 g as a result of intrauterine growth retardation and/or preterm birth.
Small for gestational age (SGA)	Designation given to a newborn whose birth weight is less than the growth expectations for gestational age; weight is below the 10th percentile or 2 standard deviations below the mean for gestational age.

CONTENT REVIEW

I. Infant morbidity and mortality

A. The focus of health assessment and care during the neonatal period is based on the understanding that

1. The origins of many adult health and personal problems are found early in life and are influenced by parental habits, their knowledge, and their care of the infant
2. Infancy is the most hazardous year of life until the age of 65—the highest mortality rate occurs during the neonatal period, the first 28 days of life
3. Gross inequities may exist in the healthcare system with regard to the care of infants—the poor, uninsured, minorities, homeless, and those living in rural areas are not afforded the same opportunities for quality health care as the more advantaged segments of the population

B. Predictors of infant morbidity and mortality

1. Maternal predictors
   a. Age—<20 years of age or >35 years of age
   b. Member of a minority group
   c. Unmarried, with a limited support system

  d. Poorly educated
  e. Inadequate health care
  f. Exposure to teratogens, including the use of tobacco, alcohol, drugs, before and during pregnancy
 2. Major infant predictor—low birth weight

C. Infant mortality statistics

1. Currently the United States ranks 24th among industrialized nations in terms of infant mortality
2. Infant mortality rate
    a. 8.9 for all infants
    b. 17.6 for black infants
    c. 7.3 for white infants
3. Neonatal mortality rate—number of infant deaths in the first 28 days of life per 1000 live births; closely associated with intrauterine events and LBW
    a. 5.6 for all infants
    b. 11.2 for black infants
    c. 4.5 for white infants
4. Postneonatal mortality rate—number of infant deaths after the first 28 days of life per 1000 live births
    a. Closely associated with inadequate social and environmental conditions resulting from poverty, unsafe or unsanitary housing, limited resources to provide for infant needs in terms of health care, nutrition, and developmental stimulation
    b. Major causes of postneonatal mortality include: SIDS, congenital anomalies, accidents, and infectious diseases
    c. Rates
        (1) 3.3 for all infants
        (2) 6.4 for black infants
        (3) 2.8 for white infants

D. Leading causes for infant mortality

1. General
    a. Congenital anomalies
    b. Sudden infant death syndrome (SIDS)
    c. Disorders related to preterm birth, LBW
    d. Respiratory distress syndrome
2. Specific
    a. White infants—congenital anomalies
    b. Black infants—disorders related to preterm birth and LBW

E. Measures identified to be effective in reducing infant mortality and improving infant health

1. Preparation for pregnancy and parenthood
   a. Parenting classes before becoming pregnant, prenatally, and after birth
   b. Family planning classes and services that assist the couple to choose the time for pregnancy and parenting that is best for them
   c. Preconception care and counseling
2. Counseling to prevent congenital anomalies
3. Comprehensive, ongoing prenatal care that begins early in pregnancy
4. Parental health habits and lifestyle that focus on health promotion and disease prevention
   a. Good nutrition
   b. Maintenance of ideal weight with a balance of good nutrition and adequate exercise
   c. Good hygienic practices
   d. Healthy stress management which balances sleep, rest and relaxation, activity or work, and recreation
   e. Avoidance of alcohol, tobacco, and drug use before, during, and after pregnancy

II. Physical assessment of the newborn

A. Guidelines

1. Use Table 17-1 as an assessment guide to determine the health status of the newborn, the adequacy of its growth in utero, and the success of its adaptation to extrauterine life
   ▼ Frequently perform physical assessments immediately after birth and during the transition period of adaptation to extrauterine life; carefully document all observations and immediately report any deviations from the norm that could indicate neonatal distress
2. Adjust the environment which should be warm, free of drafts, and well lit
3. Avoid chilling newborn by performing the assessment quickly and efficiently with all equipment available, and exposing only the areas that are being examined; a radiant heat warmer can be used to maintain body temperature during the examination
4. Employ principles of asepsis throughout examination
   a. Progress from head to toe, assessing genitalia and anus last

Table 17-1. Common Nursing Diagnoses Encountered during the Neonatal Period

Client Outcomes	Nursing Interventions	Evaluation Checklist
A. Risk for impaired gas exchange related to immature status of neonatal respiratory system and presence of mucus in the respiratory tract		
Newborn Will Exhibit		*Newborn*
Easy, full, quiet respirations at a rate of 30 to 60	Assess adequacy of oxygenation including respiratory patterns and circulatory status	Exhibited quiet, easy respirations without nasal flaring, grunting, or sternal retractions
Clear breath sounds after first few hours following birth	Maintain airway patency	Maintained respiratory rate within expected newborn range
Regular, strong apical beat at a rate of 120 to 140	Gently suction oro-nasopharynx as needed—especially when breathing and crying sound congested; use	Exhibited strong, regular apical heart beat within expected newborn range; color pink with slight acrocyanosis
Pink color of conjunctiva and oral mucus membranes	▼ Bulb syringe — Suction mouth before nose — Compress bulb before insertion — Insert along side of mouth, between cheek and gum, not over tongue; into each nostril separately — Release bulb slowly while removing — Remove syringe from mouth; compress syringe to remove contents; repeat procedure until airway is clear	Experienced small amount of clear mucus—required suctioning of mouth and nose twice using a bulb syringe, during the first 12 hours after birth
Parents of Newborn Will Identify		*Parents*
Characteristics of effective breathing in the newborn		Demonstrated correct use of bulb syringe
Measures that facilitate newborn breathing and maintain airway patency		Correctly assessed newborn's respiratory status
		Identified measures required to ensure newborn safety with regard to breathing and airway patency

Continued.

Table 17-1. Common Nursing Diagnoses Encountered during the Neonatal Period—cont'd

Client Outcomes	Nursing Interventions	Evaluation Checklist
A. Risk for impaired gas exchange related to immature status of neonatal respiratory system and presence of mucus in the respiratory tract		
	▼ Mechanical suction for more copious and tenacious secretions is set at low suction, <100 mm Hg — Lubricate sterile catheter with sterile water — Insert catheter gently without forcing and with suction off — Apply suction with removal of catheter — Suction for ≤5 sec/insertion, with rest periods in between; oxygenate if needed Suction until crying and breathing sound clear Report suspicious secretions—may require testing for infection *Position Newborn to Facilitate Drainage of Mucus, Prevent Aspiration, and Enhance Breathing*	

Side-lying with support behind back (also prevents pressure on cord and circumcision)

Reclining position at 30 to 45 degree angle or side-lying position after feeding

Avoid prone position—may interfere with expansion of chest; has been associated with SIDS

Burp well after feeding and avoid overfeeding

Avoid feeding newborn for 1 to 2 hours prior to circumcision to prevent vomiting and aspiration

Reduce Factors That Place Stress on Respiratory System

Hypoglycemia—facilitate feeding

Cold stress-hyperthermia—use measures to maintain stable temperature within normal limits

Infection—aseptic or prevention measures

Continued.

Table 17-1. Common Nursing Diagnoses Encountered during the Neonatal Period—cont'd

Client Outcomes	Nursing Interventions	Evaluation Checklist
A. Risk for impaired gas exchange related to immature status of neonatal respiratory system and presence of mucus in the respiratory tract		
	Teach Parents Signs indicative of respiratory health Use of bulb syringe Emergency care for infant who is choking, not breathing, or needs CPR Measures to prevent respiratory tract infection and injury ▼ Stop smoking, especially in proximity to the newborn ▼ Avoid contact with persons experiencing respiratory tract infections ▼ Create a safe environment (Box 17-1) ▼ Use correct feeding techniques (Boxes 17-2, 17-3) ▼ Avoid use of talc powder—use cornstarch; apply into hand then onto baby—never sprinkle onto baby	

B. Risk for altered body temperature related to immaturity of the newborn's thermoregulatory function

Newborn's temperature will stabilize between 97.7 and 99° F within 8 to 10 hours of birth Newborn will not exhibit signs of cold stress or hyperthermia *Parents Will* Demonstrate correct technique for taking newborn's temperature using the axillary or tympanic method Identify measures effective in maintaining newborn's body temperature within the normal range	Assess newborn's temperature every hour until stable and periodically thereafter; check immediately after circumcision Use radiant heat warmer and thermistor probe during transition period while temperature stabilizes ▼ Place thermistor probe over skin on upper right quadrant of abdomen, below ribs, and not over a bone or the liver ▼ Cover probe with reflective material to avoid false readings ▼ Attach thermistor to control panel and set to desired temperature; alarm will ring when temperature is reached so newborn is not overheated Advance to axillary or tympanic method once stabilized—teach parents	*Newborn* Body temperature stabilized at 98° F 7 hours after birth Experienced no signs of cold stress or hyperthermia *Parents* Demonstrated correct technique when taking an axillary temperature using an electronic thermometer Described appropriate measures to prevent overheating or chilling of newborn Demonstrated safe, effective bathing technique

Continued.

Table 17-1. Common Nursing Diagnoses Encountered during the Neonatal Period—cont'd

Client Outcomes	Nursing Interventions	Evaluation Checklist
B. Risk for altered body temperature related to immaturity of the newborn's thermoregulatory function		
	Avoid use of rectal method ▼ Danger of perforating rectum ▼ Rectal temperature remains elevated until severe cold stress is present Assess for signs of cold stress or hyperthermia Employ measures that are effective in maintaining a stable body temperature and teach applicable measures to parents Place undressed newborn under prewarmed radiant heat warmer or in a prewarmed incubator until temperature is stabilized Adjust environment: 75° F, draft free	

Keep newborn and clothing dry
- ▼ Wipe dry of amniotic fluid immediately after birth
- ▼ Change wet clothing and bedding promptly
- ▼ Perform first bath only after temperature has been stable at ≥97.7° F for at least 1 hour
- ▼ Use warm water (98 to 99° F) for bath and a warm, draft-free room
- ▼ Wash head first before unwrapping the rest of body, exposing only part to be washed
- ▼ Dry body parts immediately during bath

Avoid placing crib near heaters or windows (drafts, sunlight)

Use self as guide when dressing newborn—do not over or under dress

Wrap newborn in blanket to keep body parts together
- ▼ Decreases heat loss by reducing amount of body surface exposed to the air
- ▼ Provides a sense of comfort and security as well

Use hat to decrease heat loss

Continued.

Table 17-1. Common Nursing Diagnoses Encountered during the Neonatal Period—cont'd

Client Outcomes	Nursing Interventions	Evaluation Checklist
C. Risk for infection related to immaturity of the newborn's immunological system		
Newborn will not exhibit signs of infection Newborn's cord and/or circumcision will heal without development of infection *Parents Will* Demonstrate correct care measures for newborn's integument, cord, and circumcision Employ infection control measures in their home Identify signs indicative of newborn infection	*Assess Newborn for Signs Indicative of Infection* Temperature instability—varies >1° C or 1.8° F from one reading to another Subnormal temperatures Lethargy, restlessness, irritability Poor feeding behavior Vomiting Diarrhea—green, watery stools Decreased urine output Respiratory distress Lesions or rashes, pallor, jaundice Erythema, edema, warmth, purulent drainage at sites where skin integrity is interrupted, i.e., cord, circumcision, abrasions or cuts	*Newborn* Exhibited no signs of infection Exhibited intact skin without rashes Cord and circumcision are healing as expected with no erythema, swelling, warmth, or purulent drainage *Parents* Identified signs of infection and correctly assessed their newborn including its integument, cord, and circumcision Utilized appropriate aseptic principles when bathing, feeding, and changing diaper Performed cord and circumcision care as directed Stated that they will make arrangements with well baby clinic in their neighborhood for immunizations and health guidance

Employ measures that are effective in preventing infection and teach applicable measures to parents

Wash hands following hospital policy, before and after care

Limit contact of newborn with those who have infections, including hospital personnel, crowds

Provide newborn with its own supplies and equipment and keep all items clean including toys and pacifiers

Support breast-feeding efforts (see Box 17-2)

Prepare and store formulas correctly

Continued.

Table 17-1. Common Nursing Diagnoses Encountered during the Neonatal Period—cont'd

Client Outcomes	Nursing Interventions	Evaluation Checklist
C. Risk for infection related to immaturity of the newborn's immunological system		
	Skin care ▼ Cleanse skin with warm water, using mild soap only for very dirty areas, i.e., buttocks after a bowel movement; rinse well ▼ Bathe every other day except for essential areas of scalp, face, creases in neck, genitalia, buttocks ▼ Change diapers promptly and cleanse area thoroughly — Expose buttocks to air — Apply thin layer of vaseline, KY jelly, or A&D ointment ▼ Avoid use of powders ▼ Avoid rubbing of skin ▼ Wash clothes and bedding separately, using hot water, mild detergent, and double rinse Umbilical cord care ▼ Use alcohol or triple dye to enhance drying and prevent infection	

- Expose to air—fold diaper and shirt away from cord
- Sponge bathe until cord falls off and site heals

Eye care
- Apply erythromycin ointment within 1 hour of birth
- Wash eyes at beginning of bath with clean cloth and water, from inner to outer canthus—use separate part of cloth for each eye

Nails—cut straight across when asleep, using blunt ended scissors

Circumcision care (Box 17-4)

Administer Hepatitis B Vaccine IM as Ordered by Physician

First dose at birth (within first 12 to 24 hours), second at 1 to 2 months and third at 6 to 18 months

Recombivax HB 0.25 mcg

Engerix B 10 mcg

Teach parents importance of immunizations and make referrals as needed

Continued.

Table 17-1. Common Nursing Diagnoses Encountered during the Neonatal Period—cont'd

Client Outcomes	Nursing Interventions	Evaluation Checklist
D. Risk for alteration in nutrition—less than body requirements related to parental lack of knowledge and experience with regard to newborn nutrition and feeding technique		
Newborn Will	*Assess Nutritional Status, and Feeding Behaviors and Patterns*	*Newborn*
Lose no more than 5 to 10% of birth weight	Strength and coordination of rooting, suck, swallow; frequency of feeding	Exhibited weight loss that did not exceed 10% of birth weight during first 7 days after birth
Gain approximately 1 oz/day	Patterns of weight gain and loss	Regained weight lost by end of 2nd week
Consume approximately 100 to 150 ml/kg of fluid and 110 to 130 calories/kg each day	Signs of hydration status	Voids approximately 6 to 10 times each day by 1 week of age; urine pale yellow
Exhibit signs of hunger approximately every 3 hours	Feeding technique and skill of parents	Exhibits a flat fontanel and resilient skin turgor
Exhibit satiety after feeding by resting quietly and sleeping	Parental and newborn satisfaction with feeding method chosen	Sleeps an average of 2½ hours after feedings—awakens exhibiting signs of hunger and eagerness to feed
Parents Will	*Determine if Daily Requirement for Calories and Fluid are Being Met*	*Parents*
Demonstrate skill with the feeding method they have chosen	Calories: 110 to 130 kcal/kg (breast milk and formula contain 20 kcal/oz)	Express satisfaction and confidence with breast-feeding
Identify signs of adequate newborn nutrition and hydration	Fluid: 100 to 150 ml/kg—includes milk; may need to be increased in hot weather	Correctly assessed their newborn's nutritional and hydration status
Recognize newborn behaviors indicative of hunger and satiety		

Teach Parents

Expected frequency of feeding and amounts

Signs of hunger and satiety after feeding

Signs of adequate hydration and nutrition in terms of voiding patterns, expected weight gain, resiliency of integument, condition of anterior fontanel

Assist parents with feeding method of choice (see Boxes 17-2, 18-6)

Box 17-1. Safety Tips for Parents of Newborns and Young Infants

Hold newborn securely by supporting head, neck, and spine

Never leave newborn unattended on a flat surface without siderails such as a changing table, countertop, or bed since even newborns can roll off

- Assemble all equipment you will need ahead of time and place within easy reach
- Place hand securely on infant, if you must turn away
- Keep a bassinet or crib in which to place the newborn nearby to use in case you are suddenly called away

Place newborn in a safe crib or playpen that meets the standards of the U.S. Consumer Products Safety Commission (CPSC)

- Position crib or playpen away from draperies, blinds, or shades that have long cords
- Avoid cribs that have special carvings, nobs, indentations
- Ensure that siderail slats are no more than 2⅜" apart
- Make sure siderails can be raised and secured in place
- Use a firm mattress that fits securely or snugly in the crib; never use a water mattress; make sure matting in playpen is secured so infant cannot get under or twisted into it
- Fasten all bed linen securely so it cannot twist around newborn
- Avoid placing objects, especially ones that are soft, in the crib

Position newborn to ensure good breathing and to prevent choking

- Use side-lying position with secure back support after feeding
- Use side-lying or supine (on back) position for sleeping; do not use supine position until at least ½ hour has passed since last feeding
- Avoid prone position (on abdomen) since it may interfere with breathing and has been associated with sudden infant death syndrome (SIDS)

Learn infant CPR and first aid measures

Use measures to prevent choking

- Use only approved pacifiers
- Keep small and sharp objects such as pins, scissors, or buttons out of reach of newborn
- Do not tie anything around the newborn's neck including bibs

Use a backward facing, safety approved car seat at all times when traveling with newborn. Follow directions for its use. Car seat can be turned to face forward once the infant weighs more than 20 pounds.

Use safety straps in high chairs

Instruct other children about newborn safety

Keep emergency phone numbers next to the telephone, i.e., your healthcare provider, poison hot line, local hospital

Box 17-2. Guidelines for Successful Breast-Feeding

GOALS: Ensure adequate newborn nutrition and hydration
Preserve tissue integrity of nipples and areolas
Prevent and reduce tenderness of nipples and areolas
Enhance maternal and newborn satisfaction with breast-feeding

Recommended Breast-Feeding Technique

Initiate feeding when newborn is awake, alert, and exhibiting hunger—every 1½ to 3 hours

Assume a position of comfort in a relaxing environment. Relax newborn during feeding by making eye contact, talking, singing.

Alternate newborn breast-feeding position with each feeding—football, traditional, side-lying

Alternate starting breast (place safety pin on bra to remember)

Initiate an effective latch

- ▼ Support breast with 4 fingers on bottom and thumb on top
- ▼ Bring newborn to breast (not breast to newborn) and stimulate the rooting reflex
- ▼ Guide nipple and areola into newborn's open mouth—mouth should cover nipple and most of areola
- ▼ Observe for correct latch-on—sucking is quiet, rhythmic, with occasional brief rest periods

Remove from breast when breast is empty or newborn is finished (about 10 minutes) by releasing suction—insert finger into side of mouth

Burp newborn between breasts and at the end of the breast-feeding session

Continue process on next breast

Do not let newborn continue to suck after breast is empty

Apply small amount of milk on nipples and areolas and air dry. Use nipple shells as needed to facilitate drying.

Begin supplementation, as needed, once lactation and feeding patterns have been established in about 3 to 4 weeks. Breast milk can be collected and stored for this purpose. Use clean bottles and store in freezer or refrigerator.

Breast Massage and Manual Expression of Milk

Use gentle massage to stimulate letdown reflex, keep milk flowing during breast-feeding, and prepare breasts for expression of milk manually or with pump

Technique for breast massage (similar to BSE)

- ▼ Press pads of fingers into breast and use a circular motion
- ▼ Progress in a systematic fashion from top of breast toward areola
- ▼ Application of warm packs prior to massage may be helpful if breasts are engorged

Box 17-3. Guidelines for Successful Bottle-Feeding

GOALS: Ensure adequate nutrition and hydration
Prevent gastric distress and enhance digestion
Enhance maternal and newborn satisfaction with bottle-feeding

Recommended Bottle-Feeding Technique

Initiate feeding when newborn is awake, alert, and exhibiting hunger—every 2½ to 3 hours

Assume position of comfort in a relaxing environment. Relax newborn during feeding by making eye contact, talking, singing.

Hold newborn closely (once nipple is in mouth) in an en-face position. Change holding position with each feeding—football and traditional holds and using different arms.

Position bottle so milk fills nipple and top of bottle, thereby preventing entrance of air into the newborn's stomach

Use nipples that allow dripping of milk. Nipple hole should not be so large that milk streams out nor so small that newborn must struggle during sucking.

Stimulate rooting reflex, then place nipple into open mouth

Burp newborn after every ½ to 1 ounce of formula and at end of feeding

Never prop bottle for feeding since it increases danger of choking, may block airway, and decreases interaction with newborn

Stop feeding when newborn signals satiety (stops sucking, turns away), not when entire bottle is empty. Discard any leftover formula.

Monitor amount of formula taken at each feeding then determine amount taken daily

Formula Preparation

Use formula that is best in terms of convenience and cost—ready-to-use in bottles (most expensive), prepared formulas using powder or concentrate. Never use honey since a very dangerous botulism infection of the newborn can occur.

Follow directions exactly with regard to preparation. Never over or under dilute since serious health problems will occur, including fluid and electrolyte imbalances.

Wash hands and can opener and tops of cans or containers before opening. Use clean bottles, nipples, and equipment which have been thoroughly washed in hot water and soap and then fully rinsed.

Store formulas properly: ready-to-use and concentrates at room temperature until opened; reconstituted formulas and opened containers or cans in refrigerator

Feed newborn formula that is at room temperature or that has been warmed by placing bottle in a container of hot water. Test on wrist before feeding. *Never use microwave* to warm formula since over heating can easily occur.

Box 17-4. Circumcision Care Guidelines

Nursing Measures to Complete Prior to Circumcision

Ensure that an informed consent from one parent has been obtained; discuss procedure and options available

Do not feed newborn for 1 to 2 hours prior to the procedure to reduce the possibility of vomiting and the risk of aspiration. *Note:* check with physician and agency policy since holding the feeding prior to circumcision may not be required.

Prepare equipment for a surgical aseptic procedure: sterile instruments, gloves, gowns, vaseline gauze, anesthetics and syringes (if used)

Advocate the use of anesthesia to reduce pain experienced by newborn

Assess vital signs

Restrain newborn

Nursing Measures to Implement after Procedure

Apply vaseline gauze or neosporin ointment to the site as directed by physician. Diaper newborn. Cloth diapers may be recommended for first day or so. *Note:* if the Plastibell is used, vaseline gauze/neosporin ointment is not applied. The plastic rim remains in place for a few days while healing is occuring and then it falls off.

Assess vital signs

Wrap newborn and take to mother for feeding and comfort

Assess site for bleeding every hour for 12 hours. If active bleeding occurs apply intermittent pressure to site of bleeding and notify physician.

Change diaper promptly and cleanse thoroughly with water after elimination. Reapply vaseline gauze or neosporin to circumcision site if Plastibell was not used.

Note time of first voiding after procedure. Urination may be inhibited by edema around urethra.

Discuss expected appearance of circumcision site and care measures

- ▼ Glans will appear reddened and will become covered with a yellowish, protective exudate after the first 24 hours—exudate will disappear in 2 to 3 days and should not be removed
- ▼ Plastic rim should fall off within 8 days; if not, manual removal by healthcare provider will be required
- ▼ Apply intermittent pressure to site if active bleeding occurs and notify the physician
- ▼ Signs of infection include sustained erythema, edema, and purulent, malodorous drainage
- ▼ Change diaper promptly; cleanse site with warm water; apply ointment as appropriate. Avoid use of baby wipes until site is fully healed.
- ▼ Position on side to keep pressure off of penis

b. Wash hands before and after examination; wash during examination if they become contaminated
c. Use equipment appropriately
(1) Cleanse equipment. Example: cleanse ear pieces and diaphragm of stethoscope with alcohol swabs.
(2) Use disposable paper tape for measurement
(3) Change scale paper for each newborn
5. Make use of newborn's activity level when making observations
a. When at rest, check vital signs, posture, color, fontanels
b. When active, check musculoskeletal activity, reflexes, color changes
6. Use techniques that facilitate accuracy
a. Vital signs
(1) Accuracy of assessment is essential since vital information regarding the adequacy of the newborn's respiratory, circulatory, and thermoregulatory adaptation to extrauterine life is obtained
(2) Count apical and respiratory rate for one full minute at frequent intervals especially during the transition period following birth when newborn responses are still unstable
(3) Assess temperature using the axillary or tympanic route since the rectal route can lead to perforation of the rectum
b. Measurements
(1) Weight
(a) Weigh every day at the same time, preferably in the morning before a feeding
(b) Remove all clothing
(c) Place clean scale paper on scale for warmth and prevention of cross infection
(d) Balance scale
(e) Place newborn on scale, keeping hand hovering over top of newborn and keeping full attention on the newborn during the entire procedure—*never turn away or leave unattended!*
(2) Measurement of head, chest, abdomen, length
(a) Use nonstretchable, disposable paper tape
(b) Measure head circumference at greatest diameter of the head—across forehead at ear

level, over occiput; measurement changes as molding subsides

(c) Measure chest circumference at nipple line

(d) Measure abdominal circumference just below umbilicus

(e) Measure length from top of head to buttocks then stretch legs and measure to heels; assistance from another nurse or parent enhances accuracy

7. Involve parents and family members as a means of facilitating attachment and getting to know their baby—especially important with early discharge since parents must learn how to monitor their newborn's condition

B. Methods for data collection and assessment of the newborn

1. Review antepartal and parturition records to determine quality of fetal-newborn responses to pregnancy, labor, and birth including
   a. Physical status of mother and responses of mother and family to the pregnancy
   b. Antepartal testing performed and results
   c. Gestational age of the pregnancy and duration of labor
   d. Medications and anesthetics administered to the mother during labor
   e. Method of delivery (vaginal or cesarean), birth presentation, use of instruments, such as forceps or vacuum extractor
   f. Fetal monitoring (internal or external) during parturition including signs of fetal distress or stress
2. Apgar score performed at 1 and 5 minutes after birth
3. Full physical assessment of health status
4. Gestational age assessment and determination of adequacy of intrauterine growth
   a. Assess gestational age within 12 hours following birth by observing signs indicating degree of neuromuscular and physical maturity—compute score to determine gestational age
   b. Neuromuscular maturity assessment may be delayed for 24 hours since the newborn's nervous system is often unstable for the first 24 hours
   c. Weigh newborn and measure head and length—plot on graphs to determine adequacy of intrauterine growth

d. Describe infant:
   (1) Small for gestational age (SGA)
   (2) Appropriate for gestational age (AGA)
   (3) Large for gestational age (LGA)

5. Laboratory testing
   a. Source of specimens for testing
      (1) Cord blood at the time of birth
      (2) Heel stick is often used to obtain capillary blood for testing from the newborn
      (3) Venipuncture to obtain venous blood to recheck or confirm abnormal values. Examples: hypoglycemia, high hematocrit (Hct) and hemoglobin (Hgb).
   b. Common laboratory tests performed
      (1) Direct coombs test to determine if antibodies against Rh+ blood have been formed by an Rh– mother and transferred to her fetus via the placenta
         (a) Negative—no antibodies formed
         (b) Positive—antibodies present that can destroy an Rh+ newborn's blood cells
      (2) RPR/VDRL to determine whether intrauterine exposure to syphilis occurred
         (a) Nonreactive—no exposure
         (b) Reactive—exposed
      (3) CBC
         (a) WBC 18,000/mm
         (b) Hgb 15 to 20 g/dL
         (c) Hct 43 to 61%
      (4) Dextrostix to determine blood glucose level
         (a) Performed frequently during the first 4 to 6 hours after birth as determined by hospital policy
         (b) Should be above 45 mg/dL and increase to 60 to 70 mg/dL by day 3
      (5) Bilirubin levels (direct or indirect) to confirm presence of hyperbilirubinemia when jaundice is observed
      (6) Screening for newborn for metabolic disorders that require immediate treatment to prevent permanent damage such as mental and growth retardation; testing is often required by state law; if not performed before discharge, parents must be informed of the importance of bringing their newborn in for testing

(a) Phenylketonuria (PKU) test within 72 hours of initial feeding to detect phenylketonuria, an inborn error of protein metabolism

(b) Thyroid (T_4) testing to detect presence of hypothyroidism

(c) Additional testing for other inborn errors of metabolism (branched-chain ketonuria, galactosemia) and sickle-cell trait and disease may be required

III. Psychosocial assessment of the newborn and its family

A. Essential components

1. Quality of attachment between both newborn and parents
2. Reaction of family members to newborn
3. Stability of parental and family relationships
4. Level of parental knowledge and skill regarding newborn characteristics and care—availability of resource persons such as grandparents, friends, and healthcare providers
5. Safety and adequacy of the home environment
6. Ability to provide for the health care of the newborn
   a. Knowledge regarding importance of and frequency for regular health assessments during infancy and signs that require an emergency visit or call
   b. Arrangements made for health care (private pediatrician, clinic) and availability of health insurance
   c. Knowledge regarding the importance of immunizations

B. Methods to use for assessment

1. Observe parents and family as they care for and interact with the newborn
2. Review antepartal history
3. Interview parents prior to discharge
4. Follow-up phone calls and home visits after discharge

IV. Nursing diagnoses and interventions during the neonatal period

A. Nursing diagnoses for the healthy full-term newborn are primarily related to the newborn's risk for developing health problems as a result of

1. Physiologic systems that are not fully mature and have limited reserve capacity in times of stress

2. Parents who may be inexperienced or lack the resources to ensure the newborn's well being

B. **Priority nursing interventions**

1. Focus on early detection and prompt treatment as means of preventing more serious problems or even permanent damage or death
    a. Assess vital signs to detect early indicators of respiratory distress, cold stress
    b. Strict adherence to asepsis and universal precautions to prevent infection
    c. Administration of vitamin K using correct injection technique for newborns (Figure 17-1)—enhances clotting ability of newborn and thereby prevents excessive bleeding from cord or circumcision

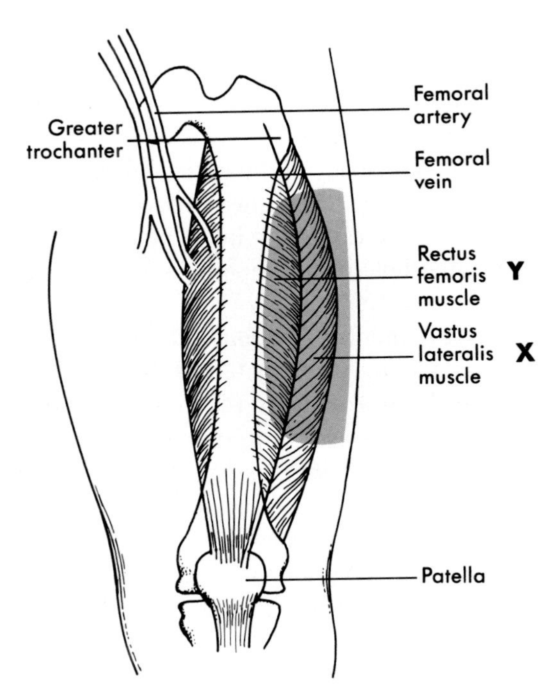

Figure 17-1. Acceptable intramuscular injection site, lateral aspect of muscle mass in middle third of distance between greater trochanter and patella. **X,** Preferred injection site in vastus lateralis muscle; **Y,** alternate injection site in rectus femoris muscle. (From Bobak IM et al: *Maternity and gynecologic care: the nurse and the family*, ed 5, St Louis, 1993, Mosby.)

2. Emphasize the education of parents
   a. Topics to include
      (1) Characteristics of newborn including what to expect and what indicates a developing problem that requires prompt attention from a healthcare provider
      (2) Newborn requirements for health care
         (a) Where and how often to go for regular health checkups, immunizations, and health guidance
         (b) Where and when to go if emergencies or signs of health problems occur
      (3) Measures to ensure
         (a) Effective breathing
         (b) Stable body temperature within normal limits
         (c) Adequate nutrient and fluid intake
      (4) Infection control techniques
      (5) How to keep their environment safe and secure as a means of preventing accidental injury (see Box 17-1)
      (6) How to stimulate the growth and development of a secure and trusting infant
   b. Methods for parental education
      (1) Group and one-on-one classes and demonstrations—a good time to teach is during the newborn's bath or when a physical assessment is being performed
      (2) Videos and written materials that can be used as references after discharge
      (3) Postpartum parenting classes and support groups
      (4) Follow-up phone calls and home visits

C. Common nursing diagnoses encountered during the neonatal period, along with selected client outcomes, nursing interventions, and evaluation criteria are described in Table 17-1

REVIEW QUESTIONS

1. Biostatistical data provide healthcare professionals with information regarding the population's health status. Which is a correct interpretation of current trends in infant mortality?

a. Neonatal and postneonatal mortality rates are approximately the same
b. The infant mortality rate for black infants is nearly double that of white infants
c. Sudden infant death syndrome (SIDS) is the leading cause of neonatal mortality
d. The major cause for both black and white infant mortality is respiratory distress syndrome

2. Weight at birth is an important factor in terms of a newborn's ability to adjust to extrauterine life. Which statement is accurate?

a. A newborn weighing <3500 g at birth is considered to be low birth weight (LBW)
b. Preterm newborns are considered to be small for gestational age (SGA)
c. The weight of a large for gestational age (LGA) newborn is at or above the 80th percentile
d. A newborn whose weight falls within 2 standard deviations of the mean for its gestational age is described as appropriate for gestational age (AGA)

3. The single most important predictor of infant morbidity and mortality is

a. Infection
b. Low birth weight (LBW)
c. Congenital anomalies
d. Race or minority status

4. A pregnant woman, age 25, is unemployed and on welfare. She smokes about ¼ pack of cigarettes each day and drinks occasionally. Six months ago, she divorced her husband and moved to another state to "get away from everyone." The factor that is LEAST likely to contribute to her risk status and to increase the chance of infant mortality would be her

a. Age
b. Economic status
c. Use of alcohol and tobacco
d. Limited support system

5. When weighing a newborn, the nurse should
   a. Leave its diaper on for comfort
   b. Place a sterile scale paper on the scale for infection control
   c. Keep hand on the newborn's abdomen for safety
   d. Weigh the newborn at the same time each day for accuracy

6. When determining the gestational age of a newborn, the nurse should
   a. Take the newborn's vital signs including BP
   b. Delay assessment of physical maturity until 24 hours after birth
   c. Assess for signs indicative of neuromuscular maturity
   d. Weigh the newborn and measure its head circumference and length

7. A newborn male, 39 weeks' gestation, would exhibit
   a. Extended posture
   b. Testes in scrotum
   c. Abundant lanugo over entire body
   d. Square window of 90 degrees

8. A newborn female, 41 weeks' gestation, would exhibit
   a. Creases over entire plantar surface of feet
   b. Prominent clitoris and labia minora
   c. Heels touch ears when legs are extended
   d. Flat areola

9. Which of the following laboratory test results would be a cause for concern if exhibited by a newborn 12 hours after birth?
   a. Direct coombs: negative
   b. Hematocrit: 58% and hemoglobin: 18 g/dL
   c. Blood glucose level: 55 g/dL
   d. RPR/VDRL: reactive

10. If the infant's chest does not rise during a rescue breath, the first action of the rescuer would be to
    a. Check mouth for an object blocking the airway
    b. Perform a chest thrust
    c. Breathe into mouth more forcefully
    d. Retilt head and try another rescue breath

ANSWERS, RATIONALES, AND TEST-TAKING TIPS

Rationales	Test-Taking Tips
1. Correct answer: b The neonatal morbidity rate is nearly twice as high as the postneonatal mortality rate. The leading cause of neonatal mortality is intrauterine events and LBW. The major cause for infant mortality among white infants is congenital anomalies while for black infants it is preterm birth and LBW.	If you have no idea of the correct response, match the key words in the question with the same words in the answer: asking about trend in "infant mortality"; the only responses with infant mortality are responses *b* and *d*. Since it is asking for a "trend" and not a cause response *b* seems to be the better answer.
2. Correct answer: d LBW is <2500 g. Preterm newborns may be SGA, AGA, or LGA depending on their gestational age and their weight. LGA newborn's weight is above the 90th percentile or 2 standard deviations above the mean for gestational age.	Response *d* seems to give the most information.
3. Correct answer: b While responses *a, c,* and *d* can have an effect on the health status of the newborn and its ability to adapt to extrauterine life, LBW, which is due to preterm birth and/or intrauterine growth retardation, is the single most important predictor for infant mortality.	Of the given responses the low birth weight would have the greatest impact on all body functions.

4. Correct answer: a

Responses *b, c,* and *d* are all risk factors and maternal predictors for infant mortality. Risk factor in terms of age would be <20 or >35 years.

Be cautious in reading this type of question since the wording is complex. Use the process of reading the question, the responses, and then reread the question. Note that in questions with "least" or "most" that all of the responses are usually correct. The approach is to list them in order of priority, reread the question and then make a selection.

5. Correct answer: d

Weigh baby undressed for accuracy with hand above, not on, the abdomen for safety. Clean scale paper is used.

If you missed the words "sterile" in response *b* and "hand on" in response *c,* you probably selected the incorrect response from reading too fast. Application of general knowledge of weighing any client can be applied here: same time, technique, and clothes daily.

6. Correct answer: c

Vital signs are not part of a gestational age assessment nor are the weight and head circumference. Physical maturity should be assessed within 12 hours of birth since exposure to the environment effects accuracy. Neuromuscular maturity assessment can be delayed for 24 hours until the neurological system stabilizes.

Cluster options *a* and *d* under physical assessment and eliminate these. Of the remaining options, *b* and *c,* option *b,* to delay assessment, is inappropriate. Select option *c,* assessment. A second method is to use the nursing process and select option *c.* The other options are interventions.

7. Correct answer: b

Responses *a, c,* and *d* are signs noted in the preterm newborn.

If you have no idea of a correct response, match the male with the testes in the scrotum since the weeks are within the normal range.

8. Correct answer: a

Responses *b, c,* and *d* are signs noted in the preterm newborn.

With the number of weeks being 41 and within normal range, select a normal finding which is response *a*.

9. Correct answer: d

A reactive RPR/VDRL indicates exposure to syphilis. The negative coombs indicates absence of antibodies against Rh+ blood. Hgb is between 15 to 20 g/dL and Hct 43 to 61%. The blood glucose level should be >45 g/dL.

Note a reactive RPR in any client is a cause of concern.

10. Correct answer: d

Never increase the force of breathing—always breathe gently. If retilting head does not work then begin the recommended procedure for the choking infant.

As with any procedure, if there are no results recheck the maneuvers and try again.

CHAPTER 18

Alterations in Adaptations of the Newborn

STUDY OUTCOMES

After completing this chapter, the reader will be able to do the following:

- Define the key terms listed.
- Describe the problems encountered by low birth weight newborns during adaptation to extrauterine life.
- Discuss treatment measures effective in the care of newborns experiencing
    - respiratory distress
    - thermoregulatory instability
    - ineffective feeding behaviors
    - hyperbilirubinemia
- Describe measures that can be used by the nurse to facilitate attachment and reduce stressors with families of newborns who are experiencing ineffective adaptation to extrauterine life.

KEY TERMS

Cold stress	Hypothermic state that increases the newborn's risk for respiratory distress, hypoxia, metabolic acidosis, and hypoglycemia.
Gavage feeding	Feeding via a gastric tube inserted through the mouth or nose and into the stomach; required when a newborn is unable to obtain sufficient nutrients and fluids orally.
Neutral thermal environment	An environment that assists the newborn to maintain a stable body temperature between 97.7 and 99.5° F (36.5 to 37.5° C) with minimal expenditure of oxygen and nutrients by using radiant heat warmers, incubators, close wrapping or bundling with coverings on hands and feet.
Phototherapy	Treatment for hyperbilirubinemia that uses a light source such as a fluorescent lightbulb panel or fiberoptic panel or blanket to facilitate bilirubin breakdown for excretion.
Respiratory distress syndrome (RDS)	Ineffective function of the newborn's respiratory system as a result of immaturity of the lungs and respiratory center and limited production of surfactant.

CONTENT REVIEW

I. Overview of altered adaptations of newborns

A. Newborns may experience difficulty adapting to extrauterine life as a result of growth and development in an unhealthy intrauterine environment that exposes them to stressors

1. Damaging teratogens including microorganisms, chemicals, drugs
2. Insufficient uteroplacental circulation
3. Inadequate supply of nutrients

B. Exposure to intrauterine stressors influences

1. Fetal growth and development leading to intrauterine growth retardation and congenital anomalies
2. Duration of pregnancy leading to a shortened period of gestation and preterm birth

C. Low birth weight newborns are those who experience intrauterine growth retardation and/or preterm birth

D. Intrauterine growth retardation results in the birth of a small for gestational age (SGA) newborn whose measurements and weight do not meet growth expectations for gestational age (fall below the 10th percentile)

1. SGA refers to size and not gestational age—these newborns can be preterm, full term, or postterm
2. SGA newborns encounter difficulty adapting to extrauterine life as a result of
   a. Hypoxic state during pregnancy which stimulates formation of greater numbers of RBCs than expected, increasing the risk for neonatal polycythemia and hyperbilirubinemia
   b. Hypoxia during labor and birth
      (1) Placenta is often smaller, limiting efficiency of gas exchange especially during intense, frequent contractions as occur in active labor
      (2) Passage of meconium may occur as a result of fetal response to hypoxia
      (3) Danger of meconium aspiration is present at the time of birth
   c. Ineffective nutrition during intrauterine life limits the formation of nutrient stores (glucose) and subcutaneous fat increasing neonatal risk for
      (1) Hypoglycemia as glucose stores are depleted with the stress of parturition and adaptation to extrauterine life
      (2) Cold stress (hypothermia)

E. Preterm newborns—born before the end of the 37th week of gestation—experience difficulty adapting to extrauterine life to the degree that they are preterm (weeks' gestation) and their organ systems are immature; Figure 18-1 illustrates some of the differences that can be seen when comparing a full-term and a preterm newborn. Major problems encountered by the preterm newborn include

1. Respiratory distress syndrome (RDS)—also known as idiopathic respiratory distress syndrome (IRDS) or hyaline membrane disease (HMD)—refers to ineffective respiratory function as a result of
   a. Immaturity of the lungs and respiratory center (regulates respiration)

Posture—The preterm infant lies in a "relaxed attitude," limbs more extended; the body size is small, and the head may appear somewhat larger in proportion to the body size. The term infant has more subcutaneous fat tissue and rests in a more flexed attitude.

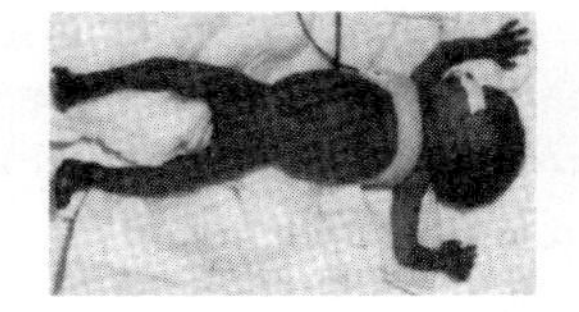

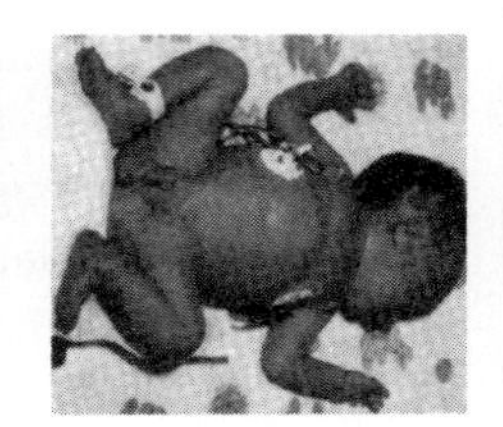

Ear—The preterm infant's ear cartilages are poorly developed, and the ear may fold easily; the hair is fine and feathery, and lanugo may cover the back and face. The mature infant's ear cartilages are well formed, and the hair is more likely to form firm, separate strands.

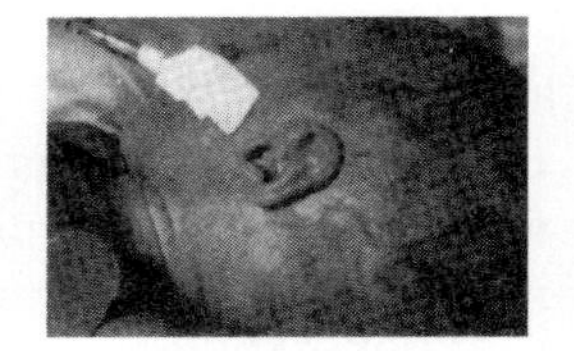

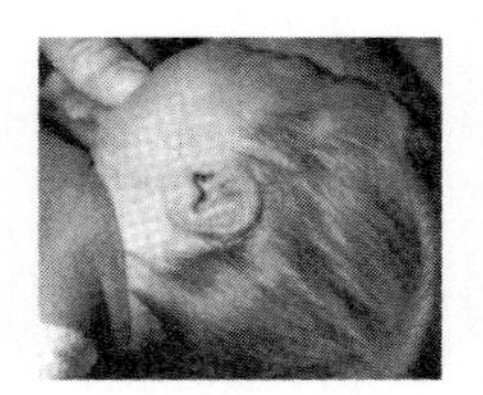

Sole—The sole of the foot of the preterm infant appears more turgid and may have only fine wrinkles. The mature infant's sole (foot) is well and deeply creased.

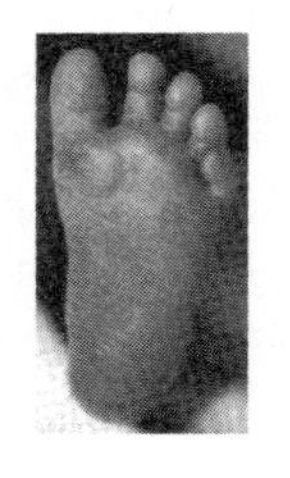

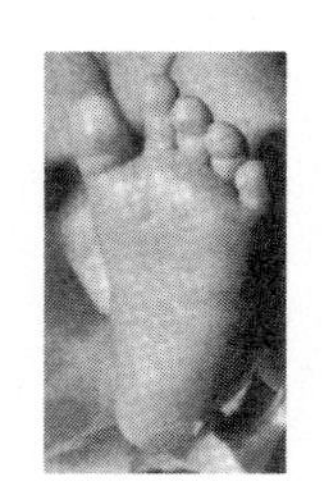

Female genitalia—The preterm female infant's clitoris is prominent, and labia majora are poorly developed and gaping. The mature female infant's labia majora are fully developed, and the clitoris is not as prominent.

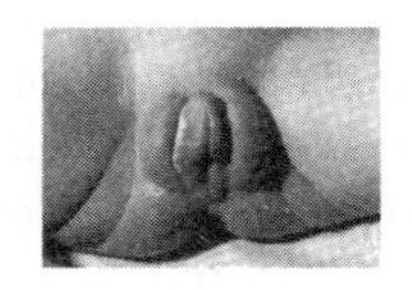

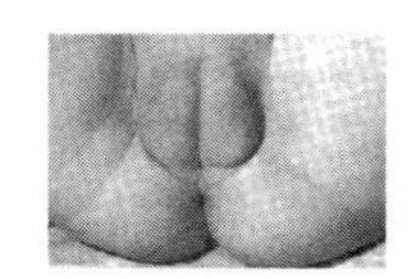

Male genitalia—The preterm male infant's scrotum is undeveloped and not pendulous; minimal rugae are present, and the testes may be in the inguinal canals or in the abdominal cavity. The term male infant's scrotum is well developed, pendulous, and rugated, and the testes are well down in the scrotal sac.

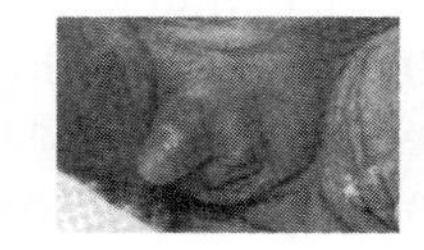

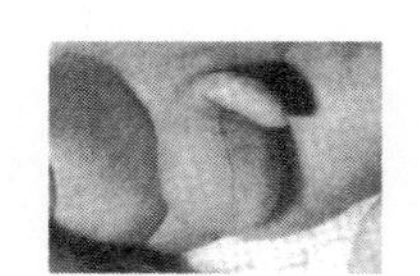

Scarf sign—The preterm infant's elbow may be easily brought across the chest with little or no resistance. The mature infant's elbow may be brought to the midline of the chest, resisting attempts to bring the elbow past the midline.

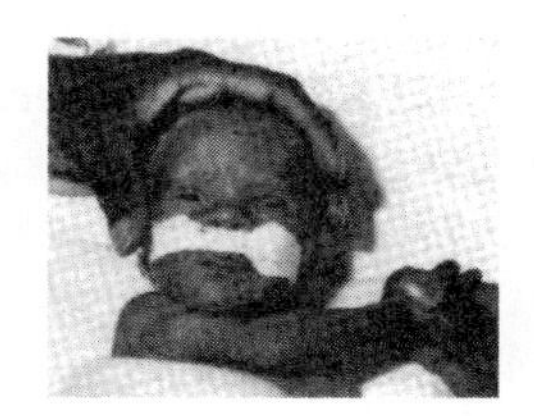

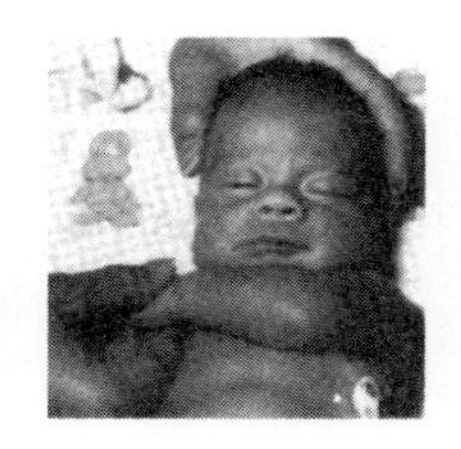

Figure 18-1. Clinical and neurologic examinations comparing preterm and full-term infants. (Data from Pierog SH, Ferrara A: *Medical care of the sick newborn*, ed 2, St Louis, 1976, Mosby. From Wong: *Whaley & Wong's nursing care of infants and children*, ed 5, St Louis, 1995, Mosby.) *(continued)*

Grasp reflex—The preterm infant's grasp is weak; the term infant's grasp is strong, allowing the infant to be lifted up from the mattress.

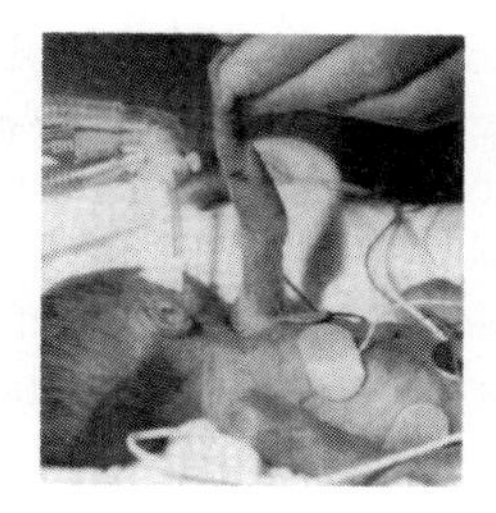

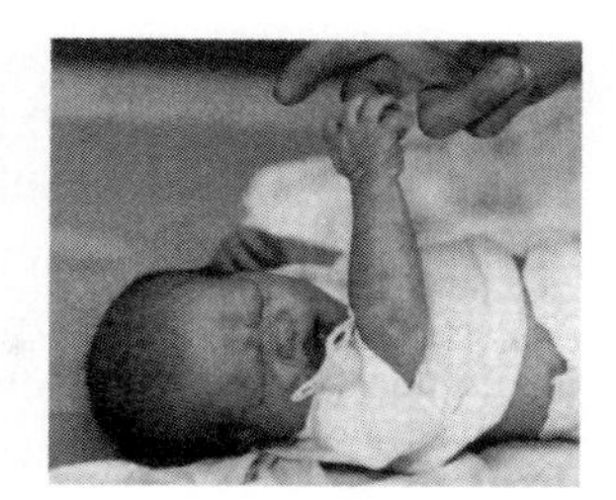

Heel-to-ear maneuver—The preterm infant's heel is easily brought to the ear, meeting with no resistance. This maneuver is not possible in the term infant since there is considerable resistance at the knee.

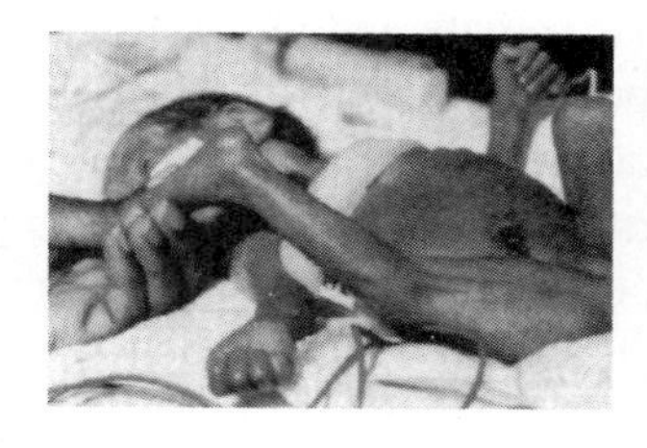

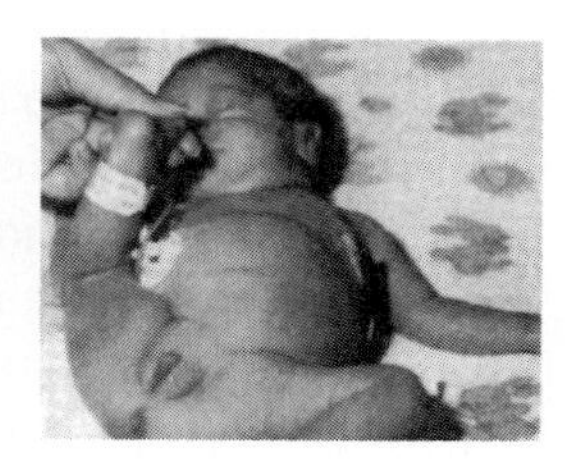

Figure 18-1. *(cont'd)* Clinical and neurologic examinations comparing preterm and full-term infants. (Data from Pierog SH, Ferrara A: *Medical care of the sick newborn*, ed 2, St Louis, 1987, Mosby. From Wong: *Whaley & Wong's nursing care of infants and children*, ed 5, St Louis, 1995, Mosby.)

   b. Limited production of surfactant
      (1) Substance that coats the lining of the alveoli and facilitates their expansion and contraction during breathing
      (2) Inadequate amounts of surfactant make alveoli stiff and difficult to expand with breathing—great effort is required for each breath to the degree that surfactant is diminished
      (3) Weak, poorly developed respiratory muscles
2. Circulatory problems as a result of
   a. Cardiovascular immaturity
   b. Limited available oxygen associated with immature respiratory function which often leads to persistent fetal circulation with the ductus arteriosus and foramen ovale failing to close
3. Risk for infection is greater than for full-term newborn as a result of
   a. Immaturity of immunological system
   b. Increased number of invasive procedures experienced
   c. Delicate, more easily traumatized integument

   d. Impaired ability to breast-feed; breast milk can be used for gavage feedings
4. Hyperbilirubinemia associated with immature hepatic function
5. Hypothermia as a result of limited
   a. Brown fat—which the newborn has, is used up more quickly when stress is experienced
   b. Glucose stores
   c. Subcutaneous fat
   d. Muscular activity and ability to assume and/or maintain a flexed posture
6. Renal immaturity which increases the risk for fluid, electrolyte, and acid-base imbalances
7. Immaturity of brain development coupled with treatment measures that may be required such as mechanical ventilation, which increase the risk for intracranial hemorrhage
8. Nutritional deficits such as hypoglycemia, hypocalcemia which are common among preterm newborns as a result of
   a. Limited gestational time to form nutrient stores
   b. Stressors encountered during parturition and extrauterine life such as hypoxia, respiratory distress, and cold stress which rapidly deplete the limited stores
   c. Limited ability to supply nutrients during extrauterine life as a result of
      (1) Immature or weak and uncoordinated suck and swallow
      (2) Weak rooting and gag reflexes
      (3) Gastrointestinal immaturity that interferes with adequate digestion of nutrients and their movement (peristalsis) and absorption through the digestive tract

F. Close observation of the extrauterine adaptation of all newborns, especially those who are at increased risk, is essential in order to accomplish early detection of a developing problem and prompt treatment before permanent damage and possible death occur

G. Treatment measures and nursing interventions for the newborn experiencing difficulty adapting to extrauterine life must emphasize

1. Supporting respiration
2. Preventing cold stress
3. Facilitating adequate nutritional intake and fluid, electrolyte, and acid-base balance

4. Detecting and reducing rising bilirubin levels
5. Preventing infection
6. Promoting attachment and reducing stressors for the newborn's family

▼ **Readers should consult a child health or high risk newborn textbook for a more in-depth discussion of the compromised newborn**

II. Respiratory distress

A. Newborns can experience respiratory distress as they adapt to extrauterine life and require assistance to varying degrees with breathing and obtaining an adequate supply of oxygen

B. Findings indicative of respiratory distress; can increase in intensity as hours pass after birth

1. Tachypnea—a respiratory rate per minute >60 progressing to 80 to 120
2. Nasal faring, expiratory grunting
3. Retractions—sternal, costal, becoming more pronounced as breathing becomes more labored
4. Crackles bilaterally over the lung fields progressing to pulmonary edema
5. Late appearing findings that indicate increased severity of respiratory distress
   a. Central cyanosis
   b. Flaccidity
   c. Diminished responsiveness to stimuli
   d. More frequent periods of apnea
   e. Diminishing breath sounds

C. Treatment measures must be instituted immediately

1. Reduce stress on the respiratory system by maintaining
   a. A neutral thermal environment thereby preventing cold stress and hyperthermia
   b. Nutrient and fluid, electrolyte, and acid-base balance thereby preventing hypoglycemia, dehydration or fluid excess, electrolyte imbalance, alkalosis-acidosis
2. Provide oxygen and assistance with breathing to prevent hypoxia
   a. Oxygen administered should be warmed and humidified
   b. Method used depends on response to treatment and degree of difficulty experienced
      (1) Plastic hood placed over newborn's head to supply humidified and warmed oxygen

(2) Continuous positive airway pressure (CPAP) provides a continuous infusion of oxygen under pressure via a nasal canula or endotracheal tube for newborns who do not respond favorably to the hood

(3) Mechanical ventilation breathes for the newborn and supplies oxygen when the hood or CPAP are ineffective in maintaining oxygenation and supporting respiration

3. Administer medications to support breathing, to facilitate respiratory treatment measures, and to prevent complications
   a. Antibiotics—prevent or treat infection
   b. Pancuronium (Pavulon)—paralyze muscles in order to facilitate effectiveness of mechanical ventilation
   c. Furosemide (Lasix)—a diuretic which facilitates fluid excretion via kidneys and reduces edema, such as pulmonary edema
   d. Vitamin E—prevents complications of oxygen administration and mechanical ventilation such as retinopathy, cranial hemorrhage, bronchopulmonary damage
   e. Surfactant therapy—prevents or treats RDS by administering surfactant via aerosol or direct instillation into the lungs
   f. Corticosteroids such as betamethasone stimulate fetal production of surfactant by administration to the pregnant woman between 28 to 32 weeks' gestation and within 1 to 7 days prior to birth
4. Observe newborn responses to treatment—status can change quickly and necessitate immediate treatment adjustments
   a. Physical assessment
   b. Blood gases
   c. Noninvasive monitoring of effectiveness of oxygenation
      (1) Transcutaneous oxygen pressure monitor assesses oxygen dissolved in plasma
      (2) Pulse oximeter assesses oxygen carried by hemoglobin; normal range is 95 to 100% saturation
5. Maintain airway patency
   a. Respiratory secretions can become tenacious, thick, and copious; may indicate dehydration
   b. Observe newborn and auscultate lungs before and after airway clearance measures

c. Use percussion and vibration (special instruments are available since hands are too big) to loosen secretions taking care to observe response of newborn and limiting length of sessions
d. Suction only after carefully assessing need since damage to delicate respiratory structures can occur with frequent suctioning

6. Change position frequently using supported side-lying or supine with slight neck extension—*never* Trendelenburg
7. Provide oral and skin care to prevent breakdown—intact skin is a barrier to infection

III. Thermoregulatory instability

A. Thermoregulation is immature in all newborns but cold stress is more likely to occur in the sick newborn, especially if LBW; it is likely to be more hazardous since compensatory mechanisms and body functions are less effective than in the full-term healthy newborn

B. Cold stress (hypothermia)—can rapidly lead to

1. Respiratory distress and hypoxia
2. Metabolic acidosis
3. Hypoglycemia

C. Measures to support thermoregulatory stability

1. Create a neutral thermal environment using
   a. Radiant heat warmer
   b. Incubator
   c. Close wrapping or bundling in blankets and covering head and feet when newborn is taken out from warmer-incubator to be fed, held, and cuddled by family
2. Keep newborn under radiant warmer-incubator until it is capable of maintaining a stable body temperature without assistance—check thermistor probe to make sure it is securely in place and covered with reflective material; assess axillary temperature periodically as a double check of the temperature recorded on the warmer control panel
3. Use a radiant warmer-incubator to facilitate assessment of newborn and performance of treatments since the newborn is undressed except for hat and sometimes foot coverings
4. Warm and humidify oxygen and air—reduces heat loss through evaporation

5. Warm all surfaces (scale, examination or treatment table) and objects (blankets, instruments, hands) that come in contact with the newborn to reduce heat loss through conduction; use of a heated water pad under the infant may assist with conservation of heat and preservation of skin integrity
6. Perform all procedures under radiant heat warmer
7. Bathe newborn judiciously
8. Assist newborn to assume and maintain a flexed posture
9. Rewarm the newborn gradually over several hours if cold stress occurs

IV. Alteration in nutrition—less than body requirements

A. Hypoglycemia—low serum glucose levels

1. Glucose levels should be determined for all newborns—more frequently, beginning at 1 hour after birth for those newborns who are at high risk
2. Testing is accomplished using a bedside glucose monitor, such as dextrostix—low readings are confirmed with laboratory testing of a blood sample
3. Glucose levels reflective of hypoglycemia
   a. Dextrostix—blood glucose <45 mg/dL
   b. Blood glucose—laboratory testing
      (1) <35 mg/dL in first 72 hours
      (2) <45 mg/dL after first 72 hours
      (3) <25 mg/dL in LBW newborn
4. Findings
   a. Jitteriness, tremors, twitching progressing to convulsions and coma
   b. Poor feeding behavior
   c. Lethargy
   d. Cyanosis and respiratory distress
   e. Weak high pitched cry
5. Prevent by beginning feedings early and reducing stressors that can deplete glucose stores
6. Treatment
   a. Increase frequency of oral feedings to at least every 2 to 3 hours and careful assessment of blood glucose levels on a regular basis such as after each feeding
   b. Administer glucose intravenously via a large vein with careful monitoring to ensure effectiveness of treatment and to prevent complications such as hyperglycemia, fluid overload, infiltration with destruction of subcutaneous tissue

B. Measures to ensure adequate nutrient and fluid intake

1. Oral feedings are preferred and should be attempted and facilitated
    a. Assess strength, coordination of suck and swallow, gag and rooting reflexes by an initial sterile water feeding
    b. Observe behaviors during feeding, tolerance for oral feeding, and amount of fluid retained
        (1) Usually feeding times are longer but should be <30 minutes
        (2) Feeding smaller amounts more frequently may be helpful for the newborn that tires easily
    c. Bottle- and breast-feeding can be attempted
        (1) Use correct technique—(see Boxes 17-3 and 17-4)
        (2) Wrap newborn securely during feeding to prevent cold stress
        (3) Provide supplemental oxygen
2. Gavage feeding
    a. Required by newborns who are unable to obtain sufficient nutrients and fluids orally
        (1) Tires during feeding and takes longer than 30 minutes to complete feeding
        (2) Suck, swallow are weak and uncoordinated
        (3) Gag reflex is weak
        (4) Respiratory distress occurs during feeding
    b. Methods
        (1) Intermittent, bolus feeding every 1 to 4 hours
            (a) Most commonly used method
            (b) Helpful for newborns who have some ability to suck yet become tired or cyanotic during feeding
            (c) Gavage and oral feedings can be alternated
        (2) Continuous drip using an infusion pump
    c. Technique (Figure 18-2)
        (1) Choose appropriate gastrointestinal tube
            (a) 15-inch no. 5 or no. 8 french catheter
            (b) Polyethylene tube—stiff, more appropriate for intermittent gavage
            (c) Polyurethane or silicone rubber—flexible, more appropriate for continuous gavage since it is less damaging to gastrointestinal tract mucosa
        (2) Wrap active newborn in a mummy restraint
        (3) Measure tube (see Figure 18-2)

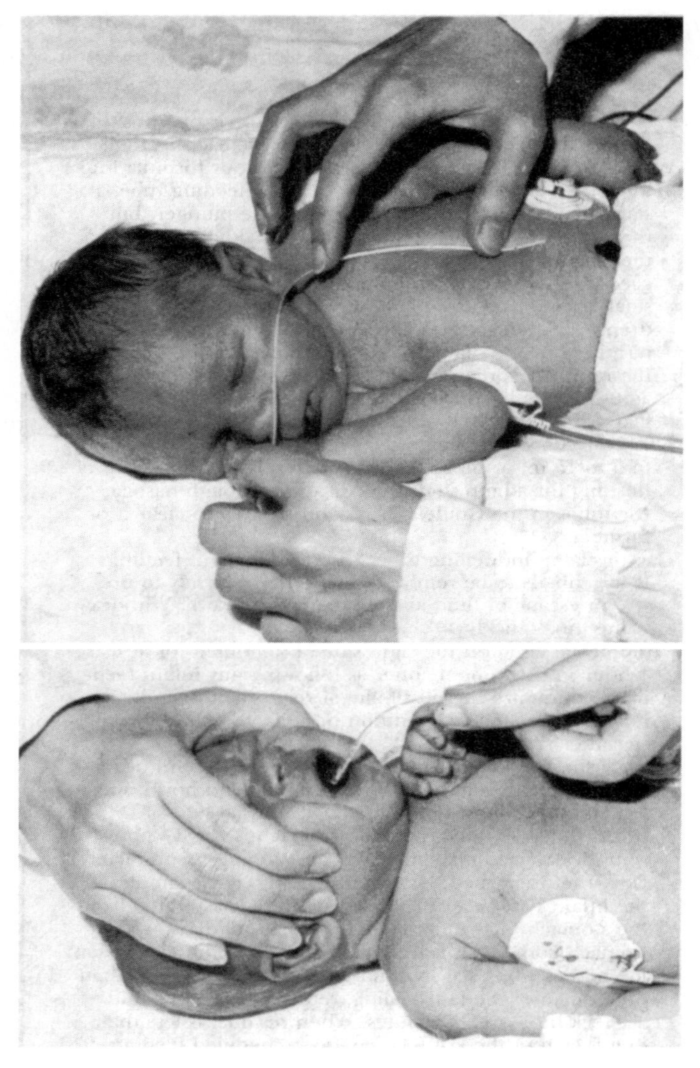

Figure 18-2. Gavage feeding. **A,** Measuring tube for nasogastric feeding from tip of nose to earlobe and to midpoint between end of xiphoid process and umbilicus. **B,** Inserting the tube. From Wong: *Whaley & Wong's nursing care of infants and children*, ed 5, St Louis, 1995, Mosby.)

(4) Lubricate tube with sterile water

(5) Insert through mouth, especially for intermittent feedings

  (a) Avoids blockage of nasal passage since newborns are nasal breathers

  (b) Stimulates sucking

(6) Tape to cheek
(7) Aspirate gastric contents and measure amount
   (a) Method of determining tube placement
   (b) Evaluates tolerance for amount of milk used by indicating residual milk in the stomach
(8) Include gastric content aspirated as part of the amount of fluid used for the feeding, unless it contains blood or mucus
(9) Use formula, breast milk, or other fluid
(10) Instill fluid by gravity flow—length of feeding should approximate the time it would take for an oral feeding (1 ml/min)
(11) Enhance tolerance for feeding and prepare for oral feeding
   (a) Allow newborn to suck on a pacifier during feeding—associates sucking with satiety
   (b) Hold and cuddle newborn—provides pleasurable physical contact that becomes associated with feeding
(12) Assess tolerance for feeding by noting
   (a) Amount taken and retained
   (b) Occurrence of vomiting or regurgitation and amount
   (c) Degree of abdominal distension
   (d) Bowel and bladder elimination

3. Total parenteral nutrition (TPN)—provision of protein (amino acids), dextrose, lipids, vitamins, and minerals intravenously via a large peripheral or central vein; used for newborns who are unable to receive oral or gavage feedings
   a. Respiratory distress (very rapid respirations)
   b. Mechanical ventilation
   c. Malabsorption syndrome, necrotizing enterocolitis (NEC)
   d. Surgery on the gastrointestinal tract
4. Determine effectiveness of nutrition method chosen
   a. Weigh daily
   b. Measure length and head circumference weekly
   c. Assess hydration status
   d. Monitor blood glucose levels
5. Observe for signs of readiness for oral feeding
   a. Strong, coordinated suck and swallow
   b. Gag and rooting reflexes present and strong
   c. Spontaneous sucking on tube, hands, pacifier

d. Signs of hunger as feeding time approaches and signs of satiety after feeding are exhibited

6. Gradually advance newborn to oral feeding—progress from TPN to gavage to oral by decreasing amount administered by one method and increasing amount administered by the other

V. Hyperbilirubinemia—increased level of unconjugated bilirubin related to the inability of the newborn's liver to break down and excrete the bilirubin produced by red blood cell (RBC) destruction

A. Types

1. Physiologic hyperbilirubinemia-jaundice appears after the first 24 hours of life especially in
   a. Low birth weight newborns
   b. Newborns of diabetic mothers
   c. Newborns who have difficulty with feeding immediately after birth, such as breast-fed newborns
2. Pathologic hyperbilirubinemia-jaundice appears during the first 24 hours of life, with levels increasing at a more rapid pace and to higher levels—associated with hemolytic disease of
   a. Rh incompatibility—Rh+ newborn is exposed to antibodies formed by an Rh– mother and transmitted to it transplacentally; antibodies destroy the newborn's Rh+ RBCs
   b. ABO blood type incompatibility—usually noted with mothers with an O blood type who have newborns who are A or B; experience less difficulty than the Rh incompatible newborn

B. Prevention

1. Initiate early and frequent feedings—stimulate gastrocolic reflex; bowel movement occurs with passage of meconium; bilirubin is excreted in the stool rather than being reabsorbed into the circulatory system
2. Administration of Rhogam to all eligible (unsensitized Rh– mothers who have an Rh+ newborn; father of baby is Rh+) mothers after any pregnancy related event that can lead to exposure of her blood to that of her fetus. Examples: abortion, amniocentesis, stillbirth, vaginal or cesarean birth.

C. Treatment measures—must be instituted promptly to reduce rising bilirubin levels and facilitate its

excretion before bilirubin level becomes so high (>20 g/dL) that bilirubin invades the brain, causing permanent damage (kernicterus)

1. Phototherapy—light source of fluorescent bulbs is placed 18 to 20 inches above the newborn to facilitate bilirubin breakdown for excretion
   a. Place undressed newborn under the lights for full skin exposure—small diaper or genital covering may be used to collect stool or urine
   b. Cover eyes completely
      (1) Close eye lids before patches are applied
      (2) Remove patches after taking newborn out from under lights in order to
         (a) Check eyes for discharge, excess pressure, corneal irritation, edema
         (b) Facilitate visual stimulation and eye contact with parents and family
   c. Do not apply any lotions, creams, or oils to the skin
   d. Feed frequently at 2- to 3-hour intervals in order to
      (1) Maintain hydration by replacing fluid lost via the skin and liquid stools
      (2) Enhance excretion of bilirubin by facilitating elimination through the gastrointestinal tract
      (3) Provide water supplementation if needed
   e. Observe stools which are often loose, green, and more frequent
   f. Assess temperature at least q 4 hr since newborn is prone to cold stress and hyperthermia
      (1) Skin is exposed to air which increases heat loss
      (2) Newborn is usually sleepy and lethargic with a decrease in heat producing muscular activity
      (3) Radiant heat warmer may be used for cold stress
      (4) Lights along with radiant heat warmer may raise body temperature
   g. Change position q 2 hr so all skin surfaces are exposed
   h. Assess effectiveness of treatment
      (1) Monitor progress of jaundice
      (2) Collect blood samples for bilirubin levels as ordered; note trend in terms of rising or decreasing levels
      (3) Treatment is usually discontinued when a downward trend in bilirubin levels is noted

i. Fiberoptic panel or blanket that wraps around newborn is now available
  (1) Newborn can be held and cuddled
  (2) Patches are not required
  (3) Home treatment is possible since unit is portable
j. Teach parents about
  (1) Why hyperbilirubinemia occurs and what effect it can have on the newborn
  (2) What treatment is used, how it works, and why it is important
  (3) Instructions are required to
    (a) Reduce parental anxiety
    (b) Prepare parents for early discharge since jaundice will appear while at home; parents need to know what to look for as well as what to do and why
k. Document all care measures, time under phototherapy, observations of status

2. Exchange transfusion—small amount (10 to 20 ml; some may use less) of newborn's blood is removed via umbilical vein and replaced slowly with a comparable amount of compatible blood using another site; process is continued thereby removing sensitized RBCs and bilirubin and correcting the anemia that occurs as a result of hemolysis; used for
  a. Severe hyperbilirubinemia usually resulting from Rh incompatibility
  b. Hyperbilirubinemia that does not respond to phototherapy where levels continue to rise
  c. Polycythemia may also be treated with exchange transfusions

VI. Nursing interventions to facilitate the attachment process and reduce stress in families experiencing a sick newborn

A. Attachment process is often delayed, inhibited by separation from or limited contact with the newborn as a result of the physical care requirements—considerations by the nurse include

1. Early attachment of parents with their newborn has long-term implications for the newborn's future growth and development and the family's relationship with the newborn

2. Newborn requires positive stimuli that promotes development
   a. Touch or physical contact with people
   b. Auditory stimuli—speaking, singing, music
   c. Visual stimuli—eye contact, mobiles
3. Parents are often unprepared to cope with the unexpected event of a newborn with health problems and therefore may experience
   a. Anxiety regarding the often changing health status of their newborn; face an uncertain future that may result in disability or death of newborn
   b. Reluctance to make an emotional investment in the newborn and establish a relationship with it since it might die (delay naming, visit infrequently, afraid to touch or participate in care); anticipatory grieving may occur
   c. Role conflict as they attempt to be there for their baby yet also try to meet the needs of each other, children at home, jobs, and themselves
   d. Guilt, blame, and anger—questions arise: why did this happen? what did we or you do wrong? what could we or you have done differently during pregnancy?
   e. Worry regarding financial situation and ability to pay bills
4. Children at home are influenced by the unexpected events concerning their anticipated sibling and may experience
   a. Disappointment that baby did not come home
   b. Worry regarding status of baby—pick up on parental anxiety
   c. A feeling of abandonment by their parents as a result of being cared for by others

B. Nursing interventions

1. Provide time for parents to communicate; encourage them to freely discuss their feelings and concerns without fear of judgement
   a. Help them to recognize the normalcy of their feelings
   b. Allow them to proceed at their own pace
2. Introduce parents to their newborn
   a. Explain purpose of all equipment, procedures
   b. Keep them informed as to the status of their newborn recognizing that teaching and explanations may need to be repeated or reinforced since anxiety can interfere with understanding and perception
   c. Help them to focus on the newborn rather than all the equipment—point out their newborn's behaviors, such as movements, breathing, opening eyes, grasp

   d. Encourage them to touch their newborn and to interact with it
   e. Provide private time for them to interact with their newborn
3. Establish flexible visiting hours and encourage parents to come in and participate in the newborn's care, even for short periods of time
   a. Collect breast milk for gavage feedings
   b. Help with procedures
   c. Bring in clothes, toys from home, pictures to help establish the newborn's identity as their baby
   d. Reinforce their efforts at caring for their newborn
4. Involve siblings
   a. Allow visitation
   b. Prepare children for intensive care environment and what they will see
   c. Encourage touch and interaction
   d. Provide explanations
5. Initiate a discharge plan as soon as newborn is admitted to the intensive care unit—earlier discharge of newborns with special needs is a growing trend
   a. Teach parents what they need to know to care for their newborn in the home; provide time for practice
   b. Discuss home preparations that may have to be made to accommodate the infant and needed equipment
   c. Involve social worker, community health nurses, homecare agencies that will be involved in the care of the infant after discharge
   d. Assist parents with financial concerns
   e. Make referrals to support groups of parents who have had similar experiences

REVIEW QUESTIONS

1. A neutral thermal environment is one that assists the newborn to maintain a stable body temperature that does not fall below
   a. 96.7° F
   b. 97.7° F
   c. 98.6° F
   d. 99.5° F

2. Small for gestational age (SGA) newborns experience difficulty adapting to extrauterine life as a result of
   a. Anemia
   b. Hyperglycemia
   c. Limited subcutaneous fat
   d. Inadequate surfactant

3. Preterm newborns
   a. Assume a flexed posture when at rest
   b. Exhibit the scarf sign
   c. Provide resistance when heel is brought to the ear
   d. Possess an abundance of brown fat

4. When caring for a preterm newborn, nurses must be alert for signs of
   a. Hypercalcemia
   b. Premature closure of the ductus arteriosus and foramen ovale
   c. Meconium aspiration syndrome
   d. Hypoglycemia

5. A preterm newborn requires intermittent gavage feeding. The nurse should
   a. Use a 10-inch, no. 12 french catheter that is flexible and soft
   b. Lubricate the tube with tap water
   c. Measure length of tube to be inserted from tip of nose to midpoint of xiphoid process
   d. Insert tube through the mouth

6. The nurse can enhance the preterm newborn's tolerance for gavage feeding by
   a. Instilling fluid at a rate of 4 ml/min
   b. Allowing the newborn to suck on a pacifier during the feeding
   c. Keeping the newborn under the radiant heat warmer during the feeding
   d. Weighing the newborn before and after the feeding

7. Pathologic hyperbilirubinemia, as indicated by the appearance of jaundice in the first 24 hours, is most likely to occur in

a. Low birth weight newborns
b. Newborns with diabetic mothers
c. Rh+ newborns who have been exposed to Rh+ antibodies from their Rh– mothers
d. Newborns who are poor feeders

8. Phototherapy has been ordered for a newborn with an elevated bilirubin level. The nurse should

a. Cover the newborn's eyes with patches
b. Place ultraviolet lights 15 inches above the newborn
c. Coat the newborn's skin with a cream such as Nivea
d. Feed the newborn every 4 hours

9. Newborns undergoing phototherapy to enhance excretion of excess bilirubin are unlikely to exhibit

a. Hyperthermia
b. Cold stress
c. Constipation
d. Fluid deficit

ANSWERS, RATIONALES, AND TEST-TAKING TIPS

Rationales	Test-Taking Tips
1. Correct answer: b	
The goal of a neutral thermal environment is to assist the newborn to stabilize its temperature between 97.7 and 99.5° F.	An educated guess would be to select the temperature about 1 degree below normal of 98.6° F.
2. Correct answer: c	
Limited subcutaneous fat increases the newborn's risk for cold stress. SGA newborns have an excess of RBCs from exposure to hypoxia in utero. Hypoglycemia occurs from poor intrauterine nutrition and formation of nutrient stores. Inadequate surfactant production is associated with prematurity.	If you have no idea of the correct response, cluster responses *a, b,* and *d* under more internal features and response *c* as most influential with external environment.
3. Correct answer: b	
Preterm newborns have limited muscle tone allowing the elbow to be brought past the midline of the chest (scarf sign) and the heel to the ear with no resistance. They tend to assume an extended posture. Brown fat is limited, thereby increasing the risk for hypothermia-cold stress.	Remember that in a premature birth the body functions are weaker and not as strong as in the term newborn. Thus, the words in the responses "flexed," "resistance when heel . . . to ear" indicate strong muscle tone not found in the preterm, and "abundance . . . fat" is absent since the newborn had insufficient time in utero.
4. Correct answer: d	
Nutritional deficits such as hypocalcemia and hypoglycemia are common because of limited gestation	Remember the association—preterm newborns typically have "hypo" clinical findings.

time to form nutrient stores. Fetal circulatory shunts must close at birth. The hypoxia experienced by inadequate respiration interferes with the closure of the shunts in the preterm newborn. Respiratory distress syndrome with limited surfactant production is most likely to occur.

5. Correct answer: d

Use a 15-inch, no. 5 or no. 8 firm french catheter and lubricate with sterile water. Measure length of tube from tip of nose to ear lobe and then to midpoint between end of xiphoid process and umbilicus. Insertion through the mouth maintains nasal patency and stimulates sucking.

Note that the client is a preterm. The best lubricant is "sterile" water. A flexible, soft catheter will be more difficult to insert. Don't forget nose to ear to xiphoid for gastric tube measurement; caution with newborns: "midpoint between xiphoid and umbilicus" vs. adults to the xiphoid.

6. Correct answer: b

Fluid should be instilled at 1 ml/min, while holding and cuddling the newborn. Weighing the newborn gives an indication of effectiveness but does not enhance tolerance for the feeding.

The question is about feeding therefore select the response that has a focus of the gastrointestinal function, sucking of newborn, which is response *b*.

7. Correct answer: c

Responses *a, b,* and *d* are primarily associated with physiologic hyperbilirubinemia, as indicated by the appearance of jaundice after the first 24 hours of life.

The important approach in this question is to slowly and carefully read the question to identify the key word pathologic. This means that there is an abnormal process occuring in the body functions. Of the given choices, option *c* is the most characteristic of this type of event.

8. Correct answer: a

Fluorescent light is used and placed 18 to 20 inches above the newborn. Creams are never applied to the skin. Feed every 2 to 3 hours to maintain hydration and enhance excretion of bilirubin.

Under any kind of light therapy the first priority is to protect the eyes. Remember that 18 to 20 inches is a good choice for most therapy, i.e., raise the irrigation or the feeding bag 18 to 20 inches above the insertion site. Recall that being under a light, even sunlight in the summertime, may result in dehydration; thus, feeding is to be more frequent than every 4 hours.

9. Correct answer: c

Responses *a, b,* and *d* are all possible side effects of phototherapy. Newborns are likely to exhibit frequent, loose, green, diarrhea-like stools.

The key word in the stem is "unlikely." If you read too fast you may misread the question.

Comprehensive Exam

COMPREHENSIVE EXAM QUESTIONS

1. The risk for constipation in the postpartum period is unrelated to
   a. Tenderness of the episiotomy
   b. Decreasing level of estrogen
   c. Decreased abdominal muscle tone
   d. Fear of pain and of ripping stitches during a bowel movement

2. A nurse is using Naegele's rule to calculate a pregnant woman's estimated date of birth (EDB). This woman reports that her last menstrual period began on September 15, 1995 and ended 5 days later. The EDB is
   a. June 27, 1996
   b. June 8, 1996
   c. June 22, 1996
   d. December 8, 1996

3. If a woman gives birth during the 41st week of her pregnancy, it would be considered what kind of birth
   a. Preterm
   b. Term
   c. Postterm
   d. Gestational

4. Which of the following, if exhibited by a pregnant woman, represents a positive change of pregnancy?
   a. Morning sickness
   b. Quickening
   c. Positive pregnancy test
   d. Fetal heart beat auscultated with doppler or fetoscope

5. When examining the umbilical cord immediately after birth, the nurse should expect to observe
   a. One artery
   b. Two veins
   c. Whitish-gray coloration
   d. Slight odor

6. Parents should expect that their newborn will spend approximately how many hours in deep sleep
   a. 2 to 3
   b. 4 to 5
   c. 12 to 15
   d. 1 to 4

7. The newborn would respond most effectively to feeding in which state?
   a. Drowsy
   b. Quiet alert
   c. Active alert
   d. Crying

8. A pregnant woman's BMI was calculated to be 28. Which of the following represents the recommended weight gain for this woman during her pregnancy?
   a. 15 to 25 pounds
   b. 25 to 35 pounds
   c. 28 to 40 pounds
   d. 40 to 50 pounds

9. An expectant woman, 40 years old, undergoes an amniocentesis to detect the presence of Down Syndrome. The fetal chromosomes are arranged and photographed to facilitate diagnosis. The picture is called what?
   a. Genotype
   b. Phenotype
   c. Chromosometype
   d. Karyotype

10. Effective therapeutic measures designed to deal with postpartum blues would include each of the following EXCEPT
    a. Involve members in identifying typical blues behaviors and implementing appropriate support measures
    b. Encourage the primiparous woman to gain self-confidence by taking care of her new baby on her own
    c. Provide positive reinforcement for the mother's efforts in caring for her baby
    d. Inform the postpartum woman about the common stressors of this period and appropriate coping mechanisms to deal with them

11. Parents should realize that which of the following sibling behaviors related to adjustment to a new baby would require evaluation by a healthcare professional?
    a. Impatience and sometimes anger when the newborn's needs take precedence over sibling's needs
    b. Rejection of their mother when she arrives home with the new baby
    c. Asking to be bottle-fed or to sleep in their parents' bedroom along with the new baby
    d. Altered living patterns such as sleeping, eating, and refusal to go to school

12. A woman diagnosed with marginal placenta previa gave birth vaginally 15 minutes ago. At the present time she is at greatest risk for

a. Hemorrhage
b. Infection
c. Urinary retention
d. Thrombophlebitis

13. Primary sites for postpartum infection would include all but which of the following?

a. Respiratory tract
b. Endometrium
c. Urinary tract
d. Breasts

14. When caring for a postpartum woman with a uterine infection, the nurse should

a. Administer an antipyretic such as aspirin when the temperature rises above 100.4° F
b. Provide at least 2000 ml of fluid/day
c. Obtain appropriate specimens for cultures before initiating antibiotic treatment
d. Reassure the woman that future reproduction will not be affected

15. A pregnant woman at 30 weeks' gestation exhibits a rise in her baseline systolic blood pressure of 32 mm Hg, a weight gain of 2 pounds since last week, and difficulty removing the rings she usually wears on her fingers. These signs are strongly suggestive of

a. Gestational hypertension
b. Preeclampsia
c. Eclampsia
d. HELLP syndrome

16. The primary pathophysiologic basis for the clinical manifestations of pregnancy induced hypertension (PIH) is

a. Fluid retention related to excessive salt intake
b. Ineffective excretion of fluid by the kidneys
c. Cardiac decompensation
d. Ineffective dilatation of the vascular network to accommodate the expanding blood volume of pregnancy

17. The fetal presenting part is described as vertex when the
   a. Face enters the pelvis first
   b. Buttocks emerge with legs extended over the abdomen
   c. Flexed head enters the pelvis first
   d. Fetal lie is longitudinal

18. A woman is using a diaphragm incorrectly if she
   a. Inserts it up to 6 hours before intercourse
   b. Applies a spermicide inside the dome and around the rim
   c. Removes it within 2 hours after last act of coitus
   d. Washes it with mild soap and water after use and then dusts it with cornstarch

19. Before her discharge at 12 hours after birth of a full-term 8 pound baby, the postpartum woman would be unlikely to exhibit which of the following characteristics related to her uterus?
   a. Consistency of fundus: firm
   b. Height of fundus: midway between the symphysis pubis and umbilicus
   c. Location of fundus: midline of the abdomen
   d. Size of uterus: about 16 weeks' gestation

20. A primiparous woman, one day postpartum, calls the nurse into her room. The woman anxiously tells the nurse that while breast-feeding, she experienced uterine cramps and a heavy gush of flow that soaked through her peripad to her bed. The nurse should initially
   a. Palpate the woman's fundus
   b. Tell the woman that this often happens when breast-feeding for the first few days after birth
   c. Administer the Methergine that was ordered PRN
   d. Assist the woman with perineal care and changing her pad

21. The lochia of a postpartum woman on the second day after birth should exhibit each of the following characteristics except
   a. Deep red and thick
   b. A few large clots
   c. Fleshy odor
   d. Moderate amount—<6" on pad after 1 hour

22. Which of the following would not be included in the care management of a pregnant woman with heart disease?
   a. Digoxin
   b. Coumadin
   c. Dietary restriction of sodium
   d. Limitation of weight gain to approximately 24 pounds

23. A pregnant woman can reduce her risk for toxoplasmosis by
   a. Avoiding the handling of cat litter, soil, or raw meat
   b. Practicing good genital hygiene
   c. Using safer sex methods such as condoms during intercourse
   d. Maintaining a nutritious diet during pregnancy

24. In order to prevent infection by the hepatitis B virus for herself and her fetus, the pregnant woman should
   a. Receive gamma globulin during the first trimester
   b. Carefully wash hands before eating or preparing food
   c. Receive the hepatitis B vaccine
   d. Take AZT during the second and third trimester

25. The physician has ordered a Ritodrine infusion to suppress the preterm labor of a pregnant woman at 27 weeks' gestation. In administering this medication the nurse should
   a. Piggyback a solution of 150 mg of Ritodrine in 500 ml of 5% dextrose in ½ normal saline to the proximal port (port closest to the IV infusion site) of the primary tubing
   b. Begin the infusion at a rate of 1 mg/min
   c. Increase the amount of Ritodrine at a rate of 0.5 mg/min every 5 minutes
   d. Do not exceed a dosage of 3 mg/min

26. When caring for a woman whose labor is being suppressed with an infusion of Ritodrine, the nurse must be alert for the appearance of intolerable side effects requiring immediate discontinuation of the infusion and notification of the physician. An intolerable side effect associated with Ritodrine would be
   a. Maternal heart rate >100
   b. Fetal heart rate >160
   c. Maternal blood pressure >140/90
   d. Crackles and rales upon auscultation of the lungs

27. A pregnant woman at 30 weeks' gestation is receiving an IV infusion of magnesium sulfate to suppress preterm labor. In administering this infusion the nurse should

a. Increase the rate of infusion at a rate of 1 mg every 10 minutes
b. Assess deep tendon reflexes once every 2 to 4 hours
c. Ensure that the serum level of magnesium does not exceed 10 mEq/L
d. Discontinue the infusion and notify the physician if the woman's respirations are <12 per minute

28. The birth weight of a breast-fed newborn was 8 pounds 4 ounces. On the third day the newborn's weight was 7 pounds 12 ounces. Based on this finding the nurse should

a. Encourage the mother to continue breast-feeding, since it is effective in meeting the newborn's nutrient and fluid needs
b. Suggest that the mother switch to bottle-feeding, since the breast-feeding is ineffective in meeting newborn needs for fluid and nutrients
c. Notify the physician, since the newborn is being poorly nourished
d. Refer the mother to a lactation consultant to improve her breast-feeding technique

29. A newborn's birth weight is 7 pounds, 8 ounces or 3409 gm. The maximum expected weight loss for this newborn would be

a. 170 gm; 6 ounces
b. 341 gm; 12 ounces
c. 511 gm; 18 ounces
d. 682 gm; 24 ounces

30. Which of the following would not be an expected sign of dehydration in the newborn?

a. Weight loss
b. Reduced turgor
c. Concentrated urine
d. Decreased frequency and amount of urine

31. A woman with severe preeclampsia is being monitored for assessment findings indicative of cerebral edema and venospasm. Which of the following is not a typical finding of the cerebral involvement associated with preeclampsia?

a. Hypotonic deep tendon reflexes
b. Headache
c. Vision changes including blurring and spots before the eyes
d. Insomnia

32. Which measure would be least effective in relieving the signs and symptoms of mild preeclampsia?

a. Low-salt diet
b. Periods of bed rest, alternating position from side to side
c. Balanced diet with protein intake at 1.5 g/kg/day
d. Relaxation techniques and diversional activities

33. A nursing measure to prevent seizures in a woman with severe preeclampsia would include which of the following?

a. Pad siderails of the bed and maintain the bed in a low position
b. Place the woman in the room next to the nurse's station for close observation
c. Reduce environmental stimuli in the woman's room by turning off the TV and telephone and dimming the lights
d. Tape a padded tongue blade to the woman's bed

34. When caring for a laboring woman with external fetal monitoring, the nurse should

a. Apply contact gel to surface of tocotransducer and ultrasound transducer before placement on the abdomen
b. Place the tocotransducer over the point of maximum intensity
c. Keep the woman in a semirecumbent position to ensure accuracy of the tracings
d. Reapply the transducer and massage reddened areas at least once every hour

35. The major potential problem associated with internal monitoring is

a. Infection
b. Bleeding from the fetal presenting part at the point of attachment of the cardiotachometer
c. Maternal fear and anxiety
d. Limitation on maternal activity such as ambulation

36. When assessing an internal monitor tracing for the quality of FHR variability, the nurse should keep in mind that

a. Alteration in variability is a late appearing sign of hypoxia
b. A preterm fetus characteristically exhibits limited variability and as a result immature function of the autonomic nervous system (ANS)
c. Long-term variability refers to the change in FHR from one beat to the next as a result of differences in the interval between consecutive heart beats
d. Short- and long-term variability are unaffected by the fetal sleep-wake cycle

37. Two hours after giving birth a primiparous woman becomes anxious and complains of intense perineal pain with a strong urge to have a bowel movement. Her fundus is firm at the umbilicus and midline. Her lochia is moderate rubra with no clots. The nurse would suspect
a. Bladder distension
b. Uterine atony
c. Constipation
d. Hematoma formation

38. The primary nursing focus of the fourth stage of labor would be to
a. Prevent infection
b. Facilitate newborn–parent interaction
c. Enhance maternal comfort and rest
d. Prevent hemorrhage and shock

39. A woman pregnant for the first time gives birth to twins at 37 weeks' gestation. The correct terms to describe this woman's obstetrical history would be
a. Multigravida, multipara
b. Primigravida, multipara
c. Primigravida, primipara
d. Multigravida, primipara

40. A pregnant woman is the mother of two children. Her first pregnancy ended in a stillbirth at 32 weeks' gestation, her second pregnancy with the birth of her daughter at 36 weeks, and her third pregnancy with the birth of her son at 41 weeks. Using the 5-digit system to describe this woman's current obstetrical history, the nurse would record
a. 4-1-2-0-2
b. 3-1-2-0-2
c. 4-2-1-0-1
d. 3-1-1-1-2

41. Following circumcision of a newborn, the nurse provides instructions to his parents regarding postcircumcision care. The nurse should tell the parents to
a. Remove the plastibell rim after 24 hours
b. Expect a yellowish exudate to cover the glans after the first 24 hours
c. Change the diaper every 2 hours and cleanse the site with soap and water or baby wipes
d. Apply constant pressure to the site if bleeding occurs and call the physician

42. During a telephone follow-up call, the nurse would recognize that a new mother understood breast-feeding instructions if she says

a. "I feed my baby every 2 hours around the clock"
b. "I always start feeding on my right breast since my baby seems to feed best on that breast"
c. "I use both the football and traditional positions for feeding"
d. "I let my baby continue to suck for a while on the second breast after it is empty"

43. Which of the following actions of a breast-feeding mother indicate the need for further instruction?

a. Holds breast with four fingers along bottom and thumb at top
b. Leans forward to bring breast toward the baby
c. Stimulates the rooting reflex then inserts nipple and areola into newborn's open mouth
d. Puts her finger into newborn's mouth before removing breast

44. Many pregnant women identify whom as the most significant and influential person in their lives?

a. The doctor who will be delivering their baby
b. Their own mother
c. The father of their baby
d. The nurse who is guiding their pregnancy

45. Which of the following would not be a priority task to be accomplished by a family in the developmental phase of childbearing and rearing?

a. Assign roles and responsibilities to family members
b. Initiate plans for retirement
c. Socialize children for entry into society
d. Hand down to their children morals, values, and family traditions

46. Expectant parents, in the first trimester of pregnancy, ask the nurse how they can prepare their 3-year-old preschool daughter for the new baby. Which of the following would be least effective in facilitating adjustment?

a. Tell the child about the pregnancy as soon as mom begins to look pregnant
b. Arrange for a few sleep overs with the person who will care for their child at the time of the birth
c. Transfer their child to her new room and bed just before the expected birth of the baby
d. Enroll their child in a sibling preparation class for young children

47. Vitamin K is given to the newborn to
   a. Reduce bilirubin levels
   b. Increase the production of red blood cells
   c. Stimulate the formation of surfactant
   d. Enhance ability of blood to clot

48. Newborns are at risk for injury if appropriate safety precautions are not implemented. Parents should be taught to
   a. Place newborn on abdomen (prone) after feeding and for sleep
   b. Avoid use of pacifiers
   c. Use a rearward facing car seat until the infant weighs at least 20 pounds
   d. Use a crib with siderail slats that are no more than 3½" apart

49. Which of the following statements is correct and can be used as a guideline for planning diets during pregnancy?
   a. An increase of 300 calories per day is required and should begin in the first trimester
   b. A 10% increase in protein above the daily requirements for a pregnant woman's age group is recommended
   c. Iron supplementation is recommended only for women whose diets lack foods high in iron
   d. The requirement for folic acid is increased by 50% over prepregnant levels

50. An expectant couple asks the nurse about intercourse during pregnancy and if it is safe for the baby. The nurse should tell the couple
   a. Intercourse should be avoided if any spotting from the vagina occurs afterwards
   b. Intercourse is safe until the third trimester
   c. Safer sex practices should be used once the membranes rupture
   d. Intercourse and orgasm are often contraindicated if a history of or signs of preterm labor are present

ANSWERS, RATIONALES, AND TEST-TAKING TIPS

Rationales	Test-Taking Tips
1. Correct answer: b Responses *a, c,* and *d* all contribute to constipation. Progesterone, not estrogen, slows peristalsis.	If you read too quickly and overlooked the key word "unrelated" you probably selected the incorrect answer. Remember: *p*rogesterone affects *p*eristalsis to make it *p*okey or slow.
2. Correct answer: c Naegele's rule: subtract 3 months and add 7 days and 1 year to the first day of the last menstrual period. 9 15 1995 –3 +7 +1 6 22 1996	Remember with this rule, that 3 comes before 7 numerically; therefore, always subtract 3 from the given month first. Immediately the responses can be narrowed to either *a, b,* or *c.* Now remember that the first day is the starter day, so that date is the one to use; add 7 and the correct answer is obvious.
3. Correct answer: b Term births occur after 37 weeks but before the end of the 42nd week; preterm births occur before the 38th week but after 20 to 24 weeks; postterm births occur after the 42nd week; gestational is not a term used to describe the time of birth.	Remember: term *b*irth may be similar to the *b*ust size of a woman at the end of pregnancy—37 to 42,—even if the bust was small to start with before pregnancy.
4. Correct answer: d Responses *a* and *b* are presumptive changes; *c* is a probable change.	Remember that hearing a pulse is a positive sign.

5. Correct answer: c

There should be two arteries and one vein. No odor should be present.

"Go with what you know." You know that an odor is probably not normal; eliminate this option. If you can't recall the number of veins or arteries, don't make a guess. You can make an educated guess that the color is whitish-gray.

6. Correct answer: b

While 4 to 5 hours are spent in deep sleep, 12 to 15 hours are spent in light sleep, 2 to 3 hours in the quiet alert state, and 1 to 4 hours between active alert and crying.

If you have no idea of the correct response, try the number approach—eliminate the highest and the lowest numbers 2 to 3 and 4 to 5 are left; then pick 4 to 5 since it is more reasonable for deep sleep.

7. Correct answer: c

It is during the active alert state that the newborn is most sensitive to discomfort, including hunger. The newborn is very eager to feed at this time and should respond well to feeding attempts.

Use a common sense approach: if one is active, then actions will be more effective.

8. Correct answer: a

A BMI >26 indicates an overweight woman, therefore a weight gain of 15 to 25 pounds is recommended. Response *b* is the recommended weight gain for a normal weight woman and *c* for an underweight woman; *d* is beyond weight gain recommendations.

Remember that the higher the BMI the lower the total weight gain should be for pregnant clients. There is an inverse relationship.

9. Correct answer: d

Genotype is the entire genetic makeup, while phenotype is the manner in which the

Remember *k*aryotype is a picture, which is a *k*eepsake.

genotype is expressed in the physical appearance. There is nothing referred to as a chromosometype.

10. Correct answer: b

Responses *a, c,* and *d* are all highly effective measures in both the prevention of postpartum blues and dealing with them if they occur. While caring for her baby will increase her self-confidence, a woman should ask for and accept help with baby care so she can have time to herself.

Cluster the responses *a, c,* and *d* under the umbrella of positive support. Note that response *b* promotes isolation of the mother which would only further feed the blues and depression. Be sure to notice the word "except" in the question—missing this word from reading too fast is a common error of multiple choice test takers.

11. Correct answer: d

Responses *a, b,* and *c* are all typical sibling reactions, especially in younger children who have more difficulty understanding the impact of a new baby. Disturbances in life activities, especially if persistent, reflect a problem with adjustment necessitating the care of a healthcare provider before more serious difficulty develops.

If you have no idea of the correct response, cluster the responses *a, b,* and *c* to be very specific situations and eliminate them. Read response *d* and note that it is different by being more general—"altered living patterns" with examples given.

12. Correct answer: a

Hemorrhage is the most immediate risk, since the lower uterine segment has limited ability to contract to reduce blood loss. Infection is a risk because of the location of the placental site

With the question worded "greatest risk," note that all of the responses will be correct. List them in order of priority and you will select the correct response. The use of basic life support principles can help—airway, breathing, circulation. No

but is not a priority concern at this time. There is no greater risk for urinary retention or thrombophlebitis than with a normally implanted placenta.

options state needs related to respiratory and response *a* directly relates to hemorrhage; select it.

13. Correct answer: a

The respiratory tract is not a major site for infection, since the parturition and postpartum periods do not provide significant risk to the system.

The most important words in the stem to guide the selection of the best response are "primary site" and "postpartum infection." Cluster the responses *b, c,* and *d* under the parts involved in pregnancy. The respiratory system is not involved.

14. Correct answer: c

Antipyretics, preferably acetaminophen (Tylenol), should be used primarily when the temperature is above 102° F and is accompanied by discomfort, since fever has a therapeutic effect. At least 3000 ml/day are required for fluid intake. There is no way to be sure that reproduction will not be affected. False reassurance should not be given. The nurse should explain treatments, progress of healing, etc.

Apply basic guidelines for antibiotic and antipyretic administration with any client of any age.

15. Correct answer: b

Gestational hypertension is not associated with edema as noted by the excessive weight gain and upper-body edema. Eclampsia is associated with seizures and HELLP with hemolysis, liver dysfunction, and low platelets.

Identify that the responses are somewhat listed in order of severity. Delete responses *a* and *d* the least and the most severe. Then select response *b* the less severe situation.

16. Correct answer: d

Failure of the vascular network to expand leads to venospasm and third spacing of fluid to interstitial spaces. Blood pressure rises and edema can occur. Sodium intake is not responsible for the findings of PIH. Renal involvement occurs when renal perfusion is eventually affected.

If you have no idea, cluster responses *a, b,* and *c* under the umbrella of specific area: salt intake, kidneys, and heart. Response *d* describes a physiology that would affect the entire body.

17. Correct answer: c

Vertex indicates that the head is fully flexed allowing the area over the parietal bones, the vertex, to present first into the pelvis. The head is extended in the situation with a face presentation. Longitudinal lie indicates that maternal spine and fetal spine are parallel to each other, with the presentation that could be breech or cephalic. Breech presentation with legs extended upward is a frank breech.

If you narrowed the responses to *a* or *c,* response *c* is better since it is the most specific.

18. Correct answer: c

It should be left in place for 6 to 8 hours but not longer than 24 hours after the last intercourse.

In general most contraceptive devices or substances need to be in place for at least 6 hours after intercourse.

19. Correct answer: b

Responses *a, c,* and *d* are all expected. The fundus should be at or 1 cm below the umbilicus within 12 hours of birth.

Think if the size of the uterus is about 16 weeks then the fundus would be near but below the umbilicus since the level of the umbilicus is at about 20 weeks.

20. Correct answer: a

Although this is an expected finding with breast-feeding, fundal massage, or ambulation, the nurse should still make sure that the fundus is firm. If firm, the nurse can then implement responses *b* and *d*. If the uterus is boggy, it should be massaged and then Methergine administered.

Use the nursing process steps: when a client has a complaint initially do further assessment of the given area before intervening.

21. Correct answer: b

Large clots are a warning sign that the uterus may not be contracting properly. Small clots are expected.

The word that is the clue to an abnormal finding is "large." If you focused on "few" instead, the incorrect answer was probably selected.

22. Correct answer: b

Coumadin crosses the placenta and is teratogenic to the fetus. Heparin is the anticoagulant of choice. Digoxin is used to strengthen the action of the heart. Salt is restricted to reduce fluid retention. Weight gain is limited to the lower end of the recommended range to reduce stress on the heart.

Remember: "*c*oumadin is *c*ontraindicated since it *c*rosses over to the fetus.

23. Correct answer: a

Toxoplasmosis is a protozoan infection transmitted by handling or eating anything contaminated with infected cat feces or eating or handling raw meat. Response *b, c,* and *d* are unrelated to the mode of transmission for toxoplasmosis.

If you have no idea of the correct response, cluster responses *b, c,* and *d* under positive statements of what to do—practice, use, and maintain. Response *a* uses a negative statement—avoid—so is likely the correct response.

24. Correct answer: c

Hepatitis B is a blood-borne infection and hepatitis B vaccine is safe to use in pregnancy, especially if the woman is at high risk. Responses *a* and *b* relate to hepatitis A. AZT is used to reduce the risk for fetal transmission if the mother is infected with HIV.

Apply general knowledge for the preventions of hepatitis B—receive the vaccine. Note the key word in the stem is "prevent." Recall that gamma globulins are given after exposure to a substance.

25. Correct answer: a

Begin the infusion at a rate of 0.05 to 0.1 mg/min and increase at a rate of 0.05 mg/min every 10 to 20 minutes. Do not exceed a rate of 0.35 mg/min.

Go with what you know—that the proximal site is the correct piggyback site and select this response if you are not sure of the correctness of the other responses.

26. Correct answer: d

Fluid volume excess is a potentially dangerous complication of Ritodrine that can lead to pulmonary edema. Other intolerable side effects include maternal heart rate >140 beats per minute, dysrrythmias, FHR >180, and hypotension with a BP <90/60.

The key word in the question is "intolerable." Note that all responses except *d* might be tolerated by the mother and infant; fluid in the lungs as a new finding requires immediate attention and may indicate that there is fluid overload and/or left heart failure. The use of the ABCs (airway, breathing, circulation) to set priorities can be used here also. In response *d,* a breathing problem takes precedent over the other given findings.

27. Correct answer: d

Infusion rate should be increased by 0.5 to 1 Gm every 30 minutes. Deep tendon reflexes should be checked once every hour.

Of the given choice of responses use of the ABCs to set priorities leads to the selection of response *d,* the breathing problem over the other selections.

The therapeutic level of magnesium in the serum is 4 to 7 mEq/L.

28. Correct answer: a

Weight loss of 8 ounces falls within the 5 to 10 % expected weight loss during the first few days of life, which for this newborn would be 6.6 to 13.2 ounces. Breast-feeding is obviously effective making responses *b, c,* and *d* inappropriate at this time.

Cluster the responses *b, c,* and *d* since they suggest that there is a problem. Select response *a* since it is different and suggests no problem is evident.

29. Correct answer: b

The range of expected weight loss is 5 to 10% of birthweight. Therefore the maximum loss is 341 gm or 12 ounces. Response *a* represents a 5% loss, response *c* a 15% loss, and response *d* a 20% loss.

The key word in the question is "maximum." Multiply 7 pounds × 16 ounces = 112 + 8 ounces = 120 ounces; then take 10% of this which is 12 ounces.

30. Correct answer: c

Responses *a, b,* and *d* are expected findings of dehydration along with a depressed anterior fontanel and an elevation in temperature. Newborns have a limited ability to concentrate urine and as a result are unable to maintain balance of fluid, electrolytes, and acid-base during times of stress such as diarrhea, vomiting.

If you narrowed it down to responses *c* and *d,* then use what you know about the newborn—that some systems are not quite mature. If the renal system is immature then it would most likely not be able to concentrate urine, yet it would put out fluid in a frequency and amount in relation to the amount of fluid available. Make an educated guess and select response *c.*

31. Correct answer: a

Deep tendon reflexes become brisk (hyperreflexia) with increased CNS involvement.

Cluster responses *b, c,* and *d* to be associated with "cerebral" and that reflexes are not related to cerebral control.

32. Correct answer: a

Salt intake is not responsible for PIH. Bed rest in a lateral position enhances renal perfusion, thereby enhancing fluid loss and placental perfusion. Relaxation techniques and diversion reduce stress. Protein is required to replace protein losses in urine and maintain fluid in the vascular bed.

Remember PIH is a hypertension and that salt has no major influence on the condition and sequela.

33. Correct answer: c

Response *a* is a protective measure and will not prevent a seizure. A room next to the nurses' station exposes woman to environmental stimuli that can precipitate a seizure. Padded tongue blades are no longer used during a seizure.

The key word in the question is "prevent" and all of the responses except *c* are actions to deal with or observe seizure activity. Refrain from focusing on preeclampsia; the question is asking about seizure prevention for any client.

34. Correct answer: d

Only the ultrasound transducer requires contact gel before application over the PMI. The tocotransducer is placed over the fundus. Maternal position should be changed, since the transducers can be readjusted as needed.

If you have no idea go with what you know—prevention of skin breakdown is important when equipment is used, so make an educated guess and select response *d.*

35. Correct answer: a

Since internal monitoring is an invasive procedure, infection is a major concern requiring scrupulous infection-control measures. Bleeding is minimal to nonexistent at point of insertion. Maternal anxiety is a concern but not the major priority. While ambulation is limited, position changes in bed are not.

Go with what you know—a major problem with any internal, invasive procedure is infection.

36. Correct answer: b

Change in variability is often the first sign of hypoxia. Response *c* defines short-term variability. There is a temporary decrease in long-term variability during the fetal sleep state.

See rationale for recall strategies.

37. Correct answer: d

Perineal pressure along with a firm fundus and moderate lochial flow are characteristic of hematoma formation. Uterine atony would result in a boggy fundus. Constipation is unlikely at this time and bladder distention would result in an elevation of the fundus above the umbilicus.

If you have no idea of the correct response, make an educated approach and select the one that might suggest bleeding since the client is two hours postbirth, which is response *d*.

38. Correct answer: d

While responses *a, b,* and *c* are all important, the woman is most vulnerable to hemorrhage at this time. Hypovolemic shock can result, which is a life threatening complication.

Important words to focus on are "primary" and "fourth stage." In listing the responses in order of concern response *d* typically takes precedent over the others as based on an airway, breathing, and circulation approach.

39. Correct answer: c

Primigravida refers to the first pregnancy, while primipara indicates completion of one pregnancy to the age of viability. Multigravida refers to two or more pregnancies and multipara indicates that more than one pregnancy have been completed to the age of viability.

The number of children born in this case does not influence the description.

40. Correct answer: a

Gravida (the first number) = 4 since she is pregnant now and was pregnant three times before. Para, (next four numbers): T: 1 term birth at 41 weeks; P: 2 preterm births at 32 and 36 weeks; A: 0 abortions; L: 2 living children.

First establish the total number of pregnancies to be 4. This narrows the responses to either *a* or *c* with the first digit representing the number of pregnancies. If you recall that the next position is the number of term births—the client has had only one—then response *a* is selected without further need to figure out the other digits.

41. Correct answer: b

Plasitbell rim should fall off spontaneously within 8 days. The diaper is changed frequently but the site is cleansed with warm water only. Intermittent pressure is applied if bleeding occurs.

Constant pressure at this site may contribute to diminished circulation. Eliminate response *c* because cleaning with soap may irritate the site. The device in response *a* is to protect the site. Thus, response *b* is the only response left.

42. Correct answer: c

Baby should be fed when alert and exhibiting signs of hunger. The initial starting breast and position should be alternated with each feeding. Nonnutritive sucking can damage the nipple and/or areola.

Key words in the responses help to eliminate them: in response *a* "every two hours" is a clue for incorrect feeding that is not client or baby centered; in response *b* "always . . . on right" is inappropriate since alternation is the key to facilitate emptying and maintaining skin integrity; in response *d* "continue to suck . . . after . . . empty" is inappropriate.

43. Correct answer: b

Responses *a, c,* and *d* are all correct actions. The baby should be brought to the breast not the breast to the baby.

Think if the breast is brought to the baby the mother may end up with a backache from leaning forward.

44. Correct answer: c

Although responses *a, b,* and *d* are all important to the pregnant woman, the father of her baby is identified by many pregnant women to be the most important and influential.

Cluster responses *a* and *d* into nonfamily and the other responses into family. Common sense reveals that family is a priority. Now decide that the father of the child is a priority over the mother and select *c* as the correct response.

45. Correct answer: b

Making retirement plans, while important, is not a priority at this time, especially compared with the other tasks described.

Cluster responses *a, c,* and *d* with the common themes of children and family. If you missed the key words in the stem, "not a priority" then your selection was probably one of these three and incorrect.

46. Correct answer: c

Responses *a, b,* and *d* are all effective measures. Any major changes involving the child should be initiated early in pregnancy not just before the birth.

Key words that are clues to response *c* being a least effective action are "new room" and "just before the expected birth."

47. Correct answer: d

Newborns have a deficiency of vitamin K until intestinal bacteria that produce vitamin

Remember vitamin K helps clotting in any client and is the antidote if too much Coumadin has been

K are formed. Vitamin K is required for the production of certain clotting factors

given. Vitamin K is found in green leafy vegetables.

48. Correct answer: c

The prone position is no longer used, since it may interfere with chest expansion and lead to SIDS. Approved pacifiers are safe to use and fulfill the newborn's need to suck. Slats should be no more than 2⅜" apart.

Recall tip: put the newborn "back to sleep"—put the newborn on their "back."

49. Correct answer: b

Calorie increases should begin in the second trimester. Iron supplementation is required for all pregnant women beginning in the second trimester, since diet alone cannot meet required increases. Folic acid requirement is twice the prepregnant requirement.

No specific test strategy applies.

50. Correct answer: d

Some spotting often occurs from the increased fragility of the cervix and the vagina. Intercourse can continue as long as the pregnancy is progressing normally. Safer sex practices are always recommended. Rupture of membranes may require abstaining from intercourse. Uterine contractions that accompany orgasm can stimulate labor.

Response *d* is the more comprehensive response when compared to other responses and therefore more likely the best response.

BIBLIOGRAPHY

Aderhold K and Perry L: Jet hydrotherapy for labor and postpartum pain relief, *MCN* 16(2):97-99, 1991.

Aderhold K and Roberts J: Phases of the second stage of labor, *Journal of Nurse Midwifery* 36(5):267, 1991.

Andrews H and Roy C: *The roy adaptation model,* Norwalk, Conn, 1991, Appleton & Lang.

Apgar V: The newborn (Apgar) scoring system: reflections and advice, *Pediatric Clinics of North America* 13(8):695, 1966.

Association of Women's Health, Obstetric, and Neonatal Nurses (AWHONN): Postpartum follow-up: a nursing practice guide, *OGN Nursing Practice Resource,* Washington, DC, 1986, The Association (formerly NAACOG).

AWHONN: Fetal heart rate auscultation, *OGN Nursing Practice Resource,* Washington, DC, 1990, The Association (formerly NAACOG).

AWHONN: Contraceptive options, *OGN Nursing Practice Resource,* Washington, DC, 1991, The Association (formerly NAACOG).

AWHONN: Physical assessment of the neonate, *OGN Nursing Practice Resource,* Washington, DC, 1991, The Association (formerly NAACOG).

Ballard J, Khoury J, Wedig K, Wang L, Eilers-Walsman B, and Lipp R: New Ballard score, expanded to include extremely premature infants, *Journal of Pediatrics* 119:417-423, 1991.

Barkauskas V, Baumann L, Stoltenberg-Allen K, and Darling-Fisher C: *Health and physical assessment,* St Louis, 1994, Mosby.

Bernat S, Woolridge P, Marecki M, and Snell L: Biofeedback-assisted relaxation to reduce stress in labor, *JOGNN* 21(4):295-303, 1992.

Biancuzzo M: Six myths of maternal posture during labor, *MCN* 18(5):264-269, 1993.

Bobak I and Jensen M: *Maternity and gynecologic care,* ed 5, St Louis, 1993, Mosby.

Bowie W, Hammerschlag M, and Martin D: STDs in '94: the new CDC guidelines, *Patient Care* 28(7):29-53, 1994.

Brouillard-Pierce C: Indications for induction of labor, *MCN* 18(suppl):14-22, 1993.

Carlson G: When grandmothers take care of grandchildren, *MCN* 18(4):206-207, 1993.

Cosner K and de Jong E: Physiologic second-stage labor, *MCN* 18(1):38-43, 1993.

Cowan M: Home care of the pregnant woman using terbutaline, *MCN* 18(2):99-105, 1993.

Crawford N and Pruss A: Preventing neonatal hepatitis B infection during the perinatal period, *JOGNN* 22(6):491-497, 1993.

Dickason E, Silver B, and Schult M: *Maternal-infant nursing care,* ed 2, St Louis, 1994, Mosby.

Doenges M and Moorehouse M: *Maternal/newborn plans of care,* ed 2, Philadelphia, 1994, FA Davis Co.

Dyson D: Prevention of preterm birth in high risk patients: the role of education and provider contact vs home uterine activity monitoring, *American Journal of Obstetrics and Gynecology* 164(3):756-762, 1991.

Evans C: Description of a home follow-up program for childbearing families, *JOGNN* 20(2)113-118, 1991.

Fleming B, Munton M, Clarke B, and Strauss S: Assessing and promoting positive parenting in adolescent mothers, *MCN* 18(1):32-37 1993.

Fortier J, Carson V, Well S, and Shubkagel B: Adjustment to newborn: sibling preparation makes a difference, *JOGNN* 20(1):73-79, 1991.

Freda M, Mikhail E, Polizzotto R, Damus K, and Merkatz I: Fetal movement counting: which method? *MCN* 18(6):314-321, 1993.

Gebauer C and Lowe N: The biophysical profile: antepartal assessment of fetal well-being, *JOGNN,* 22(2):115-124, 1993.

Gilbert E, and Harmon J: *Manual of high risk pregnancy and delivery,* St Louis, 1993, Mosby.

Goff K: Initiation of parturition, *MCN* 18(suppl):7-13, 1993.

Gorrie T, McKinney E, and Murray S: *Foundations of maternal newborn nursing,* Philadelphia, 1994, WB Saunders Co.

Griese M, and Prickett S: Nursing management of cord prolapse, *JOGNN* 22(4):311-315 1993.

Institute of Medicine: *Nutrition during pregnancy and lactation,* Washington, DC, 1992, National Academy Press.

Killion C: Pregnancy: a critical time to target STDs, *MCN* 19(3):156-161, 1994.

Knuppel R and Drukker J: *High risk pregnancy, a team approach,* ed 2, Philadelphia, 1993, WB Saunders Co.

Koniak-Griffin D: Maternal role attainment, Image: Journal of Nursing Scholarship 25(3):257-261, 1993.

Ladewig P, London M, and Olds S: *Essentials of maternal-newborn nursing,* ed 3, Redwood City, Ca, 1994, Addison-Wesley Nursing.

Lawrence R: *Breastfeeding,* ed 4, St Louis, 1994, Mosby.

Lerner H: Sleep position of infants: applying research to practice, *MCN* 18(5):275-277, 1993.

Lott J and Kenner C: Keeping up with neonatal infections: designer bugs, part I, *MCN* 19(4):207-213, 1994.

Maloni J: Bedrest during pregnancy: implications for nursing, *JOGNN* 22(5):422-426, 1993.

Mandeville L and Troiano N: *High-risk intrapartum nursing,* Philadelphia, 1992, JB Lippincott Co.

Mattson S and Smith J: *Core curriculum for maternal-newborn nursing,* Philadelphia, 1993, WB Saunders Co.

May K and Mahlmeister L: *Maternal and neonatal nursing: family-centered care,* ed 3, Philadelphia, 1994, JB Lippincott Co.

McGregor L: Short, shorter, shortest: improving the hospital stay for mothers and newborns, *MCN* 19(2):91-96, 1994.

McKay S and Barrows T: Reliving birth: maternal responses to viewing videotape of their second stage labors, *Image: Journal of Nursing Scholarship* 24(1): 27-31, 1992.

Miller A and Lorkovic M: Prostaglandin E_2 for cervical ripening, *MCN* 18(suppl):23-30, 1993.

National Center for Health Statistics: Childbearing patterns among selected racial/ethnic minority groups—United States, 1990, *Morbidity and Mortality Weekly Report* 42(20):398-403, 1993.

National Center for Health Statistics: Infant mortality—United States, 1991, *Morbidity and Mortality Weekly Report* 42(48):926-930, 1993.

National Center for Health Statistics: Teenage pregnancy and birth rates—United States, 1990, *Morbidity and Mortality Weekly Report* 42(38): 733-737, 1993.

National Center for Health Statistics: Increasing incidence of low birth weight—United States, 1981-1991, *Morbidity and Mortality Weekly Report* 43(18):335-339, 1994.

Newman V, Fullerton J, Anderson P, and Fashp P: Clinical advances in the management of severe nausea and vomiting during pregnancy, *JOGNN* 22(6):483-490, 1993.

New York Heart Association (1955). Criteria committee of New York Heart Association: *Nomenclature and Criteria for the Diagnosis of Diseases of the Heart and Blood Vessels,* 5 ed, New York: New York Heart Association.

Phipps W, Long B, Woods N, and Cassmeyer V: *Medical-surgical nursing*, ed 4, St Louis, 1991, Mosby.

Prechtl H, and Beintemia D: The neurological examination of the full-term infant, *Child development series, no. 12*, Philadelphia, 1975, JB Lippincott Co.

Rollant, P: Acing multiple choice tests, American Journal of Nursing 1994 Career Guide, 18-21, 36, American Journal of Nursing.

Rubin R: Maternal tasks in pregnancy, *Maternal Child Nursing Journal* 4:143-153, 1975.

Rubin R: *Maternal identity and the maternal experience*, New York, 1984, Springer Publishing Co.

Seidel H, Rosenstein B, and Pathak A: *Primary care of the newborn*, St Louis, 1993, Mosby.

Taylor T: Epidural anesthesia in the maternity patient, *MCN* 18(2):86-93, 1993.

Tillman J: Syphillis: an old disease, a contemporary perinatal problem, *JOGNN* 21(3):209-213, 1992.

Tucker S: *Pocket guide to fetal monitoring*, ed 2, St Louis, 1992, Mosby.

United States Department of Health and Human Services—CDC: 1993 sexually transmitted diseases treatment guidelines, *Morbidity and Mortality Weekly Report* 42(RR-14):1-99, 1993.

Whaley L and Wong D: *Nursing care of infants and children*, ed 4, St Louis, 1991, Mosby.

Williams L and Cooper M: Nurse-managed postpartum home care, *JOGNN* 22(1):25-31, 1993.

Worthington-Roberts B and Williams S: *Nutrition in pregnancy and lactation,* ed 5, St Louis, 1993, Mosby.

Wright L: Prenatal diagnosis in the 1990s, *JOGNN* 23(6):506-515, 1994.

INDEX

A

B

C

F

G

H

I

M

N

O

P

Q

R

S

T

U

V

W

Y

Z

Instructions for Disk Start-Up

DOS Version

System Requirements

A computer with at least 324K of RAM (Random Access Memory) available is needed for this program. This computer must be IBM PC or 100% compatible.

For these examples we assume that your A drive is your floppy drive, and your C drive is your hard drive. Please substitute the letter of your floppy drive for A if your floppy drive letter is different. Substitute the letter of your hard drive for C if your hard drive letter is different.

Start-up (floppy drive):

1. Turn your computer on
2. At the prompt, insert the disk into your A drive
3. Type A: and press <Enter>
4. Type MOSBY and press <Enter>
5. Follow the instructions on the screen

Start-up (hard disk):

1. Turn your computer on
2. At the prompt, insert the disk into your A drive
3. Type C: and press <Enter>
4. Type MD\MOSBY and press <Enter>
5. Type CD\MOSBY and press <Enter>
6. Type COPY A:*.* and press <Enter>

The software is now installed on your hard drive. Once the software is installed, start the software by following these directions:
1. Type CD\MOSBY and press <Enter>
2. Type MOSBY and press <Enter>
3. Follow the directions on the screen

MAC Version

System Requirements

Mac 68XXX or Power Mac with a total of at least 1 MB of RAM is needed for this program.

Start-up:

1. Create a new folder on your hard disk called MOSBY.
2. Insert the disk into your floppy drive and open it.
3. Drag all items from the disk to the new folder.

The software is now installed on your hard drive. Once the software is installed, start the software by following these directions:
1. Open the MOSBY folder.
2. Select the MOSBY program.
3. Follow the directions on the screen.

WRITE DOWN THE PASSWORD THAT YOU HAVE SELECTED.
YOUR DISK WILL BE BRANDED WITH THIS INITIAL ENTRY.